METHODS IN MOLECULAR BIOLOGY™

Series Editor
John M. Walker
School of Life Sciences
University of Hertfordshire
Hatfield, Hertfordshire, AL10 9AB, UK

For further volumes:
http://www.springer.com/series/7651

Hematological Malignancies

Edited by

Magdalena Czader

Department of Pathology and Laboratory Medicine, Indiana University School of Medicine, Indianapolis, IN, USA

Humana Press

Editor
Magdalena Czader
Department of Pathology and Laboratory Medicine
Indiana University School of Medicine
Indianapolis, IN, USA

ISSN 1064-3745 ISSN 1940-6029 (electronic)
ISBN 978-1-4939-5726-2 ISBN 978-1-62703-357-2 (eBook)
DOI 10.1007/978-1-62703-357-2
Springer New York Heidelberg Dordrecht London

Softcover reprint of the hardcover 1st edition 2013

Printed on acid-free paper

Humana Press is a brand of Springer
Springer is part of Springer Science+Business Media (www.springer.com)

Preface

The increasing knowledge on the pathogenesis of hematologic diseases has over the years been translated into diagnostic and prognostic applications. Hematopathology and laboratory hematology were among the first disciplines to embrace molecular diagnostics. As a consequence, the contemporary state-of-the-art hematopathology diagnosis relies on the integration of clinical, laboratory, morphologic, immunophenotypic, and genetic features. Increasingly however, the World Health Organization classification of hematopoietic and lymphoid neoplasms uses genetic/molecular features to separate clinically and prognostically distinct entities with similar morphologic or immunophenotypic characteristics. Hence, the majority of diagnostic entities require karyotyping and/or molecular testing to either confirm a diagnosis or to exclude a potential morphologically overlapping mimicker. This work presents the molecular-based assays frequently used in the routine diagnostic hematopathology and laboratory hematology. Many of these protocols were initially developed as research applications and were further refined as they transitioned to the diagnostic laboratory. Over the years, the field of molecular hematopathology has grown to represent a significant proportion of the routine diagnostic work. The assays, which originally existed only as research tools, were developed into commercially available tests, often packaged into ready-to-use kits. However, even the latter tests benefit from the comprehensive discussion by experts who use them in their everyday practice. The diagnostic testing is highly regulated and, optimally, is standardized among the laboratories. Towards this aim, the national and international collaborative studies led to the development of expert guidelines and international standards for the select of the presented molecular assays.

This work includes the discussion of the tests which have diagnostic, prognostic, and therapeutic implications. In the group of myeloproliferative and myelodysplastic/myeloproliferative neoplasms, detection or exclusion of *BCR-ABL1* rearrangement is critical for a precise diagnosis. Only after this step is completed, can one proceed with further subclassification. Additionally, BCR-ABL1 fusion transcript levels are used in patient follow-up and to monitor the efficacy of tyrosine kinase treatment. Patients demonstrating an increase in BCR-ABL1 transcript levels are considered for alternative therapies and tested for BCR-ABL1 kinase domain mutations. Additional mutations seen in myeloproliferative neoplasms, *JAK2*V617F and *KIT*D816V mutations, have been associated with Philadelphia chromosome-negative myeloproliferative neoplasms and mast cell disease. Both are critical for the diagnosis and are increasingly used as a therapeutic target. The molecular methods for a diagnosis and follow-up of chronic myeloid neoplasms are presented in the opening chapters. Similarly, current classification of acute myeloid and lymphoblastic leukemias relies heavily on genetic features. To bypass the delay in diagnosis typically associated with conventional karyotyping, various molecular techniques have been used to demonstrate the genetic abnormalities in acute leukemias. These tests, and immune and molecular assays, which established a niche in the posttreatment follow-up of patients with acute leukemias are presented next.

The following chapters focus on the molecular applications in lymphoid neoplasms. Initially, lymphomas lagged behind the disorders of blood and bone marrow in terms of classification based on their genetic features. However, in recent years this gap is closing and a molecular work-up is becoming increasingly important in lymphoid malignancies. Molecular tests are used for the confirmation of diagnosis, classification, and detection of residual disease. A proportion of lymphoid malignancies are associated with viral infections. Viruses are also a significant cause of morbidity and mortality in patients with hematologic malignancies who are frequently immunosuppressed. Both in situ demonstration of these pathogenic viruses and the monitoring of infection kinetics are the subjects of molecular testing.

The cornerstones of individualized therapies include the precise, clinically significant disease classification and the knowledge of individual variations in the response to different therapies. Testing of the polymorphisms in drug metabolizing genes is already an integral part of clinical management in select hematologic entities, and the field of molecular pharmacogenetics is rapidly growing due to the application of high-throughput technologies. The latter assays cannot be comprehensively discussed in a single text, and have been presented in separate publications of this series. We have elected to include the microRNA profiling due to its emerging role in hematologic malignancies.

I am indebted to all the authors who contributed to this work for sharing their expertise and for providing excellent yet practical and concise descriptions of the tests essential for contemporary laboratory diagnostics of hematological neoplasms.

Indianapolis, IN, USA ***Magdalena Czader***

Contents

Contributors

SHAOCHUN BAI • *Department of Medical and Molecular Genetics, Indiana University School of Medicine, Indianapolis, IN, USA*

DEEPA BHOJWANI • *Department of Oncology, St. Jude Children's Research Hospital, Memphis, TN, USA*

AMY CHADBURN • *Department of Pathology, Northwestern University-Feinberg School of Medicine, Chicago, IL, USA*

YUAN-YUAN CHEN • *Department of Pathology, City of Hope, Duarte, CA, USA*

LIANG CHENG • *Indiana University Health Pathology Laboratory, Department of Pathology and Laboratory Medicine, Indiana University School of Medicine, Indianapolis, IN, USA*

MAGDALENA CZADER • *Department of Pathology and Laboratory Medicine, Indiana University School of Medicine, Indianapolis, IN, USA*

SANDEEP DAVE • *Duke Institute for Genome Sciences and Policy, Duke University Medical Center, Durham, NC, USA*

ROSANNY ESPINAL-WITTER • *Department of Pathology and Laboratory Medicine, Weill Cornell Medical College, New York, NY, USA*

HONGXIN FAN • *Department of Pathology, University of Texas Health Science Center at San Antonio, San Antonio, TX, USA*

CHRISTOPHER D. GOCKE • *Department of Pathology, Johns Hopkins University School of Medicine, Baltimore, MD, USA*

MICHAEL J. HAFEZ • *Department of Pathology, Johns Hopkins University School of Medicine, Baltimore, MD, USA*

KEITH D. JACKSON • *Department of Pathology, Johns Hopkins University School of Medicine, Baltimore, MD, USA*

JONATHAN S. KUI • *Department of Pathology and Laboratory Medicine, Weill Cornell Medical College, New York, NY, USA*

CASSANDRA LOVE • *Duke Institute for Genome Sciences and Policy, Duke University Medical Center, Durham, NC, USA*

RAJYALAKSHMI LUTHRA • *Department of Hematopathology, The University of Texas MD Anderson Cancer Center, Houston, TX, USA*

FRANKLIN R. MOORE • *Department of Pathology, Baystate Medical Center/Tufts University School of Medicine, Springfield, MA, USA*

KATHLEEN M. MURPHY • *ProPath Services, Dallas, TX, USA*

KRISTIN POST • *Indiana University Health Pathology Laboratory, Department of Pathology and Laboratory Medicine, Indiana University School of Medicine, Indianapolis, IN, USA*

RICHARD D. PRESS • *Department of Pathology, Oregon Health and Sciences University, Portland, OR, USA*

KAAREN K. REICHARD • *Department of Laboratory Medicine and Pathology, Division of Hematopathology, Mayo Clinic Rochester, Rochester, MN, USA*

CAROLE B. REMPFER • *Department of Pathology, Oregon Health and Sciences University, Portland, OR, USA*

RYAN S. ROBETORYE • *Department of Laboratory Medicine and Pathology, Mayo Clinic Hospital, Phoenix, AZ, USA*
SHELDON ROBINETT • *Department of Pathology, University of New Mexico, Albuquerque, NM, USA*
RODNEY E. SHACKELFORD • *Department of Pathology and Laboratory Medicine, Tulane University School of Medicine, New Orleans, LA, USA*
KARL SOTLAR • *Institute of Pathology, University of Munich, Munich, Germany*
GAIL H. VANCE • *Department of Medical and Molecular Genetics, Indiana University School of Medicine, Indianapolis, IN, USA*
Y. LYNN WANG • *Department of Pathology and Laboratory Medicine, Weill Cornell Medical College, New York, NY, USA*
LAWRENCE M. WEISS • *Clarient Pathology Services, Inc. Aliso Viejo, CA, USA*
JANET WILSON • *Department of Pathology, Northwestern Memorial Hospital, Chicago, IL, USA*
BRENT L. WOOD • *Department of Laboratory Medicine, University of Washington, Seattle, WA, USA*
FEI YANG • *Department of Pathology, Oregon Health and Sciences University, Portland, OR, USA*
JUN J. YANG • *Department of Pharmaceutical Sciences, St. Jude Children's Research Hospital, Memphis, TN, USA*
C. CAMERON YIN • *Department of Hematopathology, The University of Texas MD Anderson Cancer Center, Houston, TX, USA*
QING ZHANG • *Department of Medical and Molecular Genetics, Indiana University School of Medicine, Indianapolis, IN, USA*

Chapter 1

Quantitative BCR-ABL1 RQ-PCR Fusion Transcript Monitoring in Chronic Myelogenous Leukemia

Franklin R. Moore, Carole B. Rempfer, and Richard D. Press

Abstract

The reciprocal Philadelphia translocation between chromosomes 9 and 22 [t(9;22)(q34;q11)] creates a BCR-ABL1 fusion protein that occurs in approximately 95% of cases of chronic myelogenous leukemia (CML), 15% of cases of adult acute lymphoblastic leukemia, and 5% of adult cases of acute myeloid leukemia. The BCR-ABL1 protein is a constitutively activated tyrosine kinase that induces and maintains the neoplastic phenotype in these leukemias. PCR-based methods to identify and quantitate the tumor-specific BCR-ABL1 RNA have been shown to be an ultrasensitive diagnostic/prognostic tool for Philadelphia-positive leukemias. A novel tyrosine kinase inhibitor (TKI), imatinib, has been confirmed as an effective targeted treatment in most CML patients. A consensus goal for TKI treatment is to achieve a major molecular response (MMR), defined as a 3-log (1,000-fold) reduction in BCR-ABL1 transcripts. Patients who achieve an MMR have been shown to have a significantly reduced risk of disease progression. Conversely, increasing post-therapy BCR-ABL1 RNA levels convey a significantly increased risk of disease progression. The early identification of these high-risk patients may allow early changes to the therapeutic strategy, before frank relapse. Thus, quantitative measurement of BCR-ABL1 transcripts in blood and bone marrow both aids in the initial diagnosis of CML and is essential for routine post-therapy minimal residual disease monitoring. We describe here a method for quantitating BCR-ABL1 transcripts in peripheral blood or bone marrow of CML patients using real-time quantitative reverse transcription PCR (RQ-PCR).

Key words Chronic myelogenous leukemia, BCR-ABL1, Philadelphia chromosome, Imatinib, Major molecular response

1 Introduction

Chronic myelogenous leukemia (CML) is a clonal hematologic stem cell malignancy associated, in ~95% of cases, with a specific chromosomal aberration. This somatically acquired tumor-specific chromosomal alteration, the Philadelphia chromosome (Ph), is detected cytogenetically as a reciprocal translocation between the long arms of chromosomes 9 and 22 [t(9;22)(q34;q11)]. The molecular consequences of the Philadelphia translocation

Magdalena Czader (ed.), *Hematological Malignancies*, Methods in Molecular Biology, vol. 999,
DOI 10.1007/978-1-62703-357-2_1, © Springer Science+Business Media New York 2013

are the physical juxtapositioning of sequences from the chromosome 22 *BCR* gene (breakpoint cluster region) adjacent to sequences from the chromosome 9 *ABL1* gene encoding a non-receptor tyrosine kinase. Depending on the precise site of the Ph translocation breakpoint, the resulting *BCR-ABL1* fusion gene is transcribed and translated into a 210 kDa (p210) or 190 kDa (p190) BCR-ABL1 fusion product with deregulated (significantly enhanced) tyrosine kinase activity (1, 2). The p210 BCR-ABL1 protein—formed by the fusion of bcr exon 2 or 3 (within the major breakpoint cluster region) to abl exons 2–11—is expressed not only in ~95% of patients with CML but also in ~15% of adult-onset cases of acute lymphoblastic leukemia (ALL) and ~5% of adults with acute myeloid leukemia (AML). The alternative p190 BCR-ABL1 product—formed by the fusion of upstream bcr exon 1 (within the minor breakpoint cluster region) to abl exons 2–11—is expressed in ~15% of adult-onset cases of ALL and in ~5% of pediatric-onset cases of ALL. Patients with these BCR-ABL1-positive (Philadelphia chromosome positive) acute leukemias have a significantly poorer prognosis than patients with acute leukemias lacking the Philadelphia chromosome (3). Approximately 5% of patients with classic (by clinical criteria) CML lack the typical Ph chromosome but express its BCR-ABL1 molecular correlate from complex translocations not detectable with routine cytogenetic methods.

A new era in the treatment of CML was initiated with the introduction of imatinib, a relatively specific small molecule inhibitor of the BCR-ABL1 tyrosine kinase (4). Imatinib binds to, and competitively inhibits BCR-ABL1's tyrosine kinase activity, and represses, but does not eradicate, the leukemic clone—without the typical toxicity of conventional chemotherapeutic agents. As imatinib induces a complete cytogenetic response (absence of detectable Philadelphia chromosomes) in over 80% of patients, more sensitive PCR-based detection methods are required to routinely monitor minimal residual disease levels and further stratify prognosis. In most centers, this is accomplished using quantitative real-time reverse transcription PCR (RQ-PCR) with a forward bcr-specific primer and a reverse abl-specific primer. Using this methodology, BCR-ABL1 RNA levels can typically be quantitated over a 5–6 log range, and consensus recommendations are to monitor these levels every 3–6 months, over at least the first 5 years of treatment (if not indefinitely) (1). The attainment of a major molecular response (MMR), defined as a 3-log reduction in BCR-ABL1 transcripts, has been shown to be an important response threshold, denoting a group of CML patients who have a very low risk of relapse (5, 6). However, even among patients with good imatinib responses, a rise in BCR-ABL1 RNA levels conveys a significantly increased risk of both ABL1 kinase domain mutations (causing imatinib resistance) and cytogenetic or hematologic disease progression (7, 8). As alternative tyrosine kinase inhibitors, with resistance profiles unique from imatinib, are now available, serial BCR-ABL1 transcript monitoring can help identify those patients requiring an adjustment of therapeutic strategy, ideally before frank relapse. On the other side of the prognostic spectrum, the optimal level of therapeutic response is the absence of detectable BCR-ABL1 RNA by RQ-PCR, deemed a complete molecular response (CMR). The achievement of a CMR, defined, in our lab, as the absence of BCR-ABL1 RNA by a more sensitive nested PCR procedure, conveys a significantly lower risk of disease progression than does the achievement of an MMR with detectable BCR-ABL1 RNA (7). Each of these various molecular response thresholds can be determined by performing routine BCR-ABL1 RQ-PCR as per the procedures outlined below. In patients with undetectable transcripts in the first RQ-PCR reaction, our lab reflexively performs a second-round nested PCR using primers internal to those used in the first PCR. This nested procedure, also described below, increases the analytical sensitivity of the overall assay approximately threefold over the single-stage RQ-PCR. Only patients with undetected transcripts in the nested assay are declared to have achieved a CMR.

2 Materials

2.1 Cell Lysis

1. Specimens: blood or bone marrow samples. For blood collected in EDTA, 20 ml is preferred (minimum 5 ml). For bone marrow, minimum 2 ml in heparinized syringe, transferred to EDTA tube.
2. Erythrocyte lysis buffer (Buffer EL Qiagen, Valencia, CA).
3. White cell lysis buffer (Bottle #3) MagNA Pure LC mRNA HS Kit (Roche, Indianapolis, IN).
4. Polypropylene centrifuge conical tubes (sizes 15, 50, and 225 ml).
5. Positive control consisting of K562 cells (BCR-ABL1 positive) diluted 1/10,000 with HeLa cells (BCR-ABL1 negative) and dissolved in white cell lysis buffer. The total cell count is 10 million per ml of lysis buffer, and the lysates are stored in 300 μl single-use aliquots in the freezer.

2.2 Automated Isolation of mRNA Using MagNA Pure Instrument (see Note 1)

1. MagNA Pure LC mRNA HS Kit (Roche, Indianapolis, IN).
2. MagNA Pure consumables, including: MagNA Pure small, medium, and large reagent tubs; large and small reaction tips; processing cartridges, and sample cartridges.
3. MagNa Pure LC 2.0 (Roche, Indianapolis, IN) automated nucleic acid extraction instrument.

2.3 Reverse Transcription of mRNA to cDNA

1. Superscript II enzyme (Invitrogen, Carlsbad, CA).
2. 5× RT Buffer (included in Superscript II package).
3. 100 mM DTT (included in Superscript II package).
4. Random hexamer primers p(dn)$_6$ (Roche, Indianapolis, IN) dissolved in 1 ml of RNase-free PCR-grade H_2O (1 mM stock).
5. PCR nucleotide mix (Roche, Indianapolis, IN); each at a concentration of 10 mM.
6. Protector RNase Inhibitor, 40 U/μl (Roche, Indianapolis, IN).
7. Microcon Centrifugal Filter Devices-YM 50 (Amicon) for large volume concentration of cDNA.

2.4 Real-Time Amplification Using LightCycler

1. LightCycler t(9;22) Quantification Kit (Roche, Indianapolis, IN) (see Note 2).
2. LightCycler Capillaries (Roche, Indianapolis, IN).
3. LightCycler Capillary Centrifuge Adapters contained in a cold block (Roche, Indianapolis, IN).
4. LightCycler Carousel Centrifuge.
5. LightCycler 1.2 real-time PCR instrument (Roche, Indianapolis, IN).

2.5 Reverse Transcription of mRNA for Nested PCR

1. All reagents listed in Subheading 2.3 above.
2. Negative control RNA, 16S- and 23S-ribosomal from E. coli MRE600 diluted to 30 ng/μl using PCR-grade, RNase-free water (Roche, Indianapolis, IN).

2.6 "First-Round" PCR for Nested PCR Assay

1. Roche Expand Hi Fidelity Taq Polymerase System.
2. PCR nucleotide mix (Roche, Indianapolis, IN); each at a concentration of 10 mM.
3. The following primers:
   (a) [bcr gene; Accession # Y00661; Nucleotide # 3153; from (9)]:
   NB1+ (F): 5′GAG CGT GCA GAG TGG AGG GAG AAC A
   (b) [abl gene; Accession # NM_005157; Nucleotide #363; from (9)]:
   ABL 3- (R): 5′GGT ACC AGG AGT GTT TCT CCA GAC TG

2.7 "Second-Round" PCR for Nested PCR Assay: Real-Time Amplification Using LightCycler

1. LightCycler DNA Master HybProbe (Roche, Indianapolis, IN).
2. The following primers:
   (a) [bcr gene; Accession # Y00661; Nucleotide # 3202; from (9)]:
   B2A (F): 5′ TTC AGA AGC TTC TCC CTG ACA T (22 nts)

(b) [abl gene; Accession # NM_005157; Nucleotide # 337; from (9)]:
CA3- (R): 5′ TGT TGA CTG GCG TGA TGT AGT TGC TTG G (28 nts)

3. The following probes (see Note 3):
   (a) (abl gene; Accession # NM_005157; Nucleotide # 289): a3-3′ HP: 5′LC Red 640-AAT GGG GAA TGG TGT GAA GCC CAA A-P (ABL exon 3). The "acceptor" probe is labeled with LC Red 640 on the 5′ end and phosphorylated on the 3′ end.
   (b) (abl gene; Accession # NM_005157; Nucleotide # 258): a3-5′ HP: 5′ TGA AAA GCT CCG GGT CTT AGG CTA TAA TCA-FLU (ABL exon 3). The "donor" probe is labeled with Fluorescein on the 3′ end.

3 Methods

Blood or bone marrow specimens from leukemic patients are subjected to an initial total leukocyte preparation (by lysing the erythrocytes). Poly-A-containing mRNA from these unfractionated leukocytes is prepared by an affinity-binding method (with oligo-dT magnetic beads) on the MagNa Pure instrument. The mRNA is reverse transcribed into cDNA with random primers in a standard reverse transcriptase reaction. The cDNA product is then split and subjected to real-time quantitative PCR of both BCR-ABL1 RNA and a control reference gene (housekeeping) transcript—G6PDH. The simultaneous quantitation of G6PDH RNA is designed to control for the amount and integrity of the labile RNA derived from occasionally suboptimally handled clinical samples. A relative ratio (in percent) of BCR-ABL1 RNA to G6PDH RNA is calculated by routine relative quantification methods using the real-time PCR-generated crossing points of each target. The sensitivity limit of the assay is approximately 1 leukemia cell in 100,000 normal cells. Quantitative levels of BCR-ABL1 RNA above this limit indicate the minimal residual disease burden and have been shown to be an excellent surrogate marker of treatment efficacy known as "molecular response." The achievement of a 3-log drop (1,000-fold) of BCR-ABL1 RNA levels suggests a "major molecular response" (MMR) and is a confirmed good prognostic indicator (6, 10). In particular, 100% of CML patients achieving an MMR within 18 months of starting imatinib therapy were free from progression to accelerated phase or blast crisis at 60 months of therapy (6). Rising levels of BCR-ABL1 RNA are also a significant predictive risk factor for both future leukemic disease progression (7) and the development of drug resistance mutations in the BCR-ABL1 kinase domain (8).

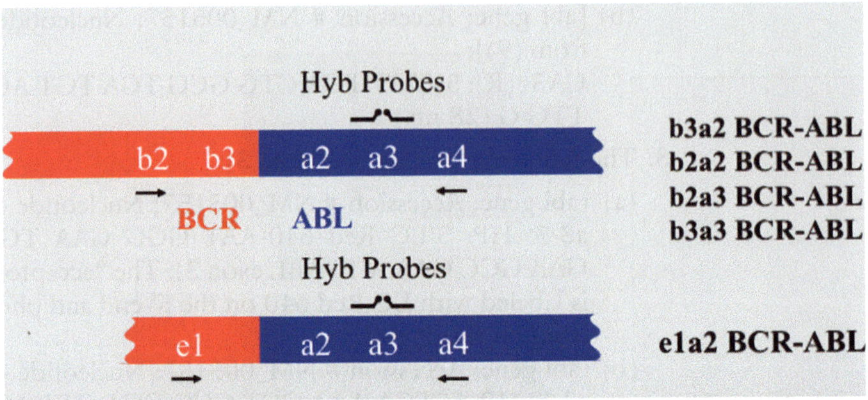

Fig. 1 Map of bcr-abl primers and probes for real-time PCR quantitation. Forward PCR primers are homologous to sequences within BCR exon b2 ("major" translocation breakpoint) and BCR exon e1 ("minor" translocation breakpoint). A common reverse primer is homologous to ABL1 exon a4. A donor and acceptor FRET probe pair are homologous to sequences within ABL1 exon a3

The BCR-ABL1 RQ-PCR assay utilizes a consensus reverse PCR primer from exon a4 of the chromosome 9 abl gene and each of two upstream primers from the chromosome 22 bcr gene, one from exon b2 (upstream of the major breakpoint cluster region) and one from upstream exon e1 (upstream of the minor breakpoint cluster region). Both the p210 (major) and p190 (minor) BCR-ABL1 fusion transcripts can thus be amplified within the same reaction tube. As all common BCR-ABL1 fusion products (b2a2, b3a2, e1a2, and the detectable rare fusion products b2a3 and b3a3) retain abl exon a3, 2 hybridization probes were designed to this conserved exon, one labeled at the 5′ end with the LC Red 640 fluorophore and the other labeled at the 3′ end with fluorescein. Only after hybridization to the synthesized PCR product (during the annealing step of the PCR reaction) do these two probes come into close physical proximity, resulting in fluorescence resonance energy transfer (FRET) between the two fluorophores. During FRET, fluorescein, the donor fluorophore, is excited by the light source of the real-time PCR instrument, and part of the excitation energy is transferred to the acceptor LC Red 640 fluorophore. The emitted fluorescence of LC Red 640 is then quantitated by the instrument in real time as a specific measure of the amount of amplified product. A map of the BCR-ABL1 primers and probes is shown in Fig. 1.

In order to maximize the sensitivity of the assay, a second "nested" PCR reaction is carried out for those initial reactions that resulted in undetectable levels of BCR-ABL1 transcript. This nested procedure is carried out on a sample of the initial PCR reaction using primers internal to the original set. The use of nested PCR results in an approximately threefold increase in analytical assay sensitivity.

3.1 Lysis of Cells from Blood or Bone Marrow

1. Count cells from the blood or bone marrow sample using an automated hematology cell counter. Alternatively, a manual cell count can be performed. Use the total leukocyte count to determine the blood or bone marrow volume necessary to achieve a total of 5.0×10^7 white blood cells.
2. After calculating the volume of bone marrow or blood to be extracted (50 million cells), transfer that volume to an appropriate tube, and add a 2× volume of Qiagen Buffer EL (erythrocyte lysis) to the sample.
3. Place the tubes on a rocking platform or gyrotory shaker for 10 min at room temperature to lyse the red blood cells. Alternatively, manually invert the sample periodically for 10 min.
4. Centrifuge the tubes at $980 \times g$ for 5 min in a table top centrifuge (with the brake off) at room temperature. After centrifuging, a white cell pellet should be visible at the bottom of the tube (corresponding to 50 million cells).
5. With a sterile pipette, carefully remove the supernatant, or pour off supernatant into a waste container, but do not disturb the pellet.
6. To eliminate any residual red blood cells that may later interfere with PCR, add an additional 5–10 ml of red cell lysis buffer (EL) to the white cell pellet, resuspend the cells, and transfer to a 15 ml conical tube.
7. Spin the sample again at $980 \times g$ for 5 min. After centrifuging, a clean white cell pellet should be visible at the bottom of the tube.
8. With a sterile pipette, carefully remove the supernatant, or pour off supernatant into a waste container, but do not disturb the pellet.
9. Based on the number of cells extracted, calculate the volume of white blood cell lysis buffer (bottle #3 in MagNA Pure mRNA HS Isolation Kit) needed to achieve a final concentration of 1.0×10^7 white cells per ml, up to a total lysis buffer volume of 5 ml for 50 million cells.
10. After removal of the red cell lysis supernatant, add the appropriate volume of WBC lysis buffer to the WBC pellet.
11. Thoroughly resuspend the white cell pellet in the lysis buffer, by pipetting up and down several times.
12. Vortex the lysate briefly, and allow the lysate to rest for 5 min.
13. After 5 min, vortex the lysate again.
14. The lysed sample may now be put directly onto the MagNA Pure for mRNA isolation, or may be frozen at −70°C for mRNA isolation at a later time.

3.2 Automated Isolation of mRNA Using Roche MagNA Pure Instrument

1. If lysates have been frozen, allow to thaw along with a 10^{-4} control (1:10,000 dilution of K562 cells into a BCR-ABL1-negative cell line, e.g., HeLa cells).
2. Programming the instrument.
   (a) Select "Start Program" on the MagNA Pure.
   (b) Select "Sample Ordering."
   (c) Under *Sample Protocol*, select "mRNA 1 cells.blk."
   (d) Under *Sample Volume*, type in the amount of cellular lysate you are starting with. This volume must be the same for all samples extracted in a given run and will usually be *300* μ*l* (*usually three million cells, to reflect lysates frozen at ten million cells per ml*).
   (e) Under *Elution Volume*, change 25 μl to 50 μl. Do not choose a *Post-E*lution Protocol.
   (f) Type in patient identifiers on "Sample Ordering" List. When the identifiers (sample numbers) have been input for each sample to be extracted, click on "Start Batch." You will see a screen which indicates the volumes of all the reagents and types of consumables needed to complete the isolation process.
3. Preparing reagents and disposables.
   (a) Remove the metal tub rack from the instrument and place the appropriate sized reagent tubs in the tub rack.
   (b) Fill the reagent tubs with the given volumes of reagents (all reagents are part of the MagNA Pure mRNA HS Kit). Be sure to put the reagent tubs in the correct order, and skip positions as indicated.
   (c) Return the tub rack to the instrument stage and close the lockbar.
   (d) Place sample processing cartridges in the heating and cooling blocks.
   (e) Place the appropriate number of processing cartridges in the correct positions, as indicated on the screen.
   (f) Insert the necessary number of large tips (blue) and small tips (yellow) into the appropriate positions.
   (g) Position a solid waste bag on the disposal chute and hold it in place with the magnet provided.
   (h) Pipette the correct volume (300 ml) of cell lysate for each sample into the appropriate wells of a *sample cartridge* and place it in the instrument. For concentrated samples (thought to have very low levels of BCR-ABL1 RNA requiring additional assay sensitivity; see Note 4), aliquot the same lysate into two separate wells for a total of 600 μl of lysate (for which the mRNA will later be pooled).

(i) Close the instrument door and click on the icon for each reagent and disposable that has been placed in the instrument.
(j) Once all icons have been selected, an "OK" button will be visible on the screen. Click on the "OK" button.
(k) The MagNA Pure will begin by slowly moving the robotic arm across the stage, to make sure that no obstacles are present. It will then begin extracting samples, eight at a time.

4. Aliquoting extracted mRNA upon program completion (see Note 5).
   (a) After the MagNA Pure instrument has completed the mRNA isolation process, mRNA samples will be in the sample cartridge in the cooling block of the instrument. Carefully aliquot the eluted mRNA (50 ml) into pre-labeled 1.5 ml tubes using pipettes designated for RNA use only.
   (b) For samples requiring a concentrated (volume-reduced) cDNA preparation (to increase RQ-PCR analytical sensitivity), pool two designated mRNA eluates (totaling 100 ml) into a single tube.
   (c) Place tubes of mRNA on ice if directly proceeding with reverse transcription, or store at −70°C for future use.
5. Dispose of consumables, and close out windows until the front screen appears. Select "Decontamination." Next, select "Start Decontamination" from the "Actions" pull-down at the top of the window. Allow the UV decontamination of the MagNa Pure to proceed for 8 h (overnight).

3.3 Reverse Transcription of mRNA

1. Make sure mRNA is kept on ice. Label 0.5 ml Eppendorf tubes with sample ID. Include a 10^{-4} control mRNA (1:10,000 dilution of K562 cells into a BCR-ABL1-negative cell line), and a water (no RNA) negative control.
2. Place the RT reagents on ice and calculate the amount of 2× RT master mix needed according to Table 1. Most likely there will be both "1×" and "concentrated" samples on the same run (see Note 4). The method used for concentration is described in Subheading 3.4. The "1×" samples will consist of 6 μl mRNA and 6 μl of master mix. "Concentrated" samples will consist of 80 μl of mRNA and 80 μl of master mix. For concentrated samples (originally 100 μl mRNA), the remaining 20 μl of mRNA is stored at −70°C for future use.
3. Prepare RT master mix and keep on ice. By preparing "$n+1$" reactions, there should be enough master mix to account for small variations in pipetting volumes.
4. When the mRNAs are completely thawed, mix gently and aliquot 6 μl into appropriately labeled 0.5 ml PCR tubes (for "1×" samples). Use 80 μl mRNA for "concentrated" samples.

Table 1
Preparation of reverse transcription master mix

Reverse transcription master mix	"Concentrated" samples (μl)	"Unconcentrated" samples (μl)	Final RT reaction concentration
5× RT Buffer (included with Superscript II)	32.0	2.4	1×
100 mM DTT (included with Superscript II)	16.0	1.2	10 mM
pd(N)$_6$ (random hexamers) (1 mM) (Roche)	8.0	0.6	50 μM
dNTP's (10 mM ea) (Roche)	16.0	1.2	1 mM ea
Superscript II (200 U/μl) (Invitrogen)	5.3	0.4	6.7 U/μl
RNase inhibitor (40 U/μl) (Roche)	2.7	0.2	0.7 U/μl
Total master mix volume (2×) (μl)	80	6	
Total RT reaction volume (μl)	160	12	

5. Denature mRNA at 65°C for 10 min.
6. After denaturation, place tubes on ice for 1 min.
7. Pipette 6 μl of master mix into "1×" tubes containing patient and control samples (80 μl for "concentrated" tubes).
8. Mix by pipetting up and down.
9. Incubate as follows: 10 min at 25°C, 50 min at 42°C, and 15 min at 70°C.
10. Proceed to next step or freeze cDNA at 20°C.

3.4 Concentration of cDNA from a Large-Scale mRNA Reverse Transcription Reaction Using Micron Centrifugal Filter Devices

1. For each "concentrated" sample, place two empty tubes (from Microcon kit) in a rack.
2. Place pink filter in one of the tubes and close.
3. Label both the top of tube containing the pink filter and the side of the empty tube with patient identifier (see Note 5).
4. Pipette the whole volume of cDNA onto the pink filter of Microcon (approx 160 μl).
5. Spin at 7,100×*g* in a microcentrifuge for 5 min to yield 10–11 μl residual volume on top of the membrane, at which point, the middle of the membrane appears dry. During spinning, the membrane allows low molecular-weight molecules (plus salt, water, etc.) to pass (isotonically) through to the "discard" side, while retaining all of the larger-sized cDNA's in a smaller volume on the membrane's "top" side.

6. If, visually, there is too much volume remaining on top of the membrane, continue spinning at small increments (30 s) until the middle of the membrane appears dry. When, visually, the middle of the membrane is dry, take the filter out of the tube and turn it upside down into the "capless" tube (to spin-transfer it to this other tube).
7. Spin for 2 min at 7,100 ×*g* to transfer the cDNA to this other tube. Place the concentrated (volume-reduced) cDNA (at least 10.5 μl) back into the original 0.5 ml Eppendorf tube (the RT reaction tube) (see Note 6).

3.5 Quantitative BCR-ABL1 t(9;22) Detection by Real-Time PCR on LightCycler Instrument

1. Check to make sure that the LightCycler Centrifuge Capillary Adapters in the cold block are in the 4°C refrigerator (do not freeze).
2. Let primer/probe mix (vials 7 and 8 from Roche t(9;22) kit) thaw in the cold block.
3. Turn on the computer and LightCycler.
4. Click on the icon "LightCycler 3.5 Front Screen."
5. When the front screen opens, click on the "Run" option.
6. Program the LightCycler according to parameters in Tables 2, 3.
7. Click on "Edit Samples."
8. Enter sample identifiers; first for G6PDH reactions (for a full rotor, rows 1–16) and then for BCR-ABL1 (rows 17–32). Typically, the first 16 capillaries (includes low positive control, negative control and 14 patient samples) are designated for G6PDH amplification, while the second 16 are designated for BCR-ABL1 amplifications.
9. At some point the computer will ask if you want to start the "LightCycler SelfTest." A Self Test should be initiated at minimum the first run of the day when using the LightCycler.
10. Check to make sure that all sample identifiers have been entered in the correct positions and either "G6PDH" or "BCR-ABL" was entered in the "notes" section on the right.
11. Save the experiment, and click "Done."
12. You will return to the previous screen. At this point the LC is ready to be loaded.
13. Return to the "Pre-PCR" section of the lab to set up the PCR master mixes.
14. Prepare enough of the following master mixes for all samples and controls (plus 1). Generally, you will have 16 G6PDH samples ($n = 17$ master mix) and 16 BCR-ABL1 samples ($n = 17$ master mix) (see Table 4).
15. When the master mixes are ready, place on ice.

Table 2
BCR-ABL LightCycler temperature parameters

Target temperature (°C)	Incubation time (s)	Temperature transition rate (°C/s)	Acquisition mode
Denaturation			
95	30	20.0	None
Amplification			
95	1	20.0	None
64	10	20.0	Single
72	26	2.0	None
Melting curve analysis			
95	0	20.0	None
45	60	20.0	None
95	0	0.2	Cont
Cooling			
40	30	20	None

Table 3
BCR-ABL LightCycler temperature parameters (The fluorescence parameters should be set as follows)

Fluorimeter gain	Value
Channel 1 (F 1)	1
Channel 2 (F 2)	15
Channel 3 (F 3)	30

Display mode: fluorescence channel *F2/F1*

16. Retrieve the cold block from the 4°C refrigerator and load it in numeric order with the appropriate number of capillaries.
17. Add 15 μl of G6PDH master mix to the top chamber of the appropriate number of capillaries (the first 16 for a full run).
18. Add 15 μl of BCR-ABL1 master mix to the remaining capillaries (the last 16 for a full run).
19. Add 5 μl of cDNA (either unconcentrated or concentrated) to each G6PDH capillary and 5 μl to each BCR-ABL1 capillary. For example, from the same tube of cDNA, 5 μl will be pipetted into capillary #1 for G6PDH and 5 μl will be pipetted into capillary #17 for BCR-ABL1 and so on. Change gloves as often as needed to prevent contamination. Carefully, cap each capillary after cDNA is added.

Table 4
Preparation of G6PDH and BCR-ABL master mixes

G6PDH PCR master mix:	
G6PDH Detection mix (vial 8)[a]	3.8 μl
PCR-grade H_2O (vial 11)	9.2 μl
10× Reaction mix (vial 6)[b]	2.0 μl
Total master mix volume[c]	15.0 μl
BCR-ABL PCR master mix:	
t(9;22) Detection mix (vial 7)[a]	6.2 μl
PCR-grade H_2O (vial 11)	6.8 μl
10× Reaction mix (vial 6)[b]	2.0 μl
Total master mix volume[c]	15.0 μl

[a]Vial numbers refer to Roche t(9;22) reagent kit. Vials 7 and 8 contain primer and probes

[b]Contains $MgCl_2$, Taq buffer, dNTPs, and Taq polymerase. Keep on ice. Avoid freeze thawing

[c]The total volume of both PCR reactions (master mix plus cDNA) is 20 μl

20. After all capillaries have been loaded and capped, gently insert capillaries into carousel and spin them in the LC carousel centrifuge.
21. Return the loaded carousel to the LC and gently close the lid.
22. At the computer, click "Run."
23. The LightCycler will begin by asking if you would like to save the run.
24. Save the run and click "Done."

3.6 Data Printout

1. If a run has just been completed (see Note 7) on the LC, the file for that run will be displayed on the monitor. If you are analyzing data from an old run, choose "Data Analysis" from the LC Front Screen. Once in Data Analysis, simply go to the correct folder and open the appropriate file.
2. The first screen you see upon beginning data analysis depicts the temperature history at the top and the amplification (fluorescence) history at the bottom.
3. Click on "Quantification." The screen will display a graph that shows the amplification of each sample. See Fig. 2 for representative amplification curves of the G6PDH reference gene and Fig. 3 for representative amplification curves of BCR-ABL1.
4. Click on "Print Summary Report" from "Report" pull-down. This will print out all crossing points. Crossing points are calculated using the second derivative maximum algorithm.
5. Highlight all *G6PDH* samples and "Print Screen."

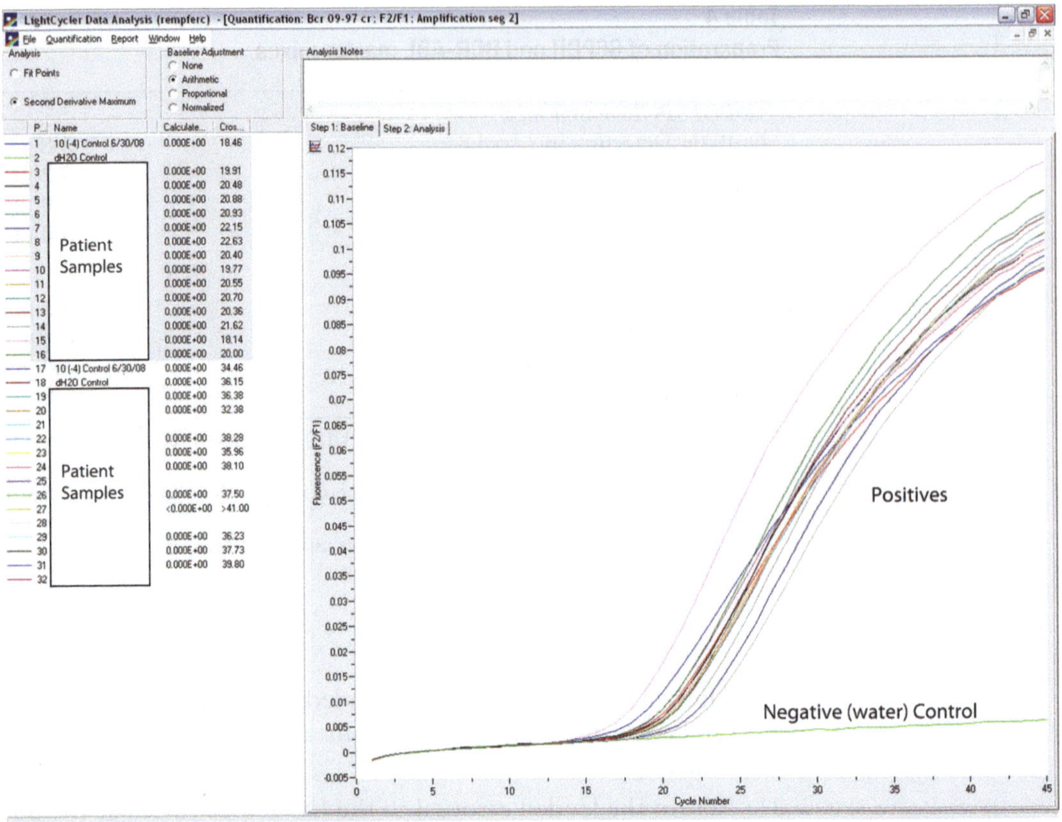

Fig. 2 Representative G6PDH amplification curves. Note the tight distribution of G6PDH reference gene crossing points of all of the samples (indicative of equivalent amounts of RNA) regardless of whether they are positive or negative for BCR-ABL1

6. Highlight a few BCR-ABL1 patients at a time and "Print Screen" (see Note 8).
7. Minimize this window to return to the previous screen.
8. Under "Select a Program" choose "Melt…" Click on "Melting Curve."
9. Click on "Extra Manual TM."
10. Select all of the positive melt BCR-ABL1 samples at one time.
11. Click and drag one of the vertical lines over to align with the peaks of all the melting curves and then print the page.
12. Deselect positives while selecting negative BCR-ABL1 samples going from first to last. This will "blow up" some of the negative and weaker melting curves.
13. Then print the page. See Fig. 4 for representative melting curves of BCR-ABL1.
14. If a sample is "negative" on the melt curve and it is not a diagnostic specimen, it will be reflexed to a more sensitive nested PCR assay to detect any low-level minimal residual disease (see Note 9).

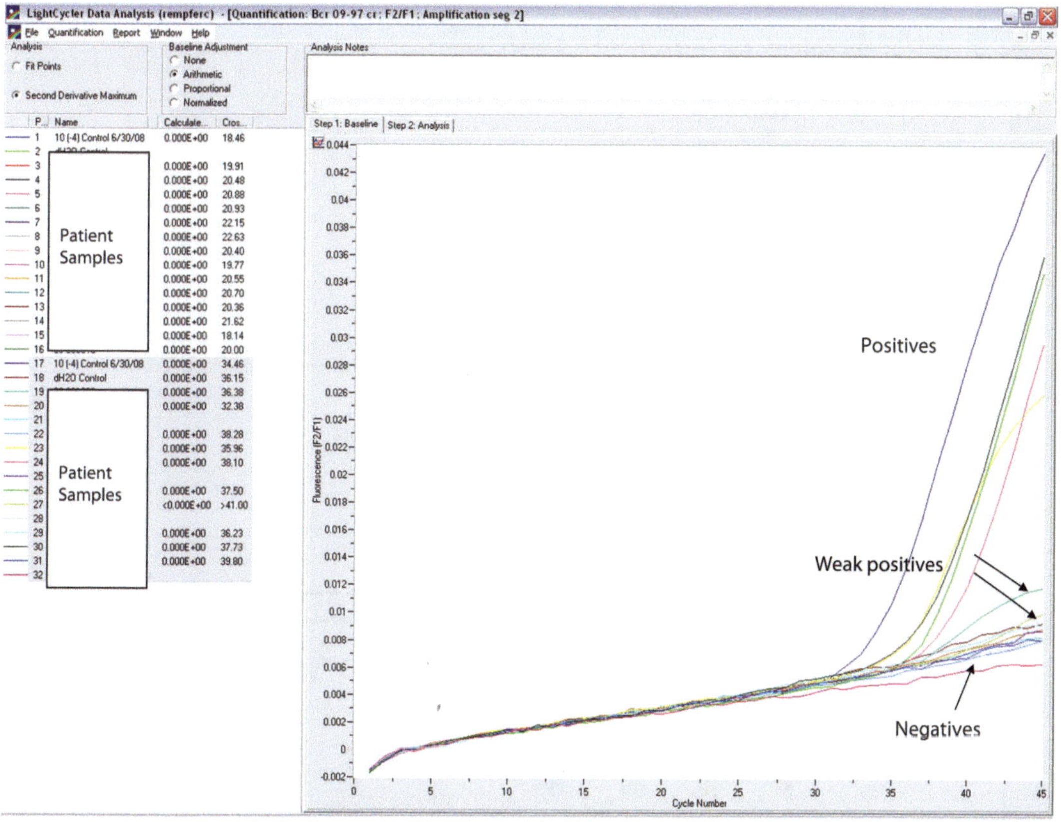

Fig. 3 Representative BCR-ABL1 amplification curves from the same experiment as Fig. 2. Note that some samples are clearly positive, some are clearly negative, and some give a "weak positive" amplification curve

3.7 Calculation of BCR-ABL1/G6PDH RNA Ratio and International Scale Value

The "RNA ratio" (in units of "percent") is calculated using the "delta Ct" method as

$$\text{Ratio}\left(\text{in units of “percent”}\right) = \frac{100}{2.0\ \exp\left(\text{BCRCp} - \text{G6Cp}\right)}$$

where BCRCp is the crossing point of BCR-ABL1 and G6Cp is the crossing point of G6PDH.

For example, if the BCRCp is 33 and the G6Cp is 22, then the "Delta" Cp value is 11. The denominator of the ratio equation would then be 2^{11} (=2,048), and the RNA ratio would be $100/2{,}048 = 0.049\%$. The "delta Ct" method can be used because the efficiencies of the BCR-ABL1 and G6PDH PCR reactions are indistinguishable.

The "international scale" (IS) (11–13) represents a standardized measurement scale (regardless of housekeeping gene or assay technology) in which an IS value of 0.1% is defined as both a 3-log drop from baseline (untreated) BCR-ABL1 RNA levels and as a "major molecular response" with an associated excellent prognosis.

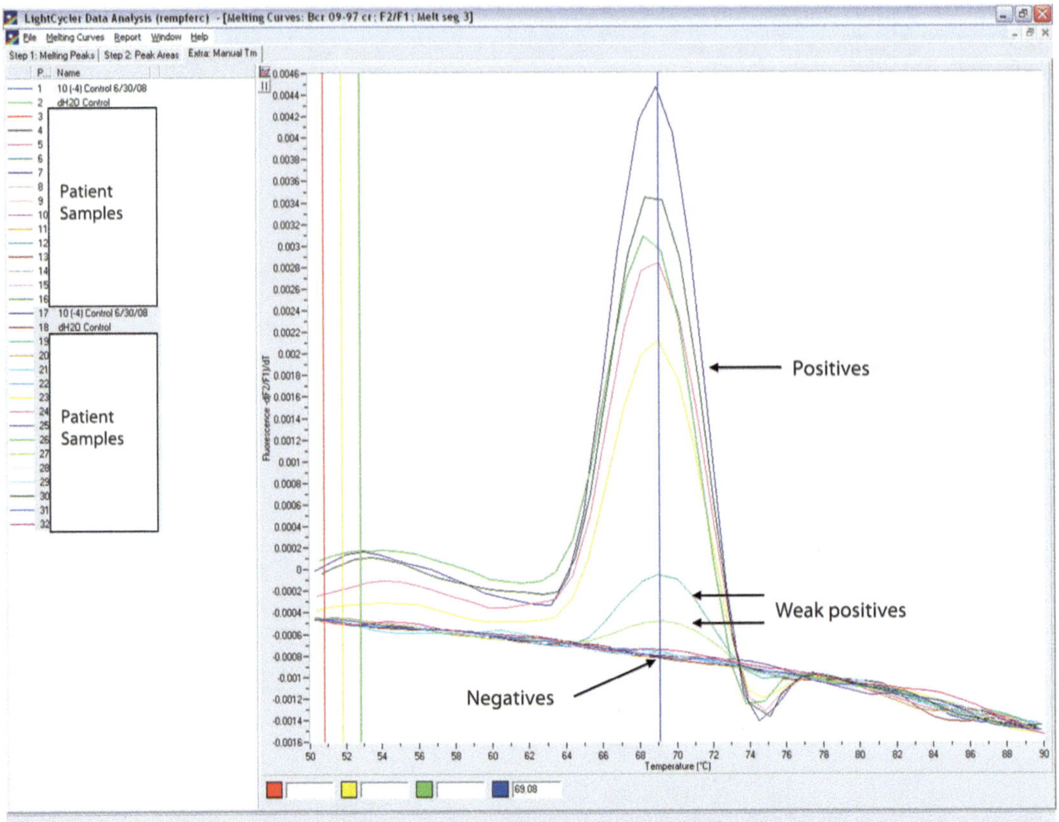

Fig. 4 Representative BCR-ABL1 melting curves from the same experiment as in Figs. 2 and 3. The BCR-ABL1-positive specimens all melt at approximately 69°C. Note that the two weak positives from Fig. 3 show a similarly weak (but positive) melting curve

In the absence of a universal BCR-ABL reference material that is tied to the IS, the calculation of an IS value requires each lab to individually determine its own "conversion factor" by sharing samples with another lab whose BCR-ABL assay is already validated on the IS (11, 13). The conversion factor is then used as a multiplier to convert lab-specific "ratio" values to IS values. For example, the conversion factor for our laboratory (which is 29) means that the 0.049% ratio from the above example (Delta Cp = 11) converts to a BCR-ABL IS value of 1.4% , which is about a 1.8 log drop from baseline [log(100/1.4) = 1.8).

3.8 Acceptable Run Parameters

1. Low positive BCR-ABL control (1:10,000 diluted K562) must yield a Ct value that abides by the lab's self-determined Westgard Rules (see Note 10).
2. Negative control sample must be negative (including melt curve) for BCR-ABL.
3. Melt peaks for BCR-ABL should be approximately 69°C.

Table 5
Preparation of reverse transcription master mix for nested PCR

Reverse transcription master mix for nested PCR	Reaction (μl)	Final concentration
5× RT Buffer (comes with Superscript II)	4.0	1×
100 mM DTT (comes with Superscript II)	2.0	10 mM
pd(N)$_6$ (1 mM) (Roche) (random hexamers)	1.0	50 μM
dNTP's (10 mM ea) (Roche)	2.0	1 mM ea
Superscript II (200 U/μl) (Invitrogen)	0.7	7 U/μl
RNase inhibitor (40 U/μl) (Roche)	0.3	0.6 U/μl
Total	10.0	

Total PCR volume = 20 μl (10 μl master mix plus 10 μl RNA)

3.9 Reverse Transcription of mRNA for Nested PCR

1. Place the mRNA samples and RT reagents on ice to thaw. Include a 10^{-4} control and a negative control.
2. Label 0.5 ml microcentrifuge tubes with patient identifiers.
3. Aliquot 10 μl of mRNA into each designated tube.
4. Master mix can be prepared while samples are denaturing in step 5. See Table 5 for master mix preparation.
5. Denature mRNA at 65°C for 10 min.
6. After denaturation, place tubes on ice for 1 min.
7. Pipette 10 μl of master mix into tubes on ice.
8. Mix by pipetting up and down.
9. Incubate as follows: 2 h at 42°C, and 10 min at 65°C.
10. Proceed to next step or freeze cDNA at −20°C (see Note 11).

3.10 "First-Round" PCR for Nested PCR Assay

1. Nested PCR is performed in triplicate. Label three tubes for each cDNA sample (see Note 12). The positive control and negative control only need to be performed in singlicate.
2. Prepare master mix (Table 6) and place on ice.
3. Aliquot 20 μl of master mix into the labeled 0.5 ml Eppendorf microcentrifuge tubes.
4. Pipette 5 μl of cDNA into each of the three patient tubes, the positive, and negative controls.
5. Amplify according to the following PCR conditions.
6. After cycling, the sample is held at 72°C for 10 min and 4°C "forever."

   (a) 30 cycles of 96°C for 1 min.
   (b) 56°Cfor 1 min.
   (c) 72°C for 1 min.

Table 6
Preparation of first-round master mix for nested PCR

First-round PCR master mix for nested PCR	Reaction (µl)	Final concentration
Vial 2: 10× Hi Fi Taq PCR Buffer w/15 mM $MgCl_2$	2.5	1× (1.5 mM $MgCl_2$)
Vial 4: 25 mM $MgCl_2$	1.0	1 mM
NB1+ primer (12.5 µM)	1.0	0.5 µM
ABL 3- primer (12.5 µM)	1.0	0.5 µM
10 mM ea dNTP's	0.5	0.2 mM ea
Hi Fi Expand Taq Polymerase (3.5 U/µl)	0.22	0.031 U/µl
dH_2O (RNase-free)	13.78	
Total	20.0	

Total PCR reaction volume = 25 µl (20 µl master mix plus 5 µl cDNA)

3.11 "Second-Round" PCR for Nested PCR Assay: Real-Time Amplification Using LightCycler

1. Prepare the master mix (Table 7) for patient samples, positive and negative controls, and a new negative control.
2. Bring tube of master mix into post-PCR room.
3. Take out the capillary cold block from the refrigerator and place in designated second-round area.
4. Place master mix in holder and (with fresh gloves) aliquot 15 µl of master mix into each capillary.
5. Add 5 µl of each first-round PCR sample to the appropriately numbered capillaries containing master mix.
6. Cap each capillary after the first-round PCR sample is added, being careful not to touch the lip of the capillary with your glove. Change gloves as often as needed to prevent contamination.
7. Turn on the computer and LightCycler.
8. Click on the icon "LightCycler 3.5 Front Screen."
9. When the front screen opens, click on the "Run" option.
10. Program the LightCycler according to parameters in Tables 2, 3.
11. Click on "Edit Samples." Enter sample identifiers.
12. At some point the computer will ask if you want to start the "LightCycler SelfTest." A Self Test should be initiated at minimum the first run of the day when using the LightCycler.
13. Check to make sure that all sample identifiers have been entered in the correct positions and "BCR-ABL" was entered in the "notes" section on the right.
14. Save the experiment, and click "Done."

Table 7
Preparation of second-round master mix for nested PCR

Second-round LC PCR master mix for nested PCR	Reaction (µl)	Final concentration
dH_2O	9.0	
25 mM $MgCl_2$ (included in LightCycler DNA Master HybProbe kit)	3.2	4 mM
B2A primer (50 µM)	0.2	0.5 µM
CA3- primer (50 µM)	0.2	0.5 µM
A3-3′ Red probe (25 µM)	0.2	0.25 µM
A3-5′ Flu probe (25 µM)	0.2	0.25 µM
LightCycler DNA Master HybProbe	2.0	1 mM $MgCl_2$
Total	15.0	

Total PCR reaction volume = 20 µl (15 µl master mix plus 5 µl first-round PCR sample)

3.12 Data Printout for Nested PCR Assay

1. If a run has just been completed on the LightCycler, the file for that run will be displayed on the monitor. If you are analyzing data from an old run, choose "Data Analysis" from the LC Front Screen. Once in Data Analysis, simply go to the correct folder and open the appropriate file.
2. The first screen you see upon beginning data analysis depicts the temperature history at the top and the amplification (fluorescence) history at the bottom. There are two vertical green lines that bracket the amplification portion of the temperature history in the top graph.
3. Click on "Quantification." The screen will display a graph that shows the amplification of each sample.
4. Click on "Print Summary Report" from "Report" pull-down. This will print out all crossing points.
5. Highlight all positive samples and "Print Screen."
6. Minimize this window to return to the previous screen.
7. Under "Select a Program" choose "Melt."
8. Click on "Melting Curve."
9. Click on "Extra Manual TM."
10. Select all of the positive melt BCR-ABL samples at one time.
11. Click on one of the vertical lines and drag it over to align with the peaks of all the melting curves and print page.
12. Select negative patient's melting curves and "Print Screen."

3.13 Acceptable Run Parameters and Resulting for Nested PCR

1. Low positive BCR-ABL control (1:10,000 diluted K562) must amplify.
2. Negative control samples must be negative (including melt curve).
3. Record melt status on "Summary Report" either "melt +" or "melt −."
   (a) If one out of three replicates is melt positive, result will be "indeterminate."
   (b) If two or three out of three are melt positive, result will be "positive."
   (c) If three out of three are melt negative, result will be "negative."

4 Notes

1. Alternatively, the Qiagen RNeasy Mini kit can be used for RNA isolation.
2. This kit contains bcr-abl-specific PCR primers homologous to BCR gene exon b2 ("major" translocation breakpoint), BCR exon e1 ("minor" translocation breakpoint), and a common reverse primer from c-ABL exon a4. Quantitative detection is accomplished with a pair of FRET hybridization probes, homologous to ABL exon a3. The prime and probe sequences are modified versions of those from Emig et al. (14). The expected BCR-ABL amplicon size is 671 bp for the "major" b3a2 translocation breakpoint, 596 bp for the "major" b2a2 translocation breakpoint, and 540 bp for the "minor" e1a2 translocation breakpoint.
3. Probes contain light-sensitive fluorescent molecules. Avoid unnecessary exposure to light.
4. The decision to concentrate a cDNA sample (i.e., volume-reduce a large-volume cDNA reaction) is based upon the expected BCR-ABL transcript load. For example, in our lab, if a patient has a history of undetected or weak positive RQ-PCR's, the sample is typically concentrated prior to PCR, with the goal of achieving a higher level of analytical sensitivity. If the sample is from an untreated or poorly responding patient and/or expected to have a high transcript level, there is no need to concentrate it. The decision to concentrate a cDNA sample is undertaken as a time-saving method—as a reflex nested PCR reaction (performed only after the initial RQ-PCR is "undetected") can often be avoided on "weak positive" samples that have undergone an initial RQ-PCR with a concentrated cDNA template.

5. RNA must be handled with extreme care. RNases are ever present on hands; therefore always wear gloves. Always keep samples on ice. Always use filtered tips. Clean work space and pipettes with "RNase Out" spray. Use a dedicated RNA pipette set. Store RNA at −70°C and avoid freeze-thawing as much as possible.
6. Cut the hinge on the empty tube while it is closed so the top can be taken off easily after next step. If the tubes are spun too long (residual volume <10.5 μl), add back some of the original flow through (i.e., liquid that has already gone through the filter) to attain a final volume of at least 10.5 μl.
7. A complete run takes approximately 1 h.
8. If an amplification curve is weak, select it together with a negative control to "blow up" the *Y*-axis. If the amplifications are weak and happen to be selected with a stronger positive, it will be hard to see exactly what the crossing point looks like (as the software sets the *Y*-axis maximum as the maximum of all of the "selected" samples).
9. The nested PCR assay used in our lab does not detect patients with the minor (p190) translocation breakpoint, E1/A2.
10. The following Westgard Rules (15) are used to determine the acceptability of a run.
    (a) Warning
    If any of the following scenarios occurs on a run (on any of the control samples), this triggers a "warning" that future runs may be rejected. Document the warning on the Levy-Jennings chart, which plots the Delta Ct value of the control samples vs. the batch run number (and date).
    - 1_{2S}—A single Ct value greater than 2SD from the mean (random error).
    - 7_{T}—Seven consecutive Ct values trending in the same direction (same side of the mean; systematic error).
    - 4_{1S}—Four consecutive values greater that 1SD on the same side of the mean (systematic error).

    (b) Rejection
    If any of the following scenarios occurs on a run (on any of the control samples), this triggers a "rejection" of the run. All rejected runs will be reviewed by the laboratory director. The laboratory director will then determine if the results are acceptable, or if the run needs to be repeated. A QC failure, as indicated by a "rejected" run, may be an indication for the need to recalibrate the assay. Document action taken on the Levy-Jennings chart.

- 1_{3S}—A single value greater than 3SD from the mean (random error).
- 2_{2S}—Two consecutive values greater than 2SD on the same side of the mean (systematic error).
- R_{4S}—Two consecutive values greater than 2SD on opposite sides of the mean (random error).
- 10_X—Ten values on the same side of the mean (systematic error).

11. It is extremely important to avoid contamination in the nested PCR assay. This is accomplished by spatial isolation of the first- and second-round reactions, and by stringent handling precautions.

    First-Round PCR: Reagents for these reactions should be prepared in batches and stored in the −20°C freezer in the "pre-PCR" area. When handling reaction tubes, be careful not to touch the underside of the caps to avoid contamination.

    Second-Round Setup (Post-PCR Area): Treat this space as a separate room. The main issue is to keep all second-round products out of the second-round setup area. Use fresh gloves. Change gloves at the slightest hint of doubt. Use filtered tips and a "second-round" designated pipette.

12. The three tubes are best labeled with three different colored markers.

References

1. Baccarani M, Saglio G, Goldman J, Hochhaus A, Simonsson B, Appelbaum F et al (2006) Evolving concepts in the management of chronic myeloid leukemia. Recommendations from an expert panel on behalf of the European Leukemianet. Blood 108:1809–1820
2. O'Hare T, Eide CA, Deininger MW (2007) Bcr-Abl kinase domain mutations, drug resistance and the road to a cure of chronic myeloid leukemia. Blood 110:2242–2249
3. Radich JP (2001) Philadelphia chromosome-positive acute lymphocytic leukemia. Hematol Oncol Clin North Am 15:21–36
4. Druker BJ, Talpaz M, Resta DJ, Peng B, Buchdunger E, Ford JM et al (2001) Efficacy and safety of a specific inhibitor of the BCR-ABL tyrosine kinase in chronic myeloid leukemia. N Engl J Med 344:1031–1037
5. Hughes TP, Kaeda J, Branford S, Rudzki Z, Hochhaus A, Hensley ML et al (2003) Frequency of major molecular responses to imatinib or interferon alfa plus cytarabine in newly diagnosed chronic myeloid leukemia. N Engl J Med 349:1423–1432
6. Druker BJ, Guilhot F, O'Brien SG, Gathmann I, Kantarjian H, Gattermann N et al (2006) Five-Year follow-up of patients receiving imatinib for chronic myeloid leukemia. N Engl J Med 355:2408–2417
7. Press RD, Galderisi C, Yang R, Rempfer C, Willis SG, Mauro MJ et al (2007) A half-log increase in BCR-ABL RNA predicts a higher risk of relapse in patients with CML with an imatinib-induced complete cytogenetic response (CCR). Clin Cancer Res 13:6136–6143
8. Press RD, Willis SG, Laudadio J, Mauro MJ, Deininger MW (2009) Determining the rise in BCR-ABL RNA that optimally predicts a kinase domain mutation in patients with chronic myeloid leukemia on imatinib. Blood 114:2598–2605
9. Cross NC, Feng L, Chase A, Bungey J, Hughes TP, Goldman JM (1993) Competitive polymerase chain reaction to estimate the number of BCR-ABL transcripts in chronic myeloid leukemia patients after bone marrow transplantation. Blood 82:1929–1936
10. Press RD, Love Z, Tronnes AA, Yang R, Tran T, Mongoue-Tchokote S et al (2006) BCR-ABL mRNA levels at and after the time of a complete cytogenetic response (CCR) predict the duration of CCR in imatinib-treated patients with CML. Blood 107:4250–4256

11. Branford S, Fletcher L, Cross NC, Muller MC, Hochhaus A, Kim DW et al (2008) Desirable performance characteristics for BCR-ABL measurement on an international reporting scale to allow consistent interpretation of individual patient response and comparison of response rates between clinical trials. Blood 112: 3330–3338
12. Hughes TP, Deininger MW, Hochhaus A, Branford S, Radich JP, Kaeda J et al (2006) Monitoring CML patients responding to treatment with tyrosine kinase inhibitors - Review and recommendations for 'harmonizing' current methodology for detecting BCR-ABL transcripts and kinase domain mutations and for expressing results. Blood 108:28–37
13. White H, Matejtschuk P, Rigsby P, Gabert J, Lin F, Wang L et al (2010) Establishment of the first World Health Organization international genetic reference panel for quantitation of BCR-ABL mRNA. Blood 116: e111–e117
14. Emig M, Saussele S, Wittor H, Weisser A, Reiter A, Willer A et al (1999) Accurate and rapid analysis of residual disease in patients with CML using specific fluorescent hybridization probes for real time quantitative RT-PCR. Leukemia 13:1825–1832
15. Westgard JO, Barry PL, Hunt MR, Groth T (1981) A multi-rule Shewhart chart for quality control in clinical chemistry. Clin Chem 27:493–501

Chapter 2

Detection of BCR-ABL1 Kinase Domain Mutations Causing Imatinib Resistance in Chronic Myelogenous Leukemia

Franklin R. Moore, Fei Yang, and Richard D. Press

Abstract

The reciprocal translocation between chromosomes 9 and 22 [t(9;22)(q34;q11), Philadelphia chromosome] creates a BCR-ABL1 fusion protein that occurs in approximately 95% of cases of chronic myelogenous leukemia (CML), 15% of cases of adult acute lymphoblastic leukemia, and 5% of adult cases of acute myeloid leukemia. The BCR-ABL1 protein is a constitutively activated tyrosine kinase that induces and maintains the neoplastic phenotype in these leukemias. PCR-based methods to identify and quantitate the tumor-specific BCR-ABL1 RNA have been shown to be an ultrasensitive diagnostic, prognostic, and monitoring tool for Philadelphia-positive leukemias. A novel tyrosine kinase inhibitor (TKI), imatinib, has been confirmed as an effective targeted treatment in most CML patients. However, a significant minority of patients being treated with imatinib develop resistance to the drug as evidenced by rising BCR-ABL1 levels. The most common mechanism of resistance in these patients is the development of mutations in the BCR-ABL1 kinase domain (KD) that abrogate binding of imatinib. Although KD mutations are quite heterogeneous, the identification of the exact mutation site is clinically important, as some mutations, but not others, can be effectively treated with second-generation TKIs. One mutation, T315I, for example, renders the leukemia resistant to all first- and second-line TKIs. Thus, DNA sequencing of the BCR-ABL1 kinase domain in resistant patients helps identify those who may benefit from a change in TKI agents, or those who should be considered for other therapeutic measures, such as stem cell transplantation. We describe here a method for sequencing the BCR-ABL1 kinase domain in peripheral blood or bone marrow of CML patients.

Key words Chronic myelogenous leukemia, Philadelphia chromosome, BCR-ABL1, Imatinib, Dasatinib, Nilotinib, Tyrosine kinase inhibitors, Major molecular response

1 Introduction

Chronic myelogenous leukemia (CML) is characterized by a reciprocal chromosome translocation between chromosomes 9 and 22. This translocation creates a fusion protein consisting of BCR and the ABL1 tyrosine kinase. The novel BCR-ABL1 protein has a deregulated, constitutively activated tyrosine kinase activity that drives the cancer phenotype. A novel class of therapeutic agents, tyrosine kinase inhibitors (TKIs), have been developed that bind and

Magdalena Czader (ed.), *Hematological Malignancies*, Methods in Molecular Biology, vol. 999,
DOI 10.1007/978-1-62703-357-2_2,

repress the activity of the ABL1 kinase domain (1). The first successful drug in this class, imatinib, significantly represses the leukemic clone without the typical toxicity of conventional nonspecific anticancer drugs, and has become the consensus first-line therapy for CML (2–6). The vast majority of imatinib-treated chronic-phase CML patients undergo a complete hematologic and cytogenetic response (3, 7, 8). However, despite these excellent initial responses, a minority of patients subsequently experience secondary (acquired) imatinib resistance as evidenced by a loss of their complete cytogenetic response (CCR). Among patients with secondary imatinib resistance, up to half harbor acquired mutations in the BCR-ABL1 kinase domain that abrogate imatinib binding to its target (9–12). Currently, over 70 mutations within the BCR-ABL1 tyrosine kinase domain have been identified (10, 13, 14). As most, but not all, of these KD mutants are sensitive to inhibition by second-generation TKIs, dasatinib and nilotinib, treatment with these second-line agents is often quite effective after imatinib failure (15). Notable exceptions, however, include some mutations that are particularly insensitive to nilotinib (Y253H, E255K/V, F359V/C), to dasatinib (F317L, V299L), or to all approved TKIs (T315I) (15). Given that the discovery of one of these mutations with dasatinib and/or nilotinib resistance would predict poor efficacy with that agent, the exact identification of BCR-ABL1 KD mutations has become a consensus method for evaluating putative drug resistance in CML (4, 5, 14). Although a variety of mutation-scanning methods can be used to detect KD mutations, the majority of labs undertake BCR-ABL1 mutation analysis by direct DNA sequencing of the entire KD (14). The unbiased direct sequencing approach allows identification of patients currently on imatinib that would benefit (or not) from second-generation TKIs. Additionally, sequencing identifies patients with the T315I mutation who may benefit from new experimental TKIs such as ponatinib (16). Other more toxic alternative therapies (e.g., stem cell transplant) could then be reserved only for those patients most likely to benefit from the additional risk. Our laboratory's protocol for direct DNA sequencing of the BCR-ABL1 kinase domain is detailed blow.

2 Materials

2.1 Cell Lysis

1. Samples for BCR-ABL kinase domain sequencing can be peripheral blood (drawn into EDTA or citrate tubes; minimum 5 ml) or bone marrow (minimum 2 ml in heparinized syringe, transferred to EDTA tube). The sample should arrive in the lab (room temperature transportation) no later than 24 h after being drawn. For the typical patient with quantitative BCR-ABL

RQ-PCR samples being evaluated in the same lab, residual RNA prepared for the same sample's RQ-PCR assay can be used (stored at −80°C).

2. Erythrocyte lysis buffer (Buffer EL Qiagen, Valencia, CA).
3. White cell lysis buffer ((Bottle #3) MagNA Pure LC mRNA HS Kit (Roche, Indianapolis, IN)).

2.2 Automated Isolation of mRNA Using Roche MagNA Pure Instrument

1. MagNA Pure LC mRNA HS Kit (Roche, Indianapolis, IN).
2. MagNA Pure consumables, including MagNA Pure small, medium, and large reagent tubs; large and small reaction tips; processing cartridges; and sample cartridges.
3. MagNa Pure LC 2.0 (Roche, Indianapolis, IN) automated nucleic acid extraction instrument.

2.3 Reverse Transcription of RNA to cDNA

1. Superscript II reverse transcriptase enzyme (Invitrogen, Carlsbad, CA).
2. 5× RT Buffer (included in Superscript II package).
3. 100 mM dithiothreitol (DTT) (included in Superscript II package).
4. Random primers $p(dn)_6$ (Roche Diagnostics, Indianapolis, IN) dissolved in 1 ml of RNase-free PCR grade H_2O (1 mM stock).
5. PCR nucleotide mix (Roche Diagnostics, Indianapolis, IN); each at a concentration of 10 mM.
6. Protector RNase Inhibitor, 40 U/μl (Roche Diagnostics, Indianapolis, IN).
7. MJ Research PTC-200 Peltier Thermal Cycler.

2.4 PCR

1. Primers:

   Forward BCR gene: ~40–60 bp's upstream of B2A2 fusion junction.

   BCR-ABL-1st-step-F (1F): 5′ c tga cca act cgt gtg tga aac t 3′ (bcr gene, Accession # Y00661; Nucleotide # 3240).

   Reverse ABL1 gene: ends ~8 bp's downstream from Glu-Thr-Met C terminus of kinase domain.

   BCR-ABL-1st-step-R: 5′ cc act tcg tct gag ata ctg gat 3′ (ABL1 gene: Accession # NM_005157; Nucleotide # 1499).

   Forward E1A2 BCR gene: starts ~200 bp's upstream of E1/A2 "minor" breakpoint (see Note 1).

   BCR-ABL-1st-F-e1a2 (1Fe1a2): 5′ acc gca tgt tcc ggg aca aaa g 3′ (bcr gene: Accession # Y00661; Nucleotide # 1675).

2. 10× Buffer 1 (1.75 mM Mg^{2+}) (included in Roche®) Expand Long Template PCR System (Roche Diagnostics, Indianapolis, IN).

3. Dimethylsulfoxide.
4. dNTPs (15 mM each).
5. Expand Long Template Taq (5 U/μl) (included in Roche®) Expand Long Template PCR System (Roche Diagnostics, Indianapolis, IN).
6. MJ Research PTC-200 Peltier Thermal Cycler.

2.5 PCR Product Visualization and Purification

1. 1% DNA agarose gel.
2. Low Mass DNA Ladder (Invitrogen, Carlsbad, CA).
3. 6× Type I gel loading dye.
4. ExoSap-IT (Affymetrix, Santa Clara, CA) (a mixture of two hydrolytic enzymes, exonuclease I and shrimp alkaline phosphatase).

2.6 Sequencing

1. BigDye® Terminator v1.1 Cycle Sequencing Kit (Applied Biosystems, Carlsbad, CA).
2. 5× Sequencing Buffer (included in BigDye kit).
3. Primers for ABL1 kinase domain sequencing (F = forward strand; R = reverse strand):

   BCR-ABL-2nd-step-F [2F]: 5′cgc aac aag ccc act gtc t 3′ (*ABL1* gene: Accession # NM_005157; Nucleotide # 661).

   BCR-ABL-1st-step-R [1R]: 5′ cc act tcg tct gag ata ctg gat 3′ (*ABL1* gene: Accession # NM_005157; Nucleotide # 1500) (see Note 2).

   Seq-BCRABL-MF [MF]: 5′cat cca cag aga tct tgc tgc c 3′ (*ABL1* gene: Accession # NM_005157; Nucleotide # 1080).

   Seq-BCRABL-MR [MR]: 5′ ccc cta cca ggc agt ttc g 3′ (*ABL1* gene: Accession # NM_005157; Nucleotide # 1102).

   ABL-R6 [Hein]: 5′ aga act tgt tgt agg cca 3 (*ABL1* gene: Accession # NM_005157; Nucleotide # 1235).

   ABL-3F: 5′ tga cag ggg aca cct aca ca 3′ (*ABL1* gene: NM_005157; Nucleotide # between 1141 and 1320).
4. MJ Research PTC-200 Peltier Thermal Cycler.
5. DyeEx 96 Kit (Qiagen, Valencia, CA).
6. Tabletop microplate centrifuge.
7. 3130 Genetic Analyzer (Applied Biosystems, Carlsbad, CA).
8. Hi-Di formamide (Applied Biosystems, Carlsbad, CA).
9. ABI 3130 septa, black plate holders, 96-well plates.
10. SeqScape sequence analysis software (Applied Biosystems, Carlsbad, CA).

3 Methods

CML patients receiving imatinib therapy are routinely monitored every 3–6 months with serial BCR-ABL1 RQ-PCR transcript levels. A rise of BCR-ABL1 RNA above a 2.6-fold optimized cutoff has been shown to be associated with a significantly increased risk of harboring a concomitant KD mutation (8). Thus, when a patient's transcript level rises, the same sample is often referred for DNA sequencing. If a mutant clone other than T315I is detected, the patient often becomes a candidate for treatment with a second-generation TKI. If the T315I mutation is detected, then, if available, a novel TKI or alternative non-pharmacologic measures such as stem transplantation are considered. Our method for quantitating BCR-ABL1 transcripts in peripheral blood or bone marrow is described in an accompanying chapter of this book. Here we detail our method for DNA sequencing the BCR-ABL1 KD from these same samples.

3.1 Lysis of Cells from Blood or Bone Marrow

1. Count cells from the raw blood or bone marrow sample using an automated hematology cell counter. Alternatively, a manual cell count can be performed. Use the total leukocyte count to determine the blood or bone marrow volume necessary to achieve a total of 5.0×10^7 white blood cells.
2. After calculating the volume of bone marrow or blood to be extracted (50 million cells), transfer that volume to an appropriate tube, and add a 2× volume of Qiagen Buffer EL (erythrocyte lysis) to the sample.
3. Place the tubes on a rocking platform or gyrotory shaker for 10 min at room temperature to lyse the red blood cells. Alternatively, manually invert the sample periodically for 10 min.
4. Centrifuge the tubes at $980 \times g$ for 5 min in a tabletop centrifuge (with the brake off) at room temperature. After centrifuging, a white cell pellet should be visible at the bottom of the tube (corresponding to 50 million cells).
5. With a sterile pipette, carefully remove the supernatant, or pour off supernatant into a waste container, but do not disturb the pellet.
6. To eliminate any residual red blood cells that may later interfere with PCR, add an additional 5–10 ml of red cell lysis buffer (EL) to the white cell pellet, resuspend the cells, and transfer to a 15 ml conical tube.
7. Spin the sample again at $980 \times g$ for 5 min. After centrifuging, a clean white cell pellet should be visible at the bottom of the tube.
8. With a sterile pipette, carefully remove the supernatant, or pour off supernatant into a waste container, but do not disturb the pellet.

9. Based on the number of cells extracted, calculate the volume of white blood cell lysis buffer (bottle #3 in MagNA Pure mRNA HS Isolation Kit) needed to achieve a final concentration of 1.0×10^7 white cells per ml, up to a total lysis buffer volume of 5 ml for 50 million cells.
10. After removal of the red cell lysis supernatant, add the appropriate volume of WBC lysis buffer to the WBC pellet.
11. Thoroughly resuspend the white cell pellet in the lysis buffer, by pipetting up and down several times.
12. Vortex the lysate briefly, and allow the lysate to rest for 5 min.
13. After 5 min, vortex the lysate again.
14. The lysed sample may now be put directly onto the MagNA Pure for mRNA isolation, or may be frozen at −70°C for mRNA isolation at a later time.

3.2 Automated Isolation of mRNA Using Roche MagNA Pure Instrument

1. If lysates have been frozen, allow to thaw along with a 10^{-4} control (1:10,000 dilution of K562 cells into a BCR-ABL-negative cell line, e.g., HeLa cells).
2. Programming the instrument.
   (a) Select "Start Program" on the MagNA Pure.
   (b) Select "Sample Ordering."
   (c) Under *Sample Protocol*, select "mRNA 1 cells.blk."
   (d) Under *Sample Volume*, type in the amount of cellular lysate you are starting with. This volume must be the same for all samples extracted in a given run, and will usually be *300 µl* (*usually three million cells, to reflect lysates frozen at ten million cells per ml*).
   (e) Under *Elution Volume*, change *25 µl* to *50 µl*. Do not choose a *Post-Elution Protocol*.
   (f) Type in patient identifiers on "Sample Ordering" List. When the identifiers (sample numbers) have been input for each sample to be extracted, click on "Start Batch." You will see a screen which indicates the volumes of all the reagents and types of consumables needed to complete the isolation process.
3. Preparing reagents and disposables.
   (a) Remove the metal tub rack from the instrument and place the appropriate sized reagent tubs in the tub rack.
   (b) Fill the reagent tubs with the given volumes of reagents (all reagents are part of the *MagNA Pure mRNA HS Kit*). Be sure to put the reagent tubs in the correct order, and skip positions as indicated.
   (c) Return the tub rack to the instrument stage and close the lockbar.

   (d) Place *sample processing cartridges* in the heating and cooling blocks.
   (e) Place the appropriate number of *processing cartridges* in the correct positions, as indicated on the screen.
   (f) Insert the necessary number of *large tips* (blue) and *small tips* (yellow) into the appropriate positions.
   (g) Position a solid waste bag on the disposal chute and hold it in place with the magnet provided.
   (h) Pipette the correct volume (300 μl) of cell lysate for each sample into the appropriate wells of a *sample cartridge* and place it in the instrument. Close the instrument door and click on the icon for each reagent and disposable that has been placed in the instrument.
   (i) Once all icons have been selected, an "OK" button will be visible on the screen. Click on the "OK" button.
   (j) The MagNA Pure will begin by slowly moving the robotic arm across the stage, to make sure that no obstacles are present. It will then begin extracting samples, eight at a time.
4. Aliquoting extracted mRNA upon program.
   (a) After the MagNA Pure instrument has completed the mRNA isolation process, mRNA samples will be in the sample cartridge in the cooling block of the instrument. Carefully aliquot the eluted mRNA (50 μl) into pre-labeled 1.5 ml tubes using pipettes designated for RNA use only.
   (b) Place tubes of mRNA on ice if directly proceeding with reverse transcription, or store at −70°C for future use.
5. Dispose of consumables, and close out windows until the front screen appears. Select "Decontamination." Next, select "Start Decontamination" from the "Actions" pull-down at the top of the window. Allow the UV decontamination of the MagNA Pure to proceed for 8 h (overnight).

3.3 Reverse Transcription

1. Start the following "RT" program on the thermocycler. Block will heat up to 65°C "forever."

   "BCR" Program (for reverse transcription)
   (a) 65°C "forever."
   (b) 25°C for 10 min.
   (c) 42°C for 50 min.
   (d) 70°C for 15 min.
   (e) 4°C "forever."
2. Place mRNA samples and RT reagents on ice to thaw. Include a positive and a negative control (see Note 3).

Table 1
Reverse transcription master mix

Reagent	Reaction (μl)	Final concentration
5× RT Buffer[a]	4	1×
100 mM DTT[a]	2	10 mM
Roche $Pd(N)_6$ (1 mM)	1	50 μM
dNTPs (10 mM ea)	1	0.5 mM ea
SuperScript II (200 U/μl)	1	10 U/μl
Roche protector RNase inhibitor (40 U/μl)	1	2 U/μl
Total volume	10 μl	

Total RT reaction = 20 μl
[a]Comes with Superscript II

3. Aliquot 10 μl of mRNA (from about 1.5 million cells) into appropriately labeled 0.5 ml tubes.
4. Place in thermal cycler to denature at 65°C and set timer for 10 min.
5. While denaturing, prepare an RT master mix as shown in Table 1 and place on ice.
6. After 10 min at 65°C, place tubes containing mRNA on ice; "proceed to next step" on thermal cycler, and press "pause," which will decrease the temperature to 25°C and hold it there.
7. Add 10 μl of master mix to tubes containing denatured mRNA (total RT reaction volume is 20 μl). Mix by pipetting up and down.
8. Place tubes in thermal cycler and resume program.
9. After RT is completed, store cDNA at 4°C short term (24 h) or −20°C long term.

3.4 PCR

1. Begin the following program on the thermocycler. Pause program when temperature reaches 95°C.

   "ABL-SEQP" Program

   (a) 95°C for 2 min.

   (b) 95°C for 20 s.

   (c) 58°C for 30 s.

   (d) 68°C for 90 s.

   (e) Repeat steps b–d, 44 times.

   (f) 68°C for 7 min.

   (g) 4°C "forever."

Table 2
PCR master mix

Reagent	Reaction (μl)	Final concentration
10× Buffer 1[a] (1.75 mM Mg^{2+})	5.0	1× w/175 μM Mg^{2+}
DMSO	5.0	
dNTPs (15 mM ea)	1.5	0.45 mM ea dNTP
Bcr-abl-1st-step-F primer (1F) 30 μM	1.0	0.6 μM
Bcr-abl-1st-step-R primer (1R) 30 μM[b]	1.0	0.6 μM
Expand Long Template Taq[a] 5 U/μl	0.75	0.075 U/μl
PCR grade H_2O	30.75	
Total volume	45	

Final PCR reaction volume = 50 μl
[a]Roche® Expand Long Template PCR System
[b]Or, try e1a2 "minor" breakpoint forward primer

2. Prepare PCR master mix as shown in Table 2 in 0.5 ml PCR tubes.
3. Aliquot 45 μl of master mix into 0.5 ml empty labeled tubes.
4. Add 5 μl cDNA to each PCR tube.
5. Place tubes in thermal cycler and resume program.
6. Place cDNA back into −20°C freezer for storage in case a repeat PCR is necessary.

3.5 Visualization of PCR Products

1. Prepare a 1% DNA agarose gel (see Note 4).
2. Load 4 μl of amplicon with 1 μl 6× Type I loading dye. For approximate quantification of product, load 4 μl of Low Mass DNA Ladder.
3. Run gel for approximately 20 min at 100 V.
4. Stain in ethidium bromide for 10 min and destain for 10 min.
5. Photograph the gel on a UV box.
6. Compare BCR-ABL1 RT-PCR product bands to the ladder (see Note 5). If sample bands (of the correct size) look to be approximately 80 ng or greater, go to Subheading 3.6 (purification/cleanup of PCR products). If the bands are weak or undetectable, and this correlates with an expectedly low-level BCR-ABL1 RNA (below ~0.3% on the international scale), then set up a nested PCR reaction, as in step Nested PCR, steps a–f. If the sample is known to have high-level BCR-ABL1 RNA and there is no visible amplicon, the presence of an alternative e1a2 "minor" translocation breakpoint is possible,

and the sample should be re-amplified using an E1/A2 forward primer, as in Minor Breakpoint E1/A2 PCR, steps a–c.

Nested PCR

(a) Prepare same PCR master mix as above, using the same primers for the nested reaction as for the first-round PCR, as in Subheading 3.4 (PCR), steps 1–6. Be sure to include two negative controls: the negative control from the first round of PCR, and a new negative control (water).

(b) Aliquot 45 μl of master mix into 0.5 ml tubes in the main lab (amplicon-free).

(c) Take the master mix to the PCR room to add 5 μl of first-round PCR product.

(d) Use the same program on the thermal cycler as for first-round PCR (see Subheading 3.4 PCR, step 1).

(e) Load the product onto a test gel again to check for a nested PCR product.

(f) If no band is visible after nested PCR, report out the case as "PCR failure" (either a technical failure or BCR-ABL1 RNA level too low to amplify for sequencing).

Minor Breakpoint E1/A2 PCR

(a) Prepare the same PCR master mix as before, but substituting "Bcr-abl-1st-F-e1a2" primer (30 μM stock) for primer 1F [see section 2.4 (PCR) for primer sequences].

(b) Run the thermal cycler program as in section 3.4 (PCR).

(c) Add 5 μl of cDNA to each 50 μl PCR reaction.

3.6 Purification/Cleanup of PCR Products Using ExoSap-IT

1. To a new PCR tube, add 6 μl of ExoSap-IT to 15 μl of PCR product. Mix well.
2. Run samples on the thermocycler with the following program:
   (a) 37°C for 15 min (to remove primers and dNTPs from PCR reaction).
   (b) 80°C for 15 min (to inactivate the ExoSAP-IT enzymes).

3.7 Setting Up Sequencing Reaction

1. Set up six separate sequencing reactions (one for each of six different sequencing primers) for each PCR product template as shown in Table 3.
2. Place in the thermocycler with the following cycle sequencing program:
   (a) 96°C for 1 min.
   (b) 24 cycles of 96°C for 10 s.
   (c) 50°C for 5 s.
   (d) 60°C for 4 min.
   (e) Hold at 4°C.

Table 3
Sequencing reaction master mix

BigDye 1.1 terminator ready mix	2 µl
5× Sequencing buffer	2 µl
3.2 µM Primer	1 µl
DNA (post ExoSap-IT PCR product)	3.5 µl
dH_2O	11.5 µl
Total volume	20 µl

3. At this point, samples can be stored at 4°C protected from light for up to 4 days.

3.8 Removal of Unincorporated Dye Terminators from Sequencing Reactions

DyeEx spin columns are pre-hydrated gel filtration columns designed to remove unincorporated dye terminators from cycle sequencing reactions.

1. Set up Qiagen DyeEx plate (see Note 6) in blue collection tray. Remove the bottom foil, then the top foil for the number of samples needed.
2. Spin plate on blue (waste) collection tray to elute pre-hydration buffer for 3 min at 750 × *g* in the tabletop microplate centrifuge.
3. Discard the flow-through and save the reusable waste collection tray.
4. Transfer the DyeEx plate on top of a clean 96-well plate that will collect the column flow-through for subsequent capillary electrophoresis.
5. Carefully load the entire sequencing reaction (20 µl) onto the DyeEx spin column resin bed (see Note 7).
6. Spin the plate stack for 3 min at 750 × *g* in a microplate centrifuge to elute the sample. The gel filtration column will retain unincorporated dye terminators from the sequencing reactions. Final elution volume will be approximately 20 µl.

3.9 ABI 3130 Capillary Electrophoresis Using 36 cm Array

1. Put the uncovered 96-well plate in the designated heat block and heat at 70°C until samples are completely evaporated (about 45 min).
2. Resuspend the dried samples in 20 µl of Hi-Di formamide.
3. Gently pipette up and down to resuspend, taking care not to introduce air bubbles (see Note 8).
4. Cover the plate with a gray septum (gasket) and denature samples at 95°C for 5 min.

5. Place the plate in a black plate holder, put on a white lid (make sure holes in lid and septum are aligned), and place this "sandwich" onto the ABI 3130 instrument.
6. On the ABI instrument, replace the anode buffer in the anode buffer jar and reservoir #1 with fresh buffer. Replace the water in reservoirs #2–4 in the instrument.
7. Set up a plate record in the ABI data collection software, link to plate, and click on ⇒ (run).
8. See Note 9 for suggested naming convention for sequencing samples.

3.10 Sequencing Data Analysis

1. Open ABI *Sequencing analysis* program.
2. Under *File*, click *Add Samples.*
3. Locate previously saved data files, click (to add the file to the analysis queue), and then click OK.
4. Click on ⇒ (run) at top of screen; this will begin basecalling (by sequence analysis software).
5. Next, click to check boxes in *P* column (for print) and click on ⇒ (run) once more. Data (electropherograms) will now be printed.
6. Under *File*, click *Save all samples.*
7. Acceptable run criteria:
   (a) Sensitivity control (also positive mutation control; BCR-ABL RNA ratio ~0.1%) must amplify and yield expected sequence.
   (b) Positive mutation control must show the expected mutation (and no others).
   (c) Negative control should not show any product on test gel (not sequenced).
8. The raw ABI-generated sequencing data can be analyzed a number of different ways (even manually), depending on the lab's needs and resources. Software for analysis of raw DNA sequencing data is available from several commercial vendors. In our lab, we use Seqscape® software from ABI, which we have internally validated as an accurate and sensitive DNA sequencing data analysis package. With Seqscape, the experimental data can be automatically compared to a reference *BCR-ABL1* sequence from Genbank, and automated reports can be generated detailing the location of putative mutations and the "quality" of the mutation determination. Seqscape's analysis settings can also be user adjusted to alter the "sensitivity" for detecting "mixed bases" when low-level variants are present. This is an important parameter for finding BCR-ABL1 kinase domain mutations that may be an evolving cause of resistance to kinase inhibitor therapy. In our lab, we set

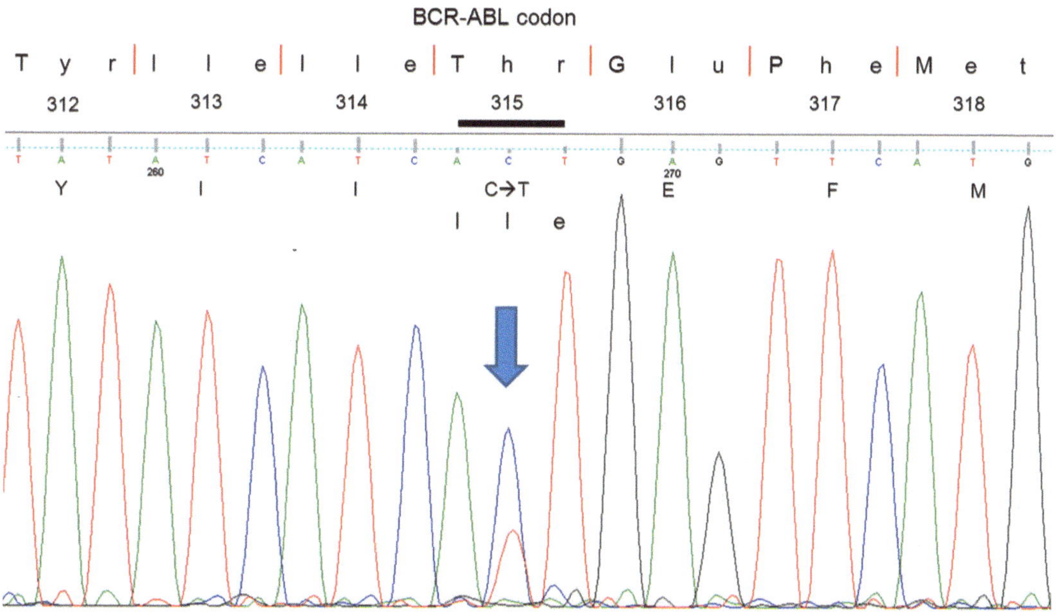

Fig. 1 A representative DNA sequencing electropherogram showing a T315I point mutation in the BCR-ABL kinase domain. The *arrow* indicates the location of a C to T single nucleotide mutation which changes a wild-type threonine amino acid (ACT) to isoleucine (ATT). The mutation appears to be expressed in only a minority of cells given the increased signal of the wild-type C nucleotide (*blue*) compared to the mutant T nucleotide (*red*)

Seqscape's "mixed base" analysis setting to 15%, which allows us to typically detect variant clones that are present at a level of approximately 15–20% in a background of wild-type BCR-ABL1. The consequence of this low mutation detection threshold setting is an increase in the number of "false-positive" mutation calls that must then be evaluated manually to discern whether or not they are "real." See Fig. 1 for a representative DNA sequencing electropherogram from a patient with a T315I point mutation. Figure 2 shows the frequency and heterogeneous distribution of mutations in the BCR-ABL1 kinase domain detected over an 8-year period at our institution.

4 Notes

1. The vast majority of patients have a p210 "major" bcr-abl breakpoint downstream of BCR exons b2 or b3. The "1F" forward primer will work in these cases. If the 1F/1R primer pair does not yield an expected 1.5–1.6 kb amplicon (and the BCR-ABL1 RNA ratio is above 0.02%), a "minor" e1a2 breakpoint is suspected—requiring the alternative 1Fe1a2 forward primer. A small minority of patients will have a p190 "minor"

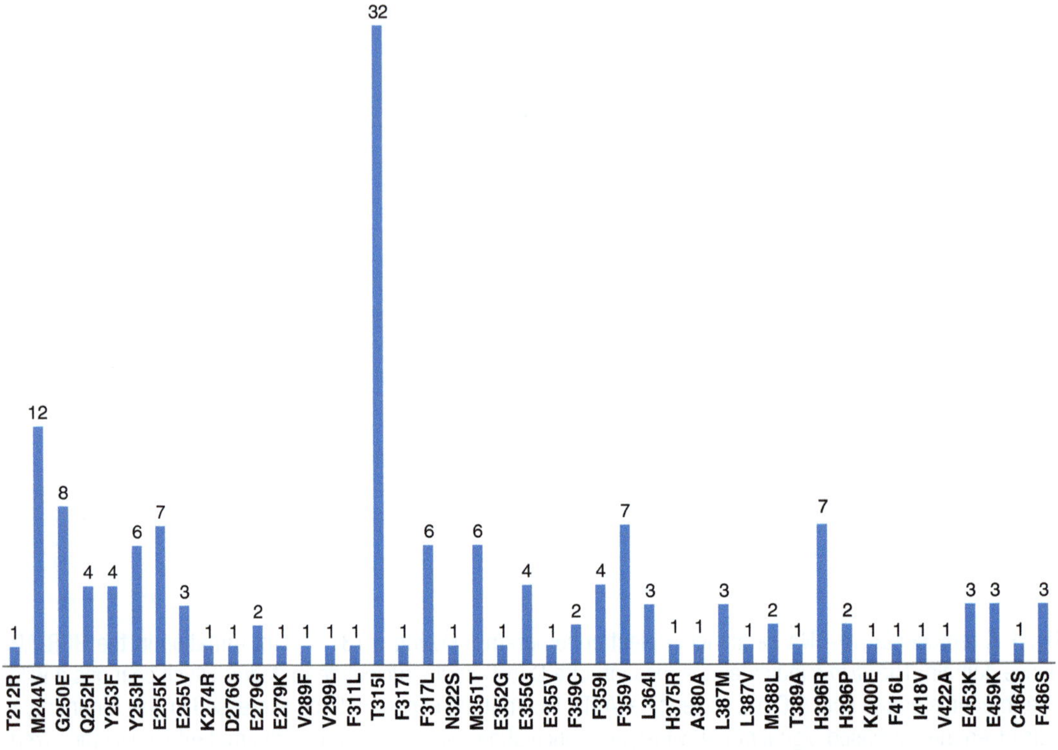

Fig. 2 The frequency of BCR-ABL kinase domain mutations in 110 leukemic patients followed at our institution. The total number of mutations sums to 153 indicative of the presence of multiple mutations in some patients. The *X*-axis depicts the BCR-ABL mutation locus using amino acid numbering as per Genbank accession number NM_005157. The *Y*-axis depicts the number of patients with each mutation. In these 110 patients, 43 distinct mutations have been detected at 34 different codons

breakpoint downstream of bcr exon e1. The exact breakpoint may or may not be known prior to sequencing.

2. The same reverse primer was used to generate the 1.5–1.6 kb BCR-ABL1 amplicon for sequencing. BCR-ABL1 RNA level must be above 0.02% (BCR-ABL1/G6PDH) to proceed with ABL1 sequencing. Levels below that cutoff will usually be insufficient to generate enough of the long BCR-ABL1 PCR product for successful sequencing.
3. For the positive mutant control, we rotate through various patient specimens previously identified as containing a mutation. For the negative control, we use water.
4. Use aerosol tips to prevent contamination when loading product onto gel.
5. PCR product (1F and 1R primers) is 1,579 bp for b3a2 and 1,504 bp for b2a2.

6. For small numbers of sequencing samples, individual DyeEx columns can be used in place of the plate method. This method follows the same procedure as above.
7. Do not touch the sides of the column or the resin bed with the tip.
8. Any bubbles that are inadvertently introduced may be removed with a pipette tip.
9. Name as sample number_primer name (e.g., n06-001014_2F, n06-001014_1R).

References

1. Savage DG, Antman KH (2002) Imatinib mesylate—a new oral targeted therapy. N Engl J Med 346:683–693
2. Druker BJ, Talpaz M, Resta DJ, Peng B, Buchdunger E, Ford JM et al (2001) Efficacy and safety of a specific inhibitor of the BCR-ABL tyrosine kinase in chronic myeloid leukemia. N Engl J Med 344:1031–1037
3. O'Brien SG, Guilhot F, Larson RA, Gathmann I, Baccarani M, Cervantes F et al (2003) Imatinib compared with interferon and low-dose cytarabine for newly diagnosed chronic-phase chronic myeloid leukemia. N Engl J Med 348:994–1004
4. Baccarani M, Saglio G, Goldman J, Hochhaus A, Simonsson B, Appelbaum F et al (2006) Evolving concepts in the management of chronic myeloid leukemia. Recommendations from an expert panel on behalf of the European Leukemianet. Blood 108:1809–1820
5. O'Brien S. NCCN clinical practice guidelines in oncology: chronic myelogenous leukemia. Version 2. 2012 (July 2011) NCCN.org. http://www.nccn.org/professionals/physician_gls/PDF/cml.pdf
6. Soverini S, Hochhaus A, Nicolini FE, Gruber F, Lange T, Saglio G et al (2011) BCR-ABL kinase domain mutation analysis in chronic myeloid leukemia patients treated with tyrosine kinase inhibitors: recommendations from an expert panel on behalf of European LeukemiaNet. Blood 118:1208–1215
7. Druker BJ, Guilhot F, O'Brien SG, Gathmann I, Kantarjian H, Gattermann N et al (2006) Five-Year follow-up of patients receiving imatinib for chronic myeloid leukemia. N Engl J Med 355:2408–2417
8. Hughes TP, Kaeda J, Branford S, Rudzki Z, Hochhaus A, Hensley ML et al (2003) Frequency of major molecular responses to imatinib or interferon alfa plus cytarabine in newly diagnosed chronic myeloid leukemia. N Engl J Med 349:1423–1432
9. Press RD, Willis SG, Laudadio J, Mauro MJ, Deininger MW (2009) Determining the rise in BCR-ABL RNA that optimally predicts a kinase domain mutation in patients with chronic myeloid leukemia on imatinib. Blood 114:2598–2605
10. O'Hare T, Eide CA, Deininger MW (2007) Bcr-Abl kinase domain mutations, drug resistance and the road to a cure of chronic myeloid leukemia. Blood 110:2242–2249
11. Jabbour E, Kantarjian H, Jones D, Talpaz M, Bekele N, O'Brien S et al (2006) Frequency and clinical significance of BCR-ABL mutations in patients with chronic myeloid leukemia treated with imatinib mesylate. Leukemia 20:1767–1773
12. Branford S, Rudzki Z, Walsh S, Parkinson I, Grigg A, Szer J et al (2003) Detection of BCR-ABL mutations in patients with CML treated with imatinib is virtually always accompanied by clinical resistance, and mutations in the ATP phosphate-binding loop (P-loop) are associated with a poor prognosis. Blood 102:276–283
13. Apperley JF (2007) Part I: mechanisms of resistance to imatinib in chronic myeloid leukaemia. Lancet Oncol 8:1018–1029
14. Jones D, Kamel-Reid S, Bahler D, Dong H, Elenitoba-Johnson K, Press R et al (2009) Laboratory practice guidelines for detecting and reporting BCR-ABL drug resistance mutations in chronic myelogenous leukemia and acute lymphoblastic leukemia. J Mol Diagn 11:4–11
15. Branford S, Melo JV, Hughes TP (2009) Selecting optimal second-line tyrosine kinase inhibitor therapy for chronic myeloid leukemia patients after imatinib failure: does the BCR-ABL mutation status really matter? Blood 114:5426–5435
16. O'Hare T, Deininger MW, Eide CA, Clackson T, Druker BJ (2011) Targeting the BCR-ABL signaling pathway in therapy-resistant Philadelphia chromosome-positive leukemia. Clin Cancer Res 17:212–221

Chapter 3

Laboratory Detection of *JAK2*^{V617F} in Human Myeloproliferative Neoplasms

Jonathan S. Kui, Rosanny Espinal-Witter, and Y. Lynn Wang

Abstract

Recently, a point mutation in the *JAK2* gene, *JAK2*^{V617F}, was discovered in several myeloid proliferative neoplasms including polycythemia vera (PV), essential thrombocythemia (ET), and primary myelofibrosis (PMF). Demonstration of the mutation and other similar mutations has now become one of the major criteria in the diagnosis of these neoplasms in the revised World Health Organization Classification of Tumors of Hematopoietic Tissues. In this chapter, we compared the advantages and disadvantages of five commonly used methods for the detection of *JAK2*^{V617F}. We explained, based on the current literature, why analytic sensitivity of the methodology is of particular importance for the detection of *JAK2*^{V617F}. A detailed laboratory procedure for the performance of an extensively optimized ARMS-PCR assay was presented. The assay shows distinct patterns for normal, mutant, and mixed genotypes. Diagnostically, it is highly sensitive, highly specific, and simple to perform with no need for any specialized equipment other than thermocyclers.

Key words JAK2^{V617F}, MPN, ARMS-PCR

1 Introduction

In 2005, five independent investigational groups described the association of a single point mutation of the *JAK2* gene with several myeloproliferative neoplasms (MPN) including polycythemia vera (PV), essential thrombocythemia (ET), and primary myelofibrosis (PMF) (1–5). JAK2 is a cytoplasmic tyrosine kinase that plays an essential role in the signaling pathways of cytokine and growth factors. Binding of a cytokine or growth factor to its receptor induces JAK2 phosphorylation and activation, phosphorylation of the receptor, and recruitment/phosphorylation of signal transducers and activators of transcription (STAT) proteins. STAT proteins by themselves, or via the subsequent activation of MAP kinase or PI3K-AKT pathway, can eventually lead to changes in gene expression, cell proliferation, and cell survival. The G>T

Magdalena Czader (ed.), *Hematological Malignancies*, Methods in Molecular Biology, vol. 999,
DOI 10.1007/978-1-62703-357-2_3,

Table 1
Frequencies of *JAK2^{V617F}* in several myeloproliferative neoplasms and the normal population

Disease	Frequencies (%)	References
Polycythemia vera	95–97	(12)
Essential thrombocythemia	~50	(12)
Primary myelofibrosis	~50	(12)
Normal individuals	~1	(33)

point mutation at nucleotide position 1849 changes conserved amino acid residue 617 from valine to phenylalanine, which renders constitutive activation of the JAK2 kinase, resulting in cytokine-/growth factor-independent cell proliferation.

The *JAK2* gene is located at chromosome 9q24. It spans ~150 kb and contains 25 exons. The encoded protein contains 1,132 amino acids and has a molecular weight of 130.7 kDa (6). JAK2 belongs to the *J*anus *K*inase family of tyrosine kinases, which includes JAK1, JAK2, JAK3, and TYK2. Similar to its family members, JAK2 possesses seven homologous domains, two of which are vital for the regulation of JAK2 function (7). The JH1 domain is a catalytic kinase domain, while the JH2 domain is a catalytically inactive pseudokinase domain which possesses an autoinhibitory function. The V617F mutation, located in exon 14 that is part of JH2, possibly abrogates the autoinhibitory function of the pseudokinase domain. Besides *JAK2^{V617F}*, more than a dozen deletions, insertions, and missense mutations involving residues 514–547 of exon 12 of the *JAK2* gene have been identified in a small fraction of PV patients (8). These mutations are functionally equivalent to the V617F mutation, causing constitutive activation of the JAK2 kinase (9, 10).

JAK2^{V617F} is an acquired somatic mutation. It is present in various myeloid hematopoietic elements including myeloid precursors but has not been identified in other tissues. As mentioned above, the *JAK2^{V617F}* mutation has been identified in three of the most common MPN. Essentially, all cases of PV are positive for *JAK2* mutations (11). In particular, the V617F mutation is present in 95–97% of PV cases, while the remaining cases have exon 12 mutations. *JAK2^{V617F}* is present in approximately 50% of ET and PMF. This mutation is also detected in a small fraction of other myeloid neoplasms such as chronic myelomonocytic leukemia, acute myeloid leukemia, and myelodysplastic syndrome (12) and ~1% of normal individuals (summarized in Table 1).

The discovery of the *JAK2* mutations has revolutionized the diagnostic approach to MPN and initiated the search for drugs targeting the JAK2 pathway (13). These diseases, previously called myeloproliferative disorders (MPD), have now been renamed to myeloproliferative neoplasms (MPN) in the 2008 version of the World Health Organization (WHO) Classification of Tumors of Hematopoietic and Lymphoid Tissues (14). In the previous 2001 version, there were multiple criteria for the diagnosis of PV: five criteria A and four criteria B. Presently, the five criteria A have been replaced by two major criteria, namely, (1) increased hemoglobin or other evidence of increased red cell volume and (2) the presence of *JAK2*^{V617F} or exon 12 mutations. All criteria B have also been replaced by three minor criteria including (1) bone marrow biopsy consistent with MPN, (2) low serum erythropoietin levels, and (3) the presence of endogenous erythroid colony formation. Currently, the diagnosis of PV requires either the existence of both major criteria and at least one minor criterion, or the presence of the first major criterion with at least two of the three minor criteria. These two diagnostic approaches decrease the effects of false positivity by molecular testing and include rare cases of PV that may have an unknown or a low level of *JAK2* mutation.

The diagnostic criteria for ET and PMF were also changed. The major changes for the diagnosis of ET include the lowering of sustained platelet count from 600×10^9/L to 450×10^9/L and the addition of a criterion for *JAK2*^{V617F} detection. The diagnosis of PMF was simplified to include three major criteria and at least two of the four minor criteria. Major criteria include (1) bone marrow histologic findings consistent with PMF, (2) demonstration of *JAK2*^{V617F} or other mutations in the MPL gene (that encodes for the thrombopoietin receptor), and (3) exclusion of other myeloid neoplasms. The minor criteria include (1) leukoerythroblastosis, (2) increased serum lactate dehydrogenase (LDH) levels, (3) anemia, and (4) palpable splenomegaly.

The new WHO criteria for diagnosis of MPN highlight the importance of molecular testing, particularly identification of *JAK2* mutations for the diagnosis of PV, ET, and PMF. In this chapter, we focus on methods for the detection of *JAK2*^{V617F} since it is the most common and best characterized mutation. As new mutations in exon 12 are still being discovered, screening methods such as sequencing, pyrosequencing, or denaturing high-pressure liquid chromatography (DHPLC) followed by sequencing are recommended for those interested in detection of exon 12 mutations.

The *JAK2*^{V617F} (1849 G>T) point mutation can be detected by various methods. When selecting a method for clinical diagnostic purposes, one should pay special attention to the analytical sensitivity of the techniques. Earlier studies using direct sequencing reported lower frequencies of the *JAK2*^{V617F} in all three entities of MPN: 65% in PV, 23% in ET, and 30% in PMF. Reevaluation using more sensitive techniques revealed higher frequencies: 95–97% in PV, ~50% in ET, and ~50% in PMF. The reason for these discrepancies is that the *JAK2* mutation is often present in a small fraction of the neoplastic cell population at the time of diagnosis. Using quantitative assessment, Vannuchi et al. reported that approximately 33%

Table 2
Analytical sensitivities, advantages, and disadvantages of various $JAK2^{V617F}$ detection methods

Method	Sensitivity (%)	Advantages/disadvantages
Direct sequencing	20–30	Insensitive
Pyrosequencing	~5	Quantitative/expensive equipment and special reagents
PCR-RFLP	4–5	Incomplete digestion generates a heterozygous pattern in a patient with only normal alleles
AS-PCR	1–3	Does not distinguish between homozygous and heterozygous mutations
ARMS-PCR	0.1–10	Simple, fast; allows demonstration of all three genotypes/insensitive

(57/173) of PV patients have <25% *JAK2*^{V617F} allele (15) and Lippert et al. reported that 21% (12/58) PV patients have <40% *JAK2*^{V617F} (16). Therefore, approximately 1/5 to 1/3 of PV patients would be falsely negative if direct sequencing were applied. Low sensitivity causes a bigger problem in ET where 3/4 (31/42) of cases carry <25% of the mutant *JAK2* (16). Listed in Table 2 are techniques widely used in clinical laboratories. The analytical sensitivity and advantages/disadvantages of each technique are summarized in the table and further discussed in detail below.

Direct sequencing is the most straightforward method for the detection of point mutations. However, it is problematic in the case of *JAK2*^{V617F} detection because of its low sensitivity. Although some laboratories reported that it may detect as low as 10% mutant in a mixture of mutant and normal alleles, most of the laboratories have 20–30% sensitivity for direct sequencing-based assays. Given that the percentage of V617F-positive cells in a PV, ET, or PMF patient can vary between 1 and 100%, this method is regarded as insensitive and generates a high percentage of false-negative results.

The technique of pyrosequencing is based on nucleotide extension by DNA polymerase. In the presence of nucleotides and several luciferase assay reagents, a primer upstream of the sequence variant site is extended by DNA polymerase. A particular nucleotide that complements the target sequence is added onto the primer and the primer is then extended by one base yielding a quantifiable light emission. As a result, one can rudimentarily measure the emission of light released upon the addition of a nucleotide that extends the mutant sequence versus the light released by extension of the wild-type sequence. The technique, therefore, is able to generate quantitative results estimating ratio of sequence

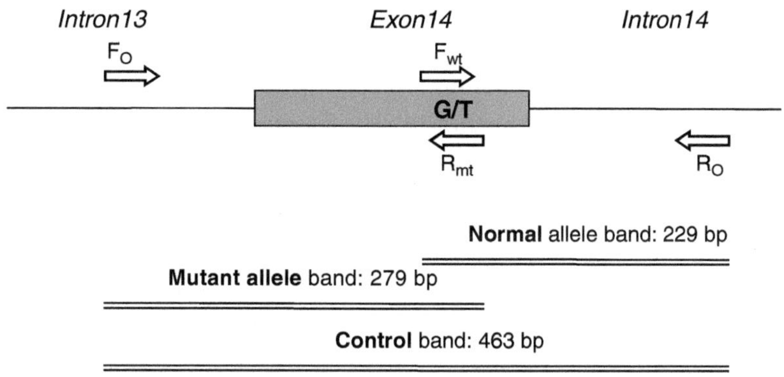

Fig. 1 *Schematic diagram of the JAK2 ARMS-PCR assay. Shaded bar* represents exon 14. G/T represents wild-type or mutant nucleotide sequence at 1849 position of the *JAK2* gene. F_0 forward outer primer, R_0 reverse outer primer, F_{wt} forward wild-type primer, and R_{mt} reverse mutant primer. Resultant amplicons are indicated by *double lines*

variants at any given nucleotide position. The analytic sensitivity of pyrosequencing can reach ~5%. However, this technique requires both expensive equipment and special reagents to perform. As a result, few hospital-based small clinical laboratories are equipped to utilize this method for routine purposes.

Restriction fragment length polymorphism (RFLP) analysis on PCR-amplified *JAK2* sequence is another method that is widely used. The amplified region is digested with BsaXI, a restriction endonuclease, whose recognition sequence hinges on the presence or absence of the 1849 G>T transversion. Although the technique has a sensitivity of 4–5%, incomplete digestion would generate a restriction fragment pattern suggesting the presence of both mutant and normal alleles in patients with only normal alleles, namely, false-positive results. In addition, the extra step of restriction digestion after PCR adds time, labor, and cost to the assay.

Conventional allele-specific PCR (AS-PCR) employs a primer that binds specifically to the mutant allele sequence. It assesses the presence of the V617F allele to a high sensitivity of 1–3%. However, because this method does not incorporate a wild-type-specific primer into its PCR design, it does not distinguish between patients carrying only the mutant allele and those carrying both normal and mutant alleles.

For the qualitative assessment of *JAK2*^{V617F} mutation, amplification refractory mutation system PCR (ARMS-PCR), a variation of AS-PCR, is recommended for routine clinical use. The ARMS-PCR method, illustrated in Fig. 1, incorporates two pairs of primers to simultaneously amplify three distinct amplicons that contain the mutant allele, the wild-type allele, and a DNA quality control. The original ARMS-PCR was published by Jones et al. (17).

The procedure has been optimized by our group, increasing its sensitivity from ~10 to 0.1% (18). A subsequent study from our group has demonstrated that the adequate analytical sensitivity of a clinical *JAK2* assay should be at the level of approximately 0.1%. With this level of sensitivity, $JAK2^{V617F}$ can be detected in almost all PV patients (11) and less than 1% of patients with non-MPN disorders (19), suggesting that the assay is highly sensitive and specific for clinical diagnostic purpose. A minor modification in primer concentrations has been added to make the assay more robust and reliable than the published method (18). The procedure is described in detail below.

2 Materials

2.1 Controls and Samples

1. Human erythrocytic leukemia (HEL) cell line (ATCC) serves as the $JAK2^{V617F}$-positive control.
2. K562, a chronic myelogenous leukemia cell line (ATCC), serves as the negative control.
3. Sensitivity controls: HEL DNA volumetrically diluted in K562 DNA to 1:500 (0.2%) and 1:1,000 (0.1%), respectively (see Subheading 2.2 for DNA extraction protocol).
4. Patient sample: peripheral blood or bone marrow (see Note 1 for alternative sample types).

2.2 Pre-analytical Cell Lysis and DNA Extraction

1. QIAamp DNA Mini Kit for DNA extraction (Qiagen, Valencia, CA), containing spin columns, proteinase K, lysis buffer AL, wash buffers AW1 and AW2, and elution buffer AE.
2. Erythrocyte lysis (EL) buffer (Qiagen, Valencia, CA).
3. Proteinase K (Invitrogen, Carlsbad, CA), 10 mg/mL stock made in 1× PCR buffer, stored at −20°C.
4. Ethanol.
5. Nuclease-Free water (Gibco, Bethesda, MD).

2.3 PCR Reagents

1. Qiagen HotStart Taq DNA polymerase and 10× PCR buffer (Qiagen, Valencia, CA).
2. dNTP mixture, 10 mM (Promega, Madison, WI).
3. Primer F_O ("forward outer"), 5′-TCC TCA GAA CGT TGA TGG CAG-3′.
4. Primer R_O ("reverse outer"), 5′-ATT GCT TTC CTT TTT CAC AAG AT-3′.
5. Primer F_{wt} ("forward wild type"), 5′-GCA TTT GGT TTT AAA TTA TGG AGT ATa TG-3′.
6. Primer R_{mt} ("reverse mutant"), 5′-GTT TTA CTT ACT CTC GTC TCC ACA aAA-3′. The intended mismatches in both F_{wt}

and R_{mt} are shown in lower case, and genotype-specific nucleotides are underlined.

7. MicroAmp reaction tubes with caps, 0.2 mL (Applied Biosystems, Carlsbad, CA).

2.4 Electrophoresis

1. Agarose (Invitrogen, Carlsbad, CA).
2. 1× TAE Buffer: 40 mM Tris acetate, 1 mM EDTA. Adjust pH to 8.3.
3. Ethidium bromide (Sigma-Aldrich, St. Louis, MO), 10 mg/mL stock solution, stored at room temperature in the dark.
4. 100 bp DNA molecular marker (Invitrogen, Carlsbad, CA).

3 Methods

A flow chart that outlines procedures involved in this assay is shown in Fig. 2. The *JAK2* ARMS-PCR assay utilizes four primers to simultaneously amplify three PCR products from a template DNA (Fig. 1). The outer primers, F_O and R_O ("forward outer" and "reverse outer"), amplify a 463-bp span of the region, flanking the 1849 G>T transversion in exon 14. Successful amplification of this control amplicon indicates that the template DNA is of sufficient quality and quantity to yield PCR products across this region. Additionally, there are two allele-specific primers included in the reaction. F_{wt} ("forward wild type") is a primer that is specific to the wild-type *JAK2* sequence, and creates a 229-bp amplicon when paired with primer R_O. R_{mt} ("reverse mutant") is a primer that is specific to the *JAK2*^{V617F} sequence, and creates a 279-bp amplicon when paired with primer F_O. The power of using this combination

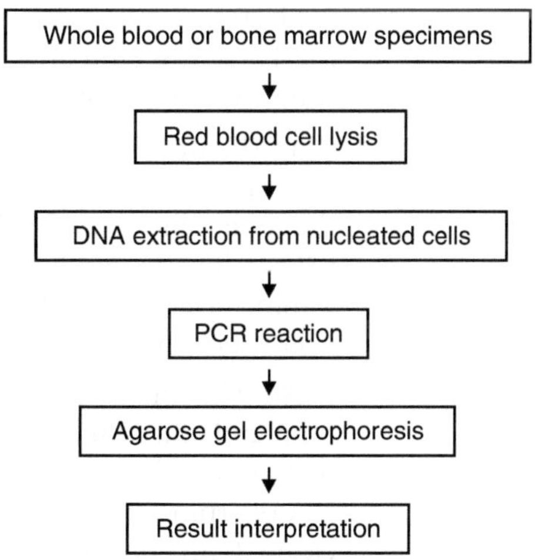

Fig. 2 Flow chart that outlines the major steps of the JAK2 ARMS-PCR assay

of primers lies both in its specificity and in its efficiency. In one PCR tube, three distinct products may be amplified simultaneously that distinguish patients who carry only *JAK2*^{V617F} from those who carry wild-type alleles and from those who carry both mixed mutant and wild-type *JAK2*^{V617F} alleles.

In the ARMS-PCR design, primer concentrations need to be delicately balanced because F_{wt} and F_O compete for R_O, and R_{mt} and R_O compete for F_O for amplification. Because F_{wt} and R_{mt} both contain mismatches to the *JAK2* genomic sequences, they would be outcompeted by F_O or R_O, respectively, if equal concentrations of the primers were employed in the reaction. In other words, if concentrations of the outer primers are too high, the kinetics of the PCR amplification will shift in favor of the control amplicon, weakening the yield of allele-specific amplicons. We have optimized the primer concentrations to allow for successful amplification of the mutant-specific amplicon when the *JAK2*^{V617F} allele is present in as low as 0.1% of total DNA.

3.1 DNA Extraction from Patient Samples

This procedure utilizes Qiagen's QIAamp DNA Mini Kit, for DNA extraction from whole blood or bone marrow specimens. Please refer to Note 2 for an alternative method for DNA preparation.

1. Lyse the red blood cells (RBC) in patient samples. Add 200 μL of whole blood or bone marrow to a 1.5 mL centrifuge tube. If a sample contains less than 200 μL, add 1× PBS to raise the sample volume to 200 μL. The manufacturer does not recommend including more than 5×10^6 cells in a lysis reaction. Add 20 μL of Qiagen proteinase K (included in the Qiagen DNA Mini Kit, concentration not indicated) and 200 μL of buffer AL to the tube. Briefly vortex and incubate at 56°C for 10 min. Briefly centrifuge the sample to remove drops from the tube lid.
2. Add 100 μL of ethanol to the sample. Mix by pulse-vortexing for 15 s. After mixing, briefly centrifuge the microcentrifuge tube to remove drops from the inside of the lid.
3. Bind the nucleic acids to the column resin. Carefully apply the mixture from step 2 to the center of a QIAamp spin column that is attached to a 2 mL collection tube (provided by the kit). Close the cap, and centrifuge at 6,000×*g* (8,000 rpm) for 1 min. Place the QIAamp spin column in a clean 2 mL collection tube, and discard the one containing the filtrate.
4. Wash with buffer AW1. Carefully open the QIAamp spin column and add 500 μL QIAamp buffer AW1 to the center of the matrix membrane. Close the cap and centrifuge at 6,000×*g* (8,000 rpm) for 1 min. Place the QIAamp spin column in a clean 2 mL collection tube, and discard the collection tube containing the filtrate.

5. Wash with buffer AW2. Carefully open the QIAamp spin column and add 500 μL QIAamp buffer AW2 to the center of the matrix membrane. Close the cap and centrifuge at full speed (20,000×*g*; or 14,000 rpm) for 3 min. Place the QIAamp spin column in a clean 1.5 mL microcentrifuge tube (not provided by the kit), and discard the collection tube containing the filtrate.
6. Elute DNA with buffer AE. Carefully open the QIAamp spin column and add 100 μL QIAamp buffer AE or nuclease-free water. Incubate at room temperature (15–25°C) for 1 min, and then centrifuge at 6,000×*g* (8,000 rpm) for 1 min. The eluate contains the purified DNA. 2.5 μL of this eluate is sufficient for use as template in the PCR reaction. While it is not necessary to measure DNA concentration, the sample may be quantified using UV spectrophotometry. 100–250 ng of template DNA may be used for PCR amplification.

3.2 Preparing Controls

1. Dilute control DNA from HEL and K562 cell lines in nuclease-free water to concentrations of 40 ng/μL.
2. Depending on frequency of usage, aliquot appropriate amount of HEL and K562 DNA into new tubes for storage at −20°C. An aliquot can be freeze/thawed a few times before being discarded.
3. Serially dilute HEL DNA in K562 DNA to final ratios of 1:500 and 1:1,000 for use as a 0.2% and 0.1% sensitivity controls, respectively. Appropriate aliquots of each of these dilutions may be stored at −20°C.

3.3 PCR Reaction

1. For each PCR reaction, reagents listed in Table 3 should be added. Creation of a PCR "master mix" to be aliquoted into separate PCR reaction tubes is recommended. To minimize the chance of cross-contamination, master mix should be added to the reaction tubes prior to the addition of sample DNA.
2. Each PCR run should include five control PCR reactions using the following as templates:
   (a) HEL DNA (positive control).
   (b) K562 DNA (negative control).
   (c) 1:500 dilution of HEL in K562.
   (d) 1:1,000 dilution of HEL in K562.
   (e) Nuclease-free water.

   To maximize the likelihood of contamination detection and minimize contamination of patient DNA with positive control DNA, addition of DNA to the PCR reaction tubes should proceed in the following order: patient DNA, HEL DNA, 0.2% control DNA, 0.1% control DNA, K562 DNA, and distilled water.

Table 3
Reagent components of the PCR reaction

Reagent (stock concentration)	Volume (μL)	Final concentration
10× DNA polymerase buffer	2.5	1×
dNTP (10 mM)	0.3	120 μM
Primer F_O (5 μM)	2.0	0.4 μM
Primer R_O (5 μM)	0.88	0.176 μM
Primer F_{wt} (5 μM)	2.5	0.5 μM
Primer R_{mt} (5 μM)	5.0	1.0 μM
Hotstart DNA polymerase (5 U/μL)	0.2	1 U
Template DNA	2.5	100 ng
H_2O	9.12	
Total volume	25	

3. Place all reaction tubes into a thermal cycler, and run the following PCR program: 95°C 15 min, 40 cycles of 94°C 30 s, 58°C 45 s, and 72°C 45 s, followed by 72°C 7 min, and hold at 4°C.

3.4 Electrophoresis and Visualization

1. Cast a 4% agarose gel. To 8.0 g of agarose powder, add 1× TAE to a volume of 200 mL. Boil and swirl gently until the molten agarose is uniformly clear. Swirling should be done carefully to avoid the introduction of air bubbles into the molten agarose.
2. Add 3 μL of 10 mg/mL ethidium bromide stock solution to the molten agarose, and gently swirl until uniform. Cast the gel into electrophoresis tray.
3. Resolve PCR products by gel electrophoresis. 10 μL of each PCR reaction is loaded onto the gel. For the HEL control reaction, as little as 2 μL may be loaded because the HEL cell line is homozygous for the *JAK2*^{V617F} allele and yields an extremely strong mutant band. The PCR products should be run with a 100 bp molecular weight marker for 45–60 min at 120 V.
4. Visualize PCR products under ultraviolet light.

3.5 Interpretation of Results

A sample gel is shown in Fig. 3. The steps below should be followed for interpretation. Expected sizes of amplicons are as follows:

Control: 463 bp.
Mutant allele: 279 bp.
Wild-type allele: 229 bp.

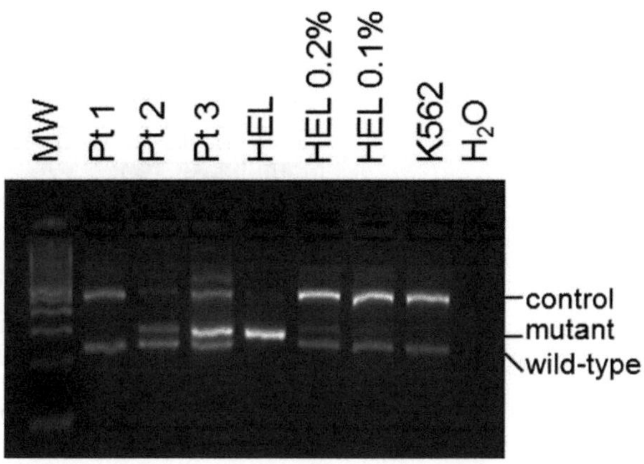

Fig. 3 *A gel picture of representative assay results.* The photo shows the wild-type pattern in patient 1 (Pt 1), and mixed mutant and wild-type patterns in patients 2 and 3, with different mutant/wild-type band ratios. The positive (HEL), sensitivity controls, negative (K562), and water controls are indicated. MW, 100 bp molecular weight marker

1. Evaluate controls to determine whether a run is acceptable. Examples of unacceptable results are described and shown in Note 3.

   Acceptable run shows the following control results:

HEL	Positive control	Mutant allele only
HEL 1:500	0.2% sensitivity control	Both normal and mutant alleles
HEL 1:1,000	0.1% sensitivity control	Both normal and mutant alleles
K562	Negative control	Normal allele only
dH_2O	Clean, no band	

2. Evaluate DNA quality for individual cases. DNA quality is determined to be adequate if the control band is present. In cases that have partial DNA degradation, the results can still be interpreted as long as the mutant band is present (see Pt. 2 and 6 in Fig. 4). If both control and mutant bands are absent, and only the wild-type band is present, the case is classified as indeterminate because DNA degradation may account for the failure to amplify the mutant amplicon, thus creating a false-negative result. Another sample should be requested if this is the case.

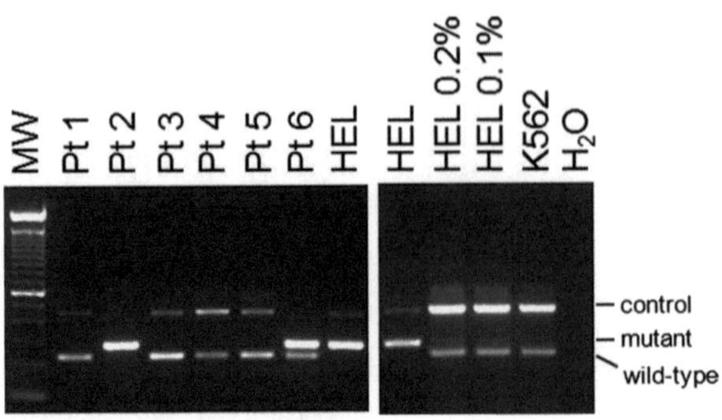

Fig. 4 *A sample gel showing unacceptable results.* Note aberrantly strong control band and weak mutant band in sensitivity controls. Pt 1, 3, 4, and 5 cannot be read as negative due to the failure of controls. Pt 2 and 6 were positive for the JAKV^{617F} mutation. The positive (HEL), sensitivity, the negative (K562), and water controls are indicated. MW, 100 bp molecular weight marker

Table 4
Interpretation of assay results

463 bp band (control)	279 bp band (mutant)	229 bp band (wild-type)	Interpretation
Present	Present	Present	Both normal and JAK2^{V617F} alleles detected
Present	Present	Absent	JAK2^{V617F} detected only
Present	Absent	Present	Normal allele detected only
Absent	Present	Present	Both normal and JAK2^{V617F} alleles detected
Absent	Present	Absent	JAK2^{V617F} detected only
Absent	Absent	Present	Indeterminant. Poor DNA quality
Absent	Absent	Absent	DNA absent or severely degraded

3. Interpret patient results. Depending on the band pattern generated, the terms in Table 4 are used for interpretation (also see Fig. 3).
4. Since *JAK2^{V617F}* mutation is a somatic mutation rather than a germ line mutation, terms such as "homozygous" and "heterozygous" are avoided. In some cases, the cells may be genetically mixed, i.e., a fraction of analyzed cells carries the mutation on one of the two alleles, and another fraction carries the mutation on both alleles through mitotic recombination, and yet another fraction carries two wild-type alleles. So the terms "homozygous" and "heterozygous" can be misleading

when describing patient samples. Cell lines are exceptions since they are derived from a single malignant clone.

5. This assay is qualitative, not quantitative (see Note 4). However, mutant-only and various mutant/normal ratios have been observed in patient samples that allow semiquantitative assessment. Despite this, semiquantitative assessment is currently of no clinical value.

4 Notes

1. Alternative sample types. The analytes for ARMS-PCR in this procedure are the DNA derived from nucleated cells in the peripheral blood or the bone marrow. Peripheral blood is used much more frequently because it is easily accessible. Purified granulocytes from the peripheral blood may be used instead of total leukocytes. Interestingly, plasma may also be used instead of the cellular component of the peripheral blood. By some recent reports, the use of plasma as the source of DNA has resulted in detection of a higher number of $JAK2^{V617F}$ cases (20, 21). Besides genomic DNA, RNA-/cDNA-based reverse transcription PCR assays (RT-PCR) have been reported to yield a higher analytical sensitivity (8). In essence, the common goal of these alternatives is to increase the analytical sensitivity of a specific method. Despite this, additional steps will involve extra time, reagents, and labor for routine analysis. It is at the discretion of the individual laboratory whether analytic sensitivity beyond 0.1% is needed for their testing. Regardless, DNA or cDNA prepared from these alternative sample types can be combined with the ARMS-PCR procedure presented here.
2. Alternative method for DNA preparation. Qiagen's QIAamp DNA Mini Kit reliably produces highly purified DNA from blood and bone marrow samples, using a simple protocol. However, some small laboratories may find this method too costly. As an alternative, our laboratory also utilizes a more cost-effective and simple method to prepare DNA for PCR. This procedure involves a red cell lysis step followed by proteinase K digestion. Proteinase K is a versatile, nonspecific endolytic protease which remains active over a wide pH range. The enzyme facilitates lysis of the leukocytes and the concomitant release of DNA of sufficient quality to yield robust and reproducible PCR amplification. The preparation steps are as follows:
   (a) RBC lysis. Add 5× of specimen volume of Qiagen erythrocyte lysis buffer (EL) to the peripheral blood or bone marrow specimen, inverting the tube several times to mix. Incubate the tube on ice for 15 min, vortexing the tube periodically during incubation.

(b) Centrifugate the specimen at $400 \times g$ for 10 min at 4°C. Aspirate and discard all but 50 μL of the supernatant, without disturbing the cell pellet. Add 2× of the original specimen volume of buffer EL to the tube, vortexing to resuspend cells. Immediately centrifuge the specimen at $400 \times g$ for 10 min at 4°C.

(c) Aspirate and discard all but 50 μL of the supernatant, without disturbing the cell pellet.

(d) Wash the cell pellet. Resuspend the pellet in 1 mL of PBS, and centrifugate the specimen at $400 \times g$ for 5 min. Aspirate and discard the supernatant.

(e) The remaining leukocyte pellet is then resuspended in 300–500 μL of proteinase K solution (0.5 mg/mL proteinase K in 1× PCR buffer) and incubated overnight at 37°C.

(f) Heat inactivate the proteinase K by incubating the lysate at 95°C for 10 min. This lysate (2.5 μL) is added to PCR reaction.

It should be noted that inexperienced workers may encounter some problems with this inexpensive method. One problem is caused by the presence of residual erythrocytes remaining after the RBC lysis step. Proteinase K-mediated lysis of these red cells releases hemoglobin into the DNA solution. Heme, a chelating substance, is a potent inhibitor of PCR, likely chelating magnesium ions that are required for the function of Taq polymerase. A good visual indicator of the presence of heme is a distinctly brown appearance of the proteinase K lysate after an overnight digestion.

One way to avoid this problem is to remove any remaining red-colored material after the PBS wash at step d. After centrifugation, the leukocytes will form a distinct white pellet occupying the bottom, while contaminating red cells will form a thin red ring or layer above the white cell pellet. This layer can be removed by pipetting.

Another potential problem of this method is deciding the proper amount of proteinase K solution to be added to the white cell pellet after RBC lysis. Because of the variability of cell counts in patient samples, 5 mL of peripheral blood from patients may yield a leukocyte pellet with a volume as low as 50 μL and as high as 500 μL. Addition of an insufficient volume of proteinase K solution often leads to failures in PCR amplification possibly because of intractably high concentrations of PCR inhibitors in the DNA solution. Based on our experience, we recommend adding ~500 μL of proteinase K solution for every 30 μL of leukocyte pellet. We have also found that adding proteinase K solution in excess is more likely to give amplifiable template than adding insufficient proteinase K. In cases where the leukocyte yield is high (>100 μL) after RBC lysis, we recommend transferring 30 μL of the pellet to a fresh microcentrifuge tube for proteinase K digestion.

3. PCR troubleshooting. The most common problem encountered with this assay is the loss of the mutant band and over-amplification of the control band. This problem is easily revealed by the sensitivity controls, particularly the 0.1% control (Fig. 4 shows such an example). The problem may be caused by one of two factors. The first is the repetitive freezing/thawing of the sensitivity control samples, which does lead to DNA degradation. Overall degradation of DNA will preferentially affect the HEL mutant DNA because of its scarcity in the sensitivity controls (0.2 and 0.1% dilutions of HEL DNA in K562 DNA). Creating a new set of controls is recommended as the first step in troubleshooting this problem.

   Another potential cause for this problem is the degradation of primers resulting from repetitive freezing/thawing. As mentioned above, a delicate balance needs to be maintained among the four primers. This degradation will result in a functional decrease in the concentration of one of the primers. As a result, the equilibrium of the PCR may shift towards a preferential amplification of one of the three amplicons. According to our experience, the 5 μM stock of primers can be freeze-thawed approximately ten times without causing problems.

4. Quantitative measurement of JAK2^{V617F} allele burden. Quantitative measurement of allele burden have been used mostly in research settings. Currently, the clinical utility of the assay remains unclear. The potential uses include:

   (a) Differential diagnosis among PV, ET, and PMF. Although ET patients have a lower level of *JAK2*^{V617F} than PV and PMF patients, there are no watershed values allowing differentiation of ET from other entities of MPN (22, 23).

   (b) Prediction of disease severity and risk-stratification of patients. Although several studies find that higher *JAK2* allele burden correlated with a higher leukocyte count, larger spleen size, and increased thrombotic events (15, 24), others did not reproduce such findings (25). Similar controversies remain in studies of ET and PMF patients (26).

   (c) Therapeutic monitoring. Clinical trials of several JAK2 inhibitors are currently ongoing. However, unlike the imatinib/*BCR-ABL* story, the *JAK2* allele burden does not seem to respond well to JAK2 inhibition (27). Several reports have suggested that *JAK2* allele burden decreases with nonspecific cytoreductive chemotherapy such as interferon alpha (28, 29) or hydroxyurea (30, 31).

However, recent studies have not confirmed that the clinical response is associated with molecular remission (24, 32). Whether such reduction would result in clinical benefit will need to be investigated further.

Although quantitative measurement of *JAK2*^{V617F} allele burden is potentially useful, published studies vary to a large degree in methods used for its determination. Studies differ in choice of specimens (BM vs. PB), cell types (granulocytes vs. total leukocytes), types of analyte (genomic DNA vs. RNA), standard curve generation (cell line vs. purified DNA vs. plasmid dilution), PCR method (AS-PCR/melting curve analysis vs. Taqman vs. pyrosequencing), and result expression (*JAK2*^{V617F}/ABL, *JAK2*/cell, or *JAK2*^{V617F}/total JAK2). Variation in these parameters make it difficult to compare different studies and also contributes significantly to discrepancies in published results regarding correlation between allele burden and clinical manifestation (23). In summary, the clinical utility of the quantitative assays needs to be further delineated and the methodologies need to be standardized, perhaps through a commercial source.

References

1. Baxter EJ, Scott LM, Campbell PJ, East C, Fourouclas N, Swanton S et al (2005) Acquired mutation of the tyrosine kinase JAK2 in human myeloproliferative disorders. Lancet 365:1054–1061
2. James C, Ugo V, Le Couedic JP, Staerk J, Delhommeau F, Lacout C et al (2005) A unique clonal JAK2 mutation leading to constitutive signalling causes polycythaemia vera. Nature 434:1144–1148
3. Kralovics R, Passamonti F, Buser AS, Teo SS, Tiedt R, Passweg JR et al (2005) A gain-of-function mutation of JAK2 in myeloproliferative disorders. N Engl J Med 352:1779–1790
4. Levine RL, Wadleigh M, Cools J, Ebert BL, Wernig G, Huntly BJ et al (2005) Activating mutation in the tyrosine kinase JAK2 in polycythemia vera, essential thrombocythemia, and myeloid metaplasia with myelofibrosis. Cancer Cell 7:387–397
5. Zhao R, Xing S, Li Z, Fu X, Li Q, Krantz SB et al (2005) Identification of an acquired JAK2 mutation in polycythemia vera. J Biol Chem 280:22788–22792
6. Cools J, Peeters P, Voet T, Aventin A, Mecucci C, Grandchamp B et al (1999) Genomic organization of human JAK2 and mutation analysis of its JH2-domain in leukemia. Cytogenet Cell Genet 85:260–266
7. James C, Ugo V, Casadevall N, Constantinescu SN, Vainchenker W (2005) A JAK2 mutation in myeloproliferative disorders: pathogenesis and therapeutic and scientific prospects. Trends Mol Med 11:546–554
8. Ma W, Kantarjian H, Zhang X, Yeh CH, Zhang ZJ, Verstovsek S et al (2009) Mutation profile of JAK2 transcripts in patients with chronic myeloproliferative neoplasias. J Mol Diagn 11:49–53
9. Scott LM, Tong W, Levine RL, Scott MA, Beer PA, Stratton MR et al (2007) JAK2 exon 12 mutations in polycythemia vera and idiopathic erythrocytosis. N Engl J Med 356:459–468
10. Scott LM, Beer PA, Bench AJ, Erber WN, Green AR (2007) Prevalence of JAK2 V617F and exon 12 mutations in polycythaemia vera. Br J Haematol 139:511–512
11. Wang YL, Vandris K, Jones A, Cross NC, Christos P, Adriano F et al (2008) JAK2 Mutations are present in all cases of polycythemia vera. Leukemia 22:1289
12. Tefferi A, Thiele J, Orazi A, Kvasnicka HM, Barbui T, Hanson CA et al (2007) Proposals and rationale for revision of the World Health Organization diagnostic criteria for polycythemia vera, essential thrombocythemia, and primary myelofibrosis: recommendations from an ad hoc international expert panel. Blood 110:1092–1097
13. Santos FP, Verstovsek S (2011) JAK2 inhibitors: what's the true therapeutic potential? Blood Rev 25:53–63
14. Swerdlow SH, Campo E, Harris NL, Jaffe ES, Pileri SA, Stein H et al (2008) WHO classification

of tumours of haematopoietic and lymphoid tissues, 4th edn. International Agency for Research on Cancer, Lyon
15. Vannucchi AM, Antonioli E, Guglielmelli P, Longo G, Pancrazzi A, Ponziani V et al (2007) Prospective identification of high-risk polycythemia vera patients based on JAK2(V617F) allele burden. Leukemia 21:1952–1959
16. Lippert E, Boissinot M, Kralovics R, Girodon F, Dobo I, Praloran V et al (2006) The JAK2-V617F mutation is frequently present at diagnosis in patients with essential thrombocythemia and polycythemia vera. Blood 108:1865–1867
17. Jones AV, Kreil S, Zoi K, Waghorn K, Curtis C, Zhang L et al (2005) Widespread occurrence of the JAK2 V617F mutation in chronic myeloproliferative disorders. Blood 106:2162–2168
18. Chen Q, Lu P, Jones AV, Cross NC, Silver RT, Wang YL (2007) Amplification refractory mutation system, a highly sensitive and simple polymerase chain reaction assay, for the detection of JAK2 V617F mutation in chronic myeloproliferative disorders. J Mol Diagn 9: 272–276
19. Wang YL, Lee JW, Kui JS, Chadburn A, Cross NC, Knowles DM et al (2007) Evaluation of JAK2 in B and T cell neoplasms: identification of JAK2(V617F) mutation of undetermined significance (JMUS) in the bone marrow of three individuals. Acta Haematol 118:209–214
20. Ma W, Kantarjian H, Verstovsek S, Jilani I, Gorre M, Giles F et al (2006) Hemizygous/homozygous and heterozygous JAK2 mutation detected in plasma of patients with myeloproliferative diseases: correlation with clinical behaviour. Br J Haematol 134:341–343
21. Ma W, Kantarjian H, Zhang X, Sun W, Buller AM, Jilani I et al (2008) Higher detection rate of JAK2 mutation using plasma. Blood 111: 3906–3907
22. Larsen TS, Pallisgaard N, Moller MB, Hasselbalch HC (2007) The JAK2 V617F allele burden in essential thrombocythemia, polycythemia vera and primary myelofibrosis—impact on disease phenotype. Eur J Haematol 79:508–515
23. Antonioli E, Guglielmelli P, Poli G, Bogani C, Pancrazzi A, Longo G et al (2008) Influence of JAK2V617F allele burden on phenotype in essential thrombocythemia. Haematologica 93:41–48
24. Silver RT, Vandris K, Wang YL, Adriano F, Jones AV, Christos PJ et al (2011) JAK2(V617F) allele burden in polycythemia vera correlates with grade of myelofibrosis, but is not substantially affected by therapy. Leuk Res 35:177–182
25. Tefferi A, Strand JJ, Lasho TL, Knudson RA, Finke CM, Gangat N et al (2007) Bone marrow JAK2V617F allele burden and clinical correlates in polycythemia vera. Leukemia 21: 2074–2075
26. Vannucchi AM, Antonioli E, Guglielmelli P, Pardanani A, Tefferi A (2008) Clinical correlates of JAK2V617F presence or allele burden in myeloproliferative neoplasms: a critical reappraisal. Leukemia 22:1299–1307
27. Tefferi A, Pardanani A (2011) JAK inhibitors in myeloproliferative neoplasms: rationale, current data and perspective. Blood Rev 25:229–237
28. Jones AV, Silver RT, Waghorn K, Curtis C, Kreil S, Zoi K et al (2006) Minimal molecular response in polycythemia vera patients treated with imatinib or interferon alpha. Blood 107:3339–3341
29. Kiladjian JJ, Cassinat B, Turlure P, Cambier N, Roussel M, Bellucci S et al (2006) High molecular response rate of polycythemia vera patients treated with pegylated interferon alpha-2a. Blood 108:2037–2040
30. Girodon F, Schaeffer C, Cleyrat C, Mounier M, Lafont I, Santos FD et al (2008) Frequent reduction or absence of detection of the JAK2-mutated clone in JAK2V617F-positive patients within the first years of hydroxyurea therapy. Haematologica 93:1723–1727
31. Theocharides A, Passweg JR, Medinger M, Looser R, Li S, Hao-Shen H et al (2008) The allele burden of JAK2 mutations remains stable over several years in patients with myeloproliferative disorders. Haematologica 93:1890–1893
32. Kuriakose E, Vandris K, Wang YL, Chow W, Jones AV, Christos PJ et al (2012) Decrease in JAK2V617F allele burden is not a prerequisite to clinical response in patients with polycythemia vera. Haematologica 97:538–542
33. Xu X, Zhang Q, Luo J, Xing S, Li Q, Krantz SB et al (2007) JAK2(V617F): prevalence in a large Chinese hospital population. Blood 109: 339–342

Chapter 4

c-kit Mutational Analysis in Paraffin Material

Karl Sotlar

Abstract

The current WHO classification of mastocytosis defines one major and four minor diagnostic criteria for systemic mastocytosis (SM). One of the minor criteria is the detection of the "gain-of-function" mutation D816V of the *c-kit* proto-oncogene in extracutaneous organs. The receptor molecule KIT is a potential therapeutic target for tyrosine kinase inhibitors. *KIT* mutations have been described in more than 80% of SM, but only in the minority of cutaneous mastocytoses (CM). Usually exon 17 amplicons generated by polymerase chain reaction are analyzed for the detection of *c-kit* mutations. Most frequently the method of restriction fragment length polymorphism (RFLP) analysis using the endonuclease *Hinf* I is used. Another well-established technique utilizes melting point analysis of amplification products with specific hybridization probes. Recently, also allele-specific PCR assays have been described. The technique used for the detection of *c-kit* mutations in mastocytosis is dependent on the kind of material to be analyzed and the laboratory equipment available. In this chapter the techniques of PNA-mediated PCR-clamping in combination with melting point analysis for the genotyping of amplification products are described for mutational analysis in total DNA and microdissected cells from formalin-fixed paraffin-embedded bone marrow trephine biopsies.

Key words Mastocytosis, PNA, PCR-clamping, Melting point analysis, FFPE, Microdissection

1 Introduction

Mastocytosis comprises a heterogeneous group of disorders characterized by accumulation of abnormal mast cells (MC) in various tissues. Two main variants of the disease exist, cutaneous and systemic forms (1, 2). Cutaneous mastocytosis typically presents as urticaria pigmentosa (UP, (3)). In systemic mastocytosis (SM), by definition, an extracutaneous tissue/organ is involved, most frequently the bone marrow (4). SM is further subdivided into an indolent variant (ISM), SM with an *a*ssociated clonal *h*ematologic *n*on-*m*ast cell lineage *d*isease (AHNMD), aggressive SM (ASM), and mast cell leukemia (MCL). For the discrimination of SM from CM and other pathologic conditions with marked increase of reactive MC, one major and four minor diagnostic

Magdalena Czader (ed.), *Hematological Malignancies*, Methods in Molecular Biology, vol. 999,
DOI 10.1007/978-1-62703-357-2_4, © Springer Science+Business Media New York 2013

criteria were defined (2). The major diagnostic criterion is the histological demonstration of multifocal compact tissue infiltrates consisting of at least 15 MC. Minor criteria include the demonstration of more than 25% spindle-shaped MC, *c-kit* mutations at codon 816, expression of CD25 and/or CD2 by MC, and a persistently elevated serum total tryptase level (exceeding 20 ng/ml). A diagnosis of SM should only be made when, either, the major criterion plus at least one minor criterion or at least three minor criteria are fulfilled (2).

The *c-kit* proto-oncogene encodes for a transmembrane tyrosine kinase receptor (*KIT*/CD117) whose ligand is the stem cell factor (*SCF*, (5, 6)). KIT is expressed on MC as well as on hemopoietic stem cells, melanocytes, and germ cells (7–12). Activated KIT mediates signals for proliferation and maturation in these cells (13, 14). Certain somatic "gain-of-function" mutations, most frequently D816V, cause ligand-independent activation of *KIT* (15, 16). The mutation is not specific for mastocytosis and, like other activating *KIT* codon 816 mutations, has also been described in testicular germ cell tumors (17). In addition, mutations in other regions of the *c-kit* gene were found in acute myeloid leukemia (AML), gastrointestinal stromal tumors (GIST), sinonasal T-cell lymphomas (18–20), and melanoma (21).

In formalin-fixed paraffin-embedded (FFPE) and decalcified tissue, like bone marrow biopsies, mRNA is widely degraded. Thus, genomic DNA has to be analyzed for mutation screening. Especially in ISM, neoplastic MCs, which are the source of *KIT* mutations, often represent only a minor fraction (less than 5%) of the nucleated bone marrow (BM) cells. Therefore, methods for the detection of *KIT* codon 816 mutations in such a large background of wild-type (WT) cells need to be highly sensitive. A number of techniques, like single-strand conformation polymorphism (SSCP), restriction fragment length polymorphism (RFLP), DNA sequencing, allele-specific amplification (ASA), or hybridization with oligonucleotide probes, have been described, which may allow detection of sequence variants in extremely small tumor cell populations in such cases.

Peptide nucleic acid (PNA) oligomers allow an enhanced allele-specific amplification of minor sequence variants (22). PNA-DNA hybrids have a higher thermal stability than DNA-DNA hybrids and PNA oligomers cannot be extended by DNA polymerases (22). These two characteristics allow the use of wild-type-specific PNA as competitors to mutation-specific primers (23, 24). A drawback of this setup is that abundant read-through from the suppressed WT may still occur, resulting in amplification products that will contain the mutation, thus making it indistinguishable from amplification products generated from the mutated alleles.

Hybridization probes consist of a pair of terminally fluorescent-labeled oligonucleotide probes designed to bind to a target strand in close proximity, enabling an energy transfer (FRET) between both fluorophores. Measurement of the fluorescence energy during a melting analysis is a sensitive monitor for base variations within the target region covered by the probes (25). Hybridization probes are widely used for the analysis of mutations, for example in the *HFE* gene in hemochromatosis or in the *N-ras* gene in cancer (26, 27). However, the analysis is restricted to see equivalent amounts of the variants or to detect the major variant only.

We have therefore combined the PNA-mediated PCR-clamping method with the subsequent online mutation detection by melting point analysis with hybridization probes (28). The method we described used a wild-type-specific PNA and mutation-specific hybridization probes for the detection of KIT^{D816V} mutations in formalin-fixed and paraffin-embedded biopsy specimens, including decalcified BM (28, 29). Recently, we introduced a locked nucleic acid (LNA) molecule instead of PNA (30, 31).

In the present chapter the method will be described in all details, including extraction of total DNA from tissue sections, PCR analysis with various amplification techniques, and genotyping by melting point analysis. In addition, the analysis of pooled singly microdissected MC is described.

2 Materials

2.1 Sample Fixation

1. Four percent neutrally buffered formalin, pH 7.0 (Sigma-Aldrich, Munich, Germany).
2. EDTA (ethylenediaminetetraacetate), pH 7.1.

2.2 DNA Extraction Using Phenol/Chloroform/IAA

1. Proteinase K buffer: 50 mM Tris–HCl, 1 mM EDTA, 0.5% Tween-20, pH 8.5. Store at 4°C.
2. Proteinase K (e.g., Qiagen, Hilden, Germany).
3. Phenol/chloroform/isoamyl alcohol (Sigma-Aldrich, Munich, Germany) is mixed at v/v/v 25:24:1. Store at room temperature in an appropriate locker under air exhausting conditions and keep away from light.
4. 8 M lithium chloride (LiCl) stock solution. Store at 4°C.
5. 100% ethanol. Store at –20°C.
6. 70% ethanol. Store at –20°C.

2.3 DNA Extraction Using Extraction Columns

1. For example, QIAamp DNA Micro Kit (Qiagen, Hilden Germany).

2.4 Determination of DNA Concentration

1. BioPhotometer plus UV/Vis Photometer (Eppendorf, Hamburg, Germany).
2. NanoDropTM 2000 (PEQlab, Erlangen, Germany). The latter one is preferable because DNA concentration may be determined from sample volume of only 1 μl.

2.5 Conventional PCR

1. Reaction tubes for preparation of DNA-free "master mixes" (e.g., Eppendorf 2.0 ml microcentrifuge tube, Eppendorf, Hamburg, Germany) and LightCycler capillaries for PCR amplification and melting point analysis (LightCycler® Capillaries (20 μl), Roche Molecular Systems, Mannheim, Germany).
2. *LightCycler® FastStart DNA Master HybProbe kit* (Roche Molecular Systems, Mannheim, Germany) containing hot-start Taq polymerase, LightCycler buffer, $MgCl_2$, and dNTPs. Store at −20°C.
3. PCR primers *c-kit 2F* (5′-CAG CCA GAA ATA TCC TCC TTA CT-3′) and *c-kit 2B* (5′-TTG CAG GAC TGT CAA GCA GAG-3′). Adjust both primers to 5 μM stock solutions and store at −20°C. Avoid repeated freezing and thawing.
4. Hybridization probes for melting point analysis: c-kit *Sensor* (5′-AGC CAG AGT CAT CAA GAA TGA TTC TA (Fl)-3′) and c-kit *Anchor* (5′-(LC) ATG TGG TTA AAG GAA ACG TGA GTA CCC A (p)-3′). Adjust both probes to 6 μM stock solutions and store at −20°C. Avoid repeated freezing and thawing. Keep away from light.

   FL, the Sensor probe is 3′ fluorescein labeled.

   LC, the Anchor probe is 5′ terminally labeled with LightCycler Red 640.

   p, the Anchor probe is 3′ terminally labeled with a phosphate group.
5. LightCycler® 1.5® or 2.0® Carousel-based System Instruments for PCR amplification and melting point analysis (Roche Molecular Systems, Mannheim, Germany). Alternatively use the high-throughput LightCycler® 480 Real-Time PCR System (Roche Diagnostics, Mannheim, Germany).

2.6 PNA-Mediated PCR-Clamping

1. DNA-free "master mixes" contain the same components as listed in Subheading 2.5, items 1–4. In addition a PNA molecule allowing PCR-clamping is added. Likewise, PCRs are performed in a final volume of 20 μl on one of the LightCycler Instruments listed above.
2. Peptide nucleic acid (PNA) for PCR-clamping: PNA molecule (5′-GCC AGA GAC ATC AAG AAT G-3′). Adjust the PNA probe to a 15 μM stock solution and store at −20°C. Avoid repeated freezing and thawing.

2.7 PNA Nested-PCR (PNA-nPCR) and Subsequent Melting Point Analysis of Amplification Products

1. Reaction tubes for preparation of DNA-free "master mixes" (e.g., Eppendorf 2.0 ml microcentrifuge tube, Eppendorf, Hamburg, Germany) and 0.2 ml PCR reaction tubes (e.g., Biozym, Hessisch Oldendorf, Germany).
2. AmpliTaq Gold® DNA polymerase kit (Applied Biosystems, Darmstadt, Germany) containing hot-start DNA polymerase, PCR buffer, and $MgCl_2$. Store at −20°C.

3. dNTP mix for PCR and nested-PCR (e.g., Fermentas GmbH, St. Leon-Rot, Germany). Adjust to 25 mM stock solution and store at −20°C.
4. PCR primers *c-kit 1F* (5′-CAC AGA GAC TTG GCA GCC AG-3′) and *c-kit 1B* (5′-CAG GAT TTA CAT TAT GAA AGT CAC GG-3′). Adjust both primers to 5 µM stock solutions and store at −20°C. Avoid repeated freezing and thawing.
5. PNA molecule (see Subheading 2.6, item 2).
6. Nested-PCR primers *c-kit 2F* and *c-kit 2B* (see Subheading 2.5, item 3).
7. Hybridization probes for melting point analysis after nested-PCR (see Subheading 2.5, item 4).
8. Thermal cycler (e.g., Veriti® 96-Well Thermal Cycler, Applied Biosystems, Darmstadt, Germany).
9. Reaction tubes for preparation of DNA-free "master mixes" (e.g., Eppendorf 2.0 ml Microcentrifuge Tube, Eppendorf, Hamburg, Germany) and LightCycler capillaries for melting point analysis (LightCycler® Capillaries (20 ml), Roche Molecular Systems, Mannheim, Germany).
10. MgCl2 solution. Use the solution supplied in excess with the LightCycler® FastStart DNA Master HybProbe kit (Roche Molecular Systems, Mannheim, Germany).
11. LightCycler® 1.5® or 2.0® Carousel-based System Instruments for melting point analysis (see Subheading 2.5, item 5).

2.8 Immunostaining of Tissue Slides for Analysis of DNA from Microdissected Pooled Single Cells

1. Deparaffinizing of tissue slides: xylol, EtOH (100, 96, 70%), sterile aqua bidest.
2. Epitope retrieval: microwave oven, min 750 W; Target Retrieval Solution pH 6.0 (Dako, Glostrup, Denmark); aqua bidest.
3. 0.5 M Tris–HCl buffer, pH 7.5.
4. Blocking of endogenous peroxidase: 7.5% H2O2.
5. Primary antibody: mast cell tryptase 1:350 (Zytomed Systems, Berlin, Germany).
6. Detection system: ImmPRESS anti-mouse Ig (peroxidase) polymer detection kit (Vector Laboratories, Burlingame, CA, USA).
7. Chromogen: AEC (Invitrogen, Darmstadt, Germany).
8. Counterstain: Hematoxylin Gill's Formula (Vector Laboratories, Burlingame, CA, USA).

2.9 Laser Pressure Catapulting (LPC) of Single Cells

1. PALM MicroBeam System (Carl Zeiss Microimaging GmbH, Munich, Germany) or an alternative system for single cell microdissection.
2. 0.2 ml PCR tubes with transparent lids (e.g., PeqLab, Erlangen, Germany).

3. Mineral oil (e.g., M5904 mineral oil, Sigma-Aldrich, Munich, Germany).
4. 10 μl pipette tips (e.g., PeqLab, Erlangen, Germany).

2.10 DNA Digestion from Microdissected Pooled Single Cells

1. Proteinase K buffer: 199 ml of 50 mM Tris–HCL/1 mM EDTA pH 8.5 (autoclaved and stored at RT) + 1 ml Tween 20. Store at 4°C.
2. Proteinase K: Dilute stock solution (Proteinase K >600 mAU/ml, Qiagen, Hilden, Germany) to 1.0 mAU/μl, prepare 50 μl aliquots. Store at −20°C.

2.11 Nested-PCR and Gel Electrophoresis for Microdissected Pooled Single Cells

1. For nested-PCR reagents and melting point analysis see Subheading 2.7.
2. 1× TBE loading buffer, pH 8.0: 10.8 g (89 mM) Tris base, 5.5 g (89 mM) boric acid, and 0.74 g (2 mM) Na2EDTA. Adjust to 1,000 ml with dH2O.
3. 2% agarose gel: mix 2 g agarose powder (SeaKem Agarose, ME Biozym, Oldendorf, Germany) and 100 ml 1× TBE buffer on a thermomixer; before casting the gel add 10 ml ethidium bromide (per 100 ml gel) and mix gently. Since EtBr is potentially mutagenic, wear gloves and work under an extractor hood; dispose gels appropriately after use.
4. Gel chamber (e.g., PerfectBlue Wide Gel System, peqlab, Erlangen, Germany).
5. Gel loading buffer (PeqLab, Erlangen, Germany). Store at 4°C.
6. Length marker Hae III digested ΦX-DNA (PeqLab, Erlangen Germany).

3 Methods

3.1 Sample Fixation and Pretreatment

Usually, tissues aimed to be investigated by histopathology are fixed in formalin and then are embedded in paraffin, allowing for the production of very thin (about 3 μm) slides. Underfixation, but especially overfixation, will impair the results of both immunohistochemical and molecular analyses. Four percent neutrally buffered (pH 7.0) formalin has turned out to be a good compromise between fixation efficiency and the option for additional molecular investigations. After fixation, bone marrow biopsies additionally have to be decalcified in EDTA overnight. EDTA should be rinsed off the trephine biopsy specimen before further processing.

3.2 DNA Extraction from Tissue Sections Using Phenol/Chloroform/IAA Method

Techniques described below are generally applicable with various sources of tissues, e.g., tissue slides mounted on glass (stained or unstained), tissue slide rolls (10–20 μm thick tissue sections will curl up and can be placed very easily into 2.0 ml reaction tubes), and smears (see Note 1).

1. For deparaffinization of tissue/paraffin rolls add at least 1,000 μl of pure xylol to each reaction tube (see Note 2), vortex vigorously for 1 min, then centrifuge for 1 min at 6,000 × *g*, and discard the supernatant (see Note 3). Repeat the procedure at least three times.
2. To wash away the xylol, add 1,000 ml pure ethanol, vortex vigorously for 1 min, then centrifuge for 1 min at 6,000 × g, and discard the supernatant. Repeat the procedure two times.
3. Place the open reaction tubes into a vacuum dryer for about 3–5 min (see Note 4).
4. Add about 300 ml of proteinase K buffer (see Note 5) and incubate for 10 min at 95°C (see Note 6).
5. Then place tubes on ice for about 5 min before adding proteinase K (1 ml proteinase K/100 ml buffer).
6. Incubate at 55°C for at least 2 h and subsequently fat 37°C overnight (see Note 7).
7. For the separation of the protein fraction from the aqueous phase add 300 ml of phenol/chloroform/isoamyl alcohol (PCI; v/v 25:24:1; see Note 8), vortex for 1 min, and centrifuge for 5 min at 13,000 × g.
8. Meanwhile, prepare a second tube with 450 ml chloroform/isoamyl alcohol (CI; v/v 24:1) for each sample.
9. After centrifugation from step 5, very carefully remove the DNA-containing upper aqueous phase from the first tube and pipette it into the second one (see Note 9).
10. To increase the amount of DNA recovery, add 150 ml dH2O (see Note 10), vortex for 1 min, and centrifuge for 5 min at 13,000 × g.
11. Again very carefully remove the upper aqueous phase and pipette it into the second tube. Then vortex the second tube for 1 min and centrifuge for 5 min at 13,000 × g.
12. Meanwhile discard the first tube and its remaining phenol phase appropriately.
13. Prepare a third tube containing 40 ml 8 M LiCl (see Note 11).
14. To precipitate the DNA, after centrifugation, carefully pipette the upper aqueous phase into the LiCl-containing third tube (see Note 12) and mix gently.
15. Add 1,200 ml ice-cold (stored at −20°C) pure ethanol, mix gently, and incubate at least 2 h at −20°C.
16. Then centrifuge at 4°C for 30 min.
17. Carefully pour the aqueous ethanol phase into a collecting tray and rinse the DNA pellet with 200 ml ice-cold 70% ethanol.

18. Pour away the ethanol completely and place the open reaction tubes into a vacuum dryer for about 5–10 min (see Note 13).
19. Resuspend the DNA pellet in 20 μl dH_2O either by intensive pipetting or in a mixer (see Note 14).

3.3 DNA Extraction with Commercial Kits (e.g., QIAamp DNA Micro Kit) (Qiagen, Hilden Germany) According to the Manufacturer's Instructions

1. Steps 1–3, Subheading 3.2.
2. Add 180 μl ATL buffer and 20 μl proteinase K to dried tissue pellet and vortex for 15 s.
3. Incubate overnight (more than 12 h) at 56°C in a thermomixer.
4. Centrifuge at 13,000 ×*g* for 10 s to detach buffer condensated at the tips of the tubes.
5. Add 200 μl AL buffer, vortex for 15 s, and centrifuge.
6. Add 200 μl pure ethanol, vortex for 15 s, then incubate for 5 min at RT, and centrifuge.
7. Transfer fluid (in total 600 μl) onto a QIAamp MinElute column (provided in the kit) and centrifuge at 6,000 ×*g* for 1 min.
8. Place columns into fresh collecting tubes and discard flow-through adequately.
9. Add 500 μl AW1 washing buffer to the columns and centrifuge at 6,000 ×*g* for 1 min, and then transfer column to a third collecting tube.
10. Add 500 μl AW2 washing buffer to the columns and centrifuge at 6,000 ×*g* for 1 min, and then transfer column to a fourth collecting tube.
11. Centrifuge at "full speed" (20,000 ×*g*) for 3 min to dry the membrane of the column.
12. Transfer columns into new sterile 1.5 ml safe lock tubes; make sure that tubes carry appropriate identifiers.
13. Pipette 15–25 μl (depending on the amount of tissue/the size of the dried tissue pellet) dH_2O onto the center of the column membrane and incubate at room temperature for 15 min.
14. Centrifuge at 20,000 ×*g* for 5 min at room temperature with open lids (see Note 15). Discard columns.

3.4 Determination of DNA Concentration

1. Determine the DNA concentration with a photometer according to the manufacturer's instructions (e.g., Eppendorf BioPhotometer plus UV/Vis Photometer, Hamburg Germany; NanoDrop™ 2000, PEQlab, Erlangen Germany).
2. If necessary (and possible) adjust the DNA concentration to 25–50 ng/μl.

3.5 Conventional Polymerase Chain Reaction (PCR) Technique

To avoid contamination, see recommendations in Note 16!

DNA-free "master mixes" contain reagents of the *LightCycler® FastStart DNA Master HybProbe kit*, i.e., Taq polymerase, LightCycler buffer, and dNTPs, as well as 3 mmol/l $MgCl_2$, 5 pmol (0.25 μM) of primers c-kit 2F and c-kit 2B, and 6 pmol (0.3 μM) of both hybridization probes c-kit *Sensor* and c-kit *Anchor* (see Note 17). PCRs are performed in a final volume of 20 μl on the capillary-based LightCycler 1.5®, on 2.0® Carousel-based System Instruments, or the high-throughput LightCycler 480 Real-Time PCR System.

1. Assemble 18 μl of PCR master mix according to the following pipetting schema:
   (a) 8.8 μl dH_2O.
   (b) 2.0 μl Roche *FastStart DNA Master* (*containing hot-start DNA polymerase, dNTPs, 10× buffer, and 10 mM MgCl2*).
   (c) 3.2 μl $MgCl_2$.
   (d) 1.0 μl primer c-kit 2F (final concentration, 0.25 μM).
   (e) 1.0 μl primer c-kit 2B (final concentration, 0.25 μM).
   (f) 1.0 μl probe c-kit Mutation (final concentration, 0.3 μM).
   (g) 1.0 μl probe c-kit Sensor (final concentration, 0.3 μM).
2. Add 2 μl sample DNA (given volumes of PCR master mix are to be multiplied with the number of samples; see Notes 18 and 19).
3. For PCR conditions, see Subheading 3.6, step 3.
4. For genotyping see Subheading 3.6, step 3.

3.6 PNA-Mediated PCR-Clamping (Fig. 1)

DNA-free "master mixes" contain the same components as listed in Subheading 3.5 (see Note 16). In addition PNA molecules allowing PCR-clamping are added. Likewise, PCRs are performed in a final volume of 20 μl on one of the LightCycler Instruments listed above.

1. Assemble of 18 ml of PCR master mix according to the following pipetting schema:
   (a) 7.8 μl dH_2O.
   (b) 2.0 μλ Roche *FastStart DNA Master*.
   (c) 3.2 μl $MgCl_2$.
   (d) 1.0 μl primer c-kit 2F (final concentration, 0.25 μM).
   (e) 1.0 μl primer c-kit 2B (final concentration, 0.25 μM).
   (f) 1.0 μl probe c-kit Mutation (final concentration, 0.3 μM).
   (g) 1.0 μl probe c-kit Sensor (final concentration, 0.3 μM).
   (h) 1.0 μl PNA (final concentration, 0.75 μM).

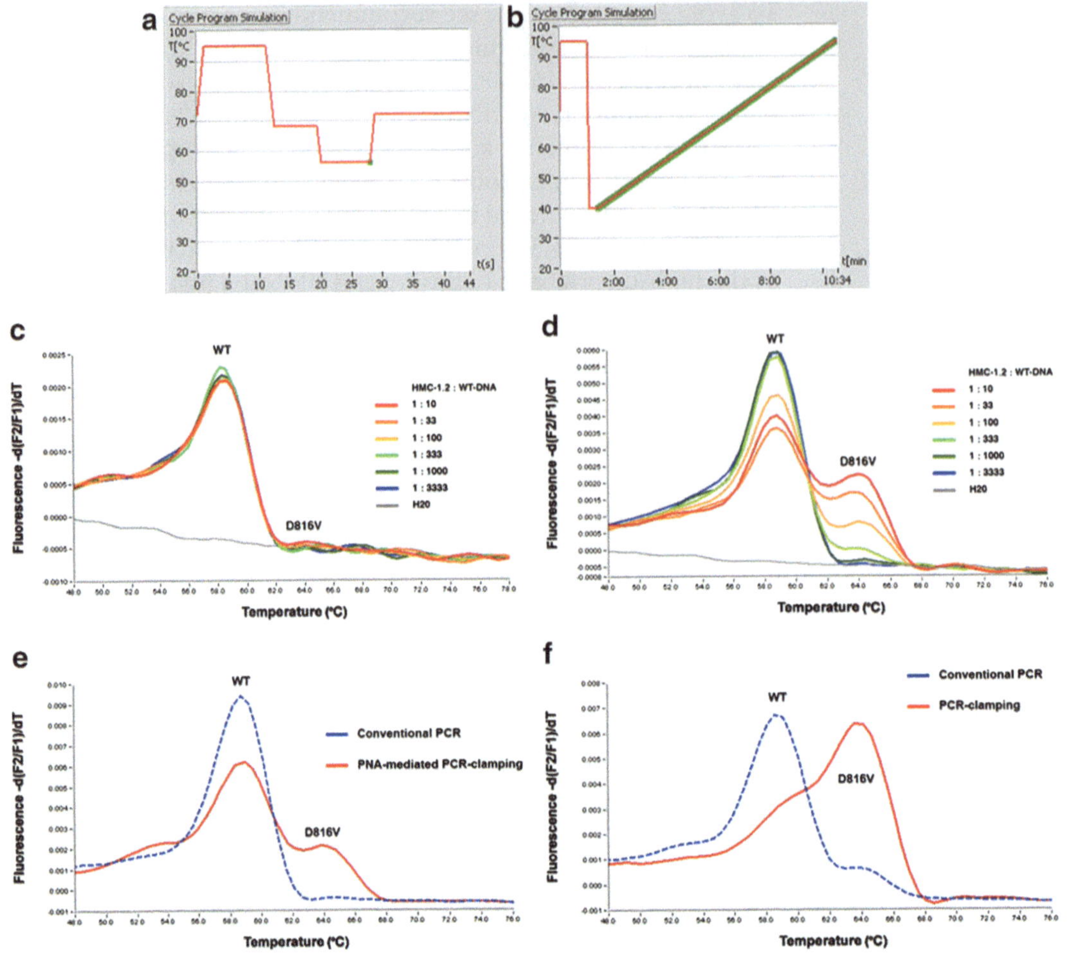

Fig. 1 Temperature profile of PNA-PCR. (**a**) Temperature profile for amplification cycles. (**b**) Temperature profile during melting point analysis. Note that green dots in both figures indicate time points for measurement of fluorescent signals. Effects of PNA-mediated PCR-clamping in dilution series of constant levels of WT-DNA (25 ng) and decreasing amounts of HMC-1 DNA (human mast cell leukemia cell line heterozygous for the mutation c-kit 816 V). (**c**) Melting point analysis of conventionally amplified DNA results in a very weak mutation-specific signal at a 1:10 dilution (red line). (**d**) Highly increased detection level after PNA-mediated PCR-clamping with a clear mutation-specific signal at 1:333 dilution (light green line) and weak mutation-specific signal at 1:1,000 dilution (dark green line). PNA-mediated PCR-clamping in systemic mastocytosis. (**e**) Indolent systemic mastocytosis (ISM) with <5% mast cells in a bone marrow biopsy specimen. KIT D7816V is only detectable by PNA-mediated PCR-clamping. (**f**) Aggressive systemic mastocytosis (ASM) with 40% mast cells. KIT D816V is already detectable by melting point analysis after conventional amplification

2. Add 2 μl sample DNA (given volumes to be multiplied with the number of samples, see Subheading 3.5, Note 17):
3. PCR conditions for simultaneous investigation of sample pairs, one amplified by conventional PCR, the other one by PNA-mediated PCR-clamping (see Note 19).

(a) Denaturation of DNA and activation of "hot-start" DNA polymerase:
- 10 min at 95°C.

(b) Amplification by 40 cycles consisting of:
- 10 s at 95°C; denaturation.
- 8 s at 68°C; PNA annealing.
- 10 s at 56°C; primer annealing.
- 10 s at 72°C; primer extension.

(c) Final extension:
- 5 min at 72°C.

(d) Melting point analysis:
- 5 min at 95°C; denaturation of amplification products.
- Immediate cooling of samples to 40°C.
- Continuous temperature increase of 0.3°C/s up to 95°C.

3.7 PNA Nested-PCR (PNA-nPCR) and Subsequent Melting Point Analysis of Amplification Products

To further increase the diagnostic sensitivity of the method, PNA-mediated PCR-clamping with primers c-kit 1F/1B (see Subheading 2.7, item 4) and subsequent conventional nested-PCR amplification with primers c-kit 2F/2B (see Subheading 2.5, item 3) may be performed. Aliquots of the nested-PCR products are used for genotyping by melting point analysis on a LightCycler Instrument. Both rounds of amplification may be performed in a conventional thermal cycler (e.g., Veriti® 96-Well Thermal Cycler, Applied Biosystems, Darmstadt, Germany).

1. First-round amplification by PNA-PCR in a final volume of 25 µl (see Note 20).

   Pipetting schema (given volumes to be multiplied with the number of samples; see Notes 21 and 22):

   (a) 15.9 µl dH_2O.

   (b) 2.5 µl 10× PCR buffer (containing $MgCl_2$ to a final concentration of 1.5 mM).

   (c) 0.2 µl dNTP mix.

   (d) 1.5 µl primer c-kit 1F.

   (e) 1.5 µl primer c-kit 1B.

   (f) 1.25 µl PNA.

   (g) 0.15 µl Taq polymerase.

   Total volume: 23 µl.

2. Add 2 µl of template DNA, i.e., 50–100 ng.

3. Cycling conditions for PNA-PCR amplification on a conventional thermal cycler (see Note 23):
   (a) Denaturation of DNA and activation of “hot-start” DNA polymerase:
      - 45 s at 95°C.
   (b) Amplification by 40 cycles consisting of:
      - 30 s at 95°C; denaturation.
      - 20 s at 68°C; PNA annealing.
      - 30 s at 56°C; primer annealing.
      - 45 s at 72°C; primer extension.
   (c) Final extension:
      - 4 min at 72°C.
4. Conventional nested-PCR using 1 μl of the PNA-PCR product as template (see Note 20) in a final volume of 25 μl.
   Pipetting schema (given volumes to be multiplied with the number of samples; see Notes 21 and 22):
   (a) 18.15 μl dH_2O.
   (b) 2.5 μl 10× PCR buffer (containing $MgCl_2$ to a final concentration of 1.5 mM).
   (c) 0.2 μl dNTP mix.
   (d) 1.5 μl primer c-kit 2F.
   (e) 1.5 μl primer c-kit 2B.
   (f) 0.15 μl Taq polymerase (5 U/μl).
5. Cycling conditions for nested-PCR amplification on a conventional thermal cycler (see Note 23).
   (a) Denaturation of DNA and activation of “hot-start” DNA polymerase:
      - 45 s at 95°C.
   (b) Amplification by 40 cycles consisting of:
      - 30 s at 95°C; denaturation.
      - 30 s at 56°C; primer annealing.
      - 45 s at 72°C; primer extension.
   (c) Final extension:
      - 4 min at 72°C.
6. Melting point analysis of 10 μl of nested-PCR products:
   Pipetting schema (given volumes to be multiplied with the number of samples; see Notes 21 and 22):
   (a) 6.4 ml dH_2O.
   (b) 1.0 μl c-kit Mutation probe.

   (c) 1.0 µl c-kit Sensor probe.
   (d) 1.6 µl 25 mM $MgCl_2$.
   Total volume: 10 µl.
7. Add 10 µl of the nested-PCR product.
8. Melting point analysis (see Subheading 3.6, step 3).

3.8 Immunostaining of Tissue Slides for Analysis of DNA from Microdissected Pooled Single Cells

1. For deparaffinization place slides into xylol twice for 2× 15 min, followed by washing twice each in 100% alcohol, 96% alcohol, and 70% alcohol. Afterward wash in distilled water three to four times (see Note 24).
2. Pretreatment is performed by incubating slides in Target Retrieval Solution in a microwave oven for 15 min twice at 750 W consumption (see Note 25). Then chill down solution at room temperature (RT) for 20 min with open cuvette lid.
3. Wash slides in Tris buffer (pH 7.5) for 5 min twice.
4. Block endogenous peroxidase in 7.5% H2O2 at RT for 10 min and for additional 10 min under cold running water.
5. Wash slides again in Tris buffer (pH 7.5) for 5 min twice.
6. Incubate slides in two drops (ca. 100 ml) "blocking serum" for 20 min at RT. Carefully tilt the supernatant and pat the slide dry.
7. Apply primary antibody (e.g., anti-mast cell tryptase, 1:350 dilution) and incubate for 60 min at RT.
8. Wash slides in Tris buffer (pH 7.5) for 5 min twice.
9. Apply detection system with anti-mouse Ig ("ready to use") and incubate for 30 min at RT.
10. Wash slides again in Tris buffer (pH 7.5) for 5 min twice.
11. Apply 100 ml AEC (aminoethylcarbazole) chromogen and incubate for 10 min at RT.
12. Afterwards wash slides under cold running water for 10 min.
13. Counterstain slides by quick (!) dipping into hematoxylin.
14. Wash slides again under cold running water for 10 min.
15. Let slides dry at RT.

3.9 Laser Pressure Catapulting (LPC) of Single Cells (Fig. 2)

1. Mark individual 0.2 ml PCR tubes at their sides with a waterproof pencil.
2. Cut off the lid leaving the hinge at the lid (see Note 26).
3. Dispense PCR oil in the lid of the PCR tube with a pipette tip (see Note 27).
4. Place the lid into the lid holder of the PALM MicroBeam system and move it carefully as close as possible to the surface of the glass slide with the immunostained tissue.

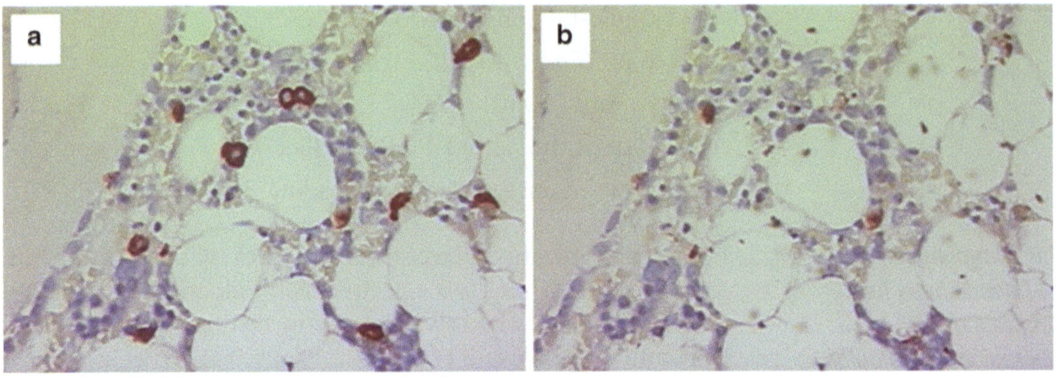

Fig. 2 Bone marrow with loosely scattered mast cells immunostained with anti-tryptase. (**a**) Before laser pressure catapulting (LPC) of single cells. (**b**) After LPC. Note that the tissue architecture of the remaining cells is nicely preserved

5. Use the software tools provided with the PALM MicroBeam system to electronically mark the cells of interest (about 100) and start the "laser pressure catapulting" procedure.
6. Place the lid on its individual tube and number the lid with a waterproof pencil (see Note 28).
7. Repeat steps 4–6 until enough cells are microdissected (see Note 29).

3.10 DNA Digestion from Microdissected Pooled Single Cells

1. Pipette 8 μl TE buffer into the lid of the PCR tube and dissolve the catapulted cells by gentle pipetting. Then close the PCR tube with belonging lid (see Note 27).
2. Place PCR tubes upside down onto a heater plate and incubate at 95°C for 20–30 min. Then centrifuge at maximum speed (e.g., 15,000 × *g*).
3. Add 2 μl of proteinase K and mix gently. Then incubate at 55°C overnight in a conventional thermal cycler with a cover plate heater.
4. Centrifuge at maximum speed, e.g., 15,000 × *g*.

3.11 Nested-PCR with Microdissected Cells

Given the low amount of template DNA obtained from 50 to 100microdissected cells from FFPE tissues, nested-PCR amplification is needed to ensure successful amplification of the *c-kit* target region. To avoid the generation of unspecific amplicons, first-round amplification is performed as "time-release" PCR (see Note 28). Apart from that, the same conditions and primers are used as described in Subheading 3.7.

1. First-round amplification in a final volume of 50 μl:
   Pipetting schema (given volumes to be multiplied with the number of samples; see Notes 27 and 28):
   (a) 28.3 μl dH_2O.

(b) 5.0 μl 10× PCR buffer (containing $MgCl_2$ to a final concentration of 1.5 mM).

(c) 0.4 μl dNTP mix.

(d) 3.0 μl primer c-kit 1F.

(e) 3.0 μl primer c-kit 1B.

(f) 0.3 μl Taq polymerase.

Total volume: 40 μl.

2. Add 10 μl of digested microdissected cells.
3. Cycling conditions for "time-release" PCR on a conventional thermal cycler (see Note 28).

   (a) Amplification by 50 cycles consisting of:
   - 30 s at 95°C; denaturation.
   - 20 s at 68°C; PNA annealing.
   - 30 s at 56°C; primer annealing.
   - 45 s at 72°C; primer extension.

   (b) Final extension:
   - 4 min at 72°C.
4. Conventional nested-PCR utilizing 1 μl of the PCR product as template *in a final volume of 25 μl*.

   Pipetting schema (given volumes to be multiplied with the number of samples; see Notes 2 and 3):

   (a) 18.2 μl dH_2O.

   (b) 2.5 μl 10× PCR buffer (containing $MgCl_2$ to a final concentration of 1.5 mM).

   (c) 0.2 μl dNTP mix.

   (d) 1.5 μl primer c-kit 2F.

   (e) 1.5 μl primer c-kit 2B.

   (f) 0.15 μl Taq polymerase.

   Total volume: 24 μl.
5. Add 1 μl of the PNA-PCR product.
6. For cycling conditions for nested-PCR amplification on a conventional thermal cycler see Subheading 3.7, step 5.
7. Melting point analysis of 10 μl of nested-PCR products as in Subheading 3.7, steps 6 and 7, and Subheading 3.6, step 3.

3.12 Gel Electrophoresis

Successfully amplified samples are identified by electrophoresis in 2% agarose gels and will be further investigated by melting point analysis. Since ethidium bromide is toxic, perform steps 1–3 under an extractor hood.

1. To generate 100 ml of 2% agarose gel, dissolve 2 g of agarose powder in about 100 ml 1× TBE buffer with a magnetic hot plate stirrer.

2. Add 10 μl of ethidium bromide to the hot gel while still stirring (see Note 29).
3. Cast the gel.
4. While the gel is cooling down, mix 2 μl of 2× loading buffer with 10 μl of the PCR product (see Note 30).
5. When the gel has cooled down, fill the gel chamber with 1× TBE buffer and remove the comb.
6. Load the samples and at least one lane of length standard into the gel pockets and run electrophoresis for 30 min at 70 V.
7. After electrophoresis, take a picture of the gel and select the successfully amplified samples for melting point analysis.

3.13 Melting Point Analysis as in Subheading 3.7, steps 6–8

4 Notes

1. We prefer to receive about 5–10 tissue rolls because they allow to directly proceed to Subheading 3.2. Tissue slides already mounted on glass have to be scratched off. To avoid electric charging, the tissue should be overlaid with proteinase K buffer. Glass slides for conventional stainings are preferable because scratching off the tissue is easier. Cells of dried smears should carefully be dissolved in proteinase K buffer by gentle pipetting.
2. Use 2 ml reaction tubes (e.g., Eppendorf 2 ml Microcentrifuge Tube, Eppendorf, Hamburg, Germany) because (a) they have a wide bottom and thus allow to place 5–10 tissue/paraffin rolls into one tube very easily and (b) they allow to add greater volumes of xylol (up to 2 ml) for an easier and more complete deparaffinization.
3. Open the reaction tube and pour the aqueous phase carefully into a collecting tray.
4. Drying time will depend on the amount of tissue and the amount of xylol left in the reaction tube. Therefore use a 100–200 μl pipette to remove as much as possible of the remaining xylol after you have discarded the vast majority from the tube. With the tip of the pipette you can lift the tissue pellet out of the fluid and adhere it to the tube wall. That will ease pipetting xylol reminder and help to avoid sucking of tissue pieces.
5. Volume of proteinase K buffer depends on the amount of tissue, which should be completely covered by buffer. Please

note that 300–400 µl of proteinase K buffer is the maximum amount that will allow addition of up to 1,200 µl of EtOH in step 12.

6. Proteolysis of cellular membranes and histone proteins will be intensified through this "boiling" step.
7. Effect of protein digestion is largely increased when a thermomixer (e.g., Eppendorf Thermomixer R®) is used!
8. Equal volume as the proteinase K buffer.
9. Centrifugation will unravel the tissue/proteinase K buffer/PCI mixture into two phases: a DNA-containing upper aqueous phase and a lower phenol phase containing the protein fraction; the latter phase contains a more or less defined milky rim at its top. Take great care to avoid carrying over parts of this protein-containing thin milky interphase into the second tube!
10. 1/2 of the PCI volume.
11. 10 µl LiCl per 100 µl of the two aqueous phases (300 µl proteinase K buffer and 150 µl dH_2O from the second washing step). Note that you will not be able to remove the total volume of 450 µl of the aqueous phase due to careful pipetting and avoiding a carryover of the PCI/CI phases.
12. Centrifugation will unravel the CI/dH_2O mixture into two lucent phases: a DNA-containing upper aqueous phase and a lower chloroform/isoamyl alcohol phase. Again take care to avoid carrying over parts of the lower phase into the third tube!
13. Careful bottom-up tapping of the open tube onto a paper towel will remove most for the fluid very effectively. After the vacuum-drying step you may visualize the lucent DNA pellet, looking like a small shrunken spot of dried adhesive.
14. Depending on the initial amount of tissue. For small biopsies 20 µl of dH_2O is enough; larger volumes will reduce the DNA concentration too much.
15. Closed lids will reduce the flow-through with the eluted DNA drastically.
16. As with all PCRs, to avoid contamination, it is highly recommended to perform the following tasks in a DNA- *and* amplicon-free lab: storage of all PCR "master mix" components listed below, storage of all tubes needed (tubes for "master mixes" and PCR tubes), generation of the PCR "master mix," and pipetting of "master mixes" into designated PCT tubes.
17. All reagents should be thawed on ice. The two c-kit probes labeled with fluorescent dyes must be protected from light. Consequently, the completed "master mix" should be used for PCR immediately.

18. Don't forget to add a negative (e.g., DNA-free) and a positive control (e.g., HMC-1.2 DNA, mast cell leukemia cell line heterozygous for the mutation *c-kit* 816 V). Considering pipetting inaccuracies, it can be recommended to calculate the volumes of the "master mix" components on a 10 + 1 basis, i.e., for each ten samples to be investigated create a "master mix" for 11 samples.
19. For a direct comparison of conventional amplification and PCR-clamping results, simultaneous investigation of samples is recommended in the same PCR run. Conventional amplification will demonstrate the structural integrity of extracted DNA, while PNA-based PCR-clamping will identify mutated samples. Using the capillary-based LightCycler Instrument with 32 positions, 16 samples, including one negative and one positive control, can be investigated simultaneously.
20. The hinge works like a handle bar which allow to hold the lids without touching (and possibly contaminating) the inside while you are pipetting.
21. Putting the pipette tip into PCR oil will suck some μl of the oil into the tip; moving this tip around in the PCR lid by adhesive surface forces will dispense a very thin oil film in the lid that is used as an adhesive for catapulted single cells.
22. It is highly recommended to list the case ID, type of microdissected cells (e.g., 100 tryptase-positive cells; 100 CD15-positive cells; 100 megakaryocyte nuclei, etc.).
23. Every fifth tube, we amplify a lid without microdissected cells as a "negative control."
24. Wash carefully to completely remove alcohol rests. Otherwise alcohol remnants will change the pH of the Target Retrieval Solution which may result in reduced target retrieval.
25. The microwave oven should be filled with cuvette dishes filled with distilled water to ensure an equal temperature distribution; leave the "water cuvettes" open, and the cuvette containing the slides has to be closed to avoid loss of fluid during boiling. After 15 min of microwave cooking control the amount of buffer and, in the event of buffer loss, replace buffer to fully cover the slides.
26. The hinge works like a handle bar which allow to hold the lids without touching (and possibly contaminating) the inside while you are pipetting.
27. Volumes of less than 8–9 μl will form a small drop at the border of the tip and will not cover the interior of the tip entirely.
28. Time release: The initial activation step (10 min incubation at 95°C) of the "hot-start" DNA polymerase is omitted and ten additional amplification cycles (50 cycles in total) are added.

This results in a slow increase of active DNA polymerase adapted to the small amount of template DNA.

29. When the heated agarose powder/TBE mixture becomes transparent and starts fuming, turn off the heater, add the ethidium bromide, and continue stirring until the fluid gel stops fuming. Then it is ready to be casted.

30. To charge a gel with a single pipette very comfortably, use a strip of parafilm where you bring forward a drop (about 2 μl) of the 2× loading buffer for each PCR sample. Then mix an aliquot (10 μl) of the PCR product with the loading buffer (use a different pipette tip for each sample!). Pipette the mixture into the gel chambers. If you rinse the pipette tip in the gel running buffer you can use the same pipette tip to load all the samples.

References

1. Valent P, Horny H-P, Li CY, Longley BJ, Metcalfe DD, Parwaresch RM et al (2001) Mastocytosis (Mast cell disease). In: Jaffe ES, Harris NL, Stein H, Vardiman JW (eds) World Health Organization (WHO) classification of tumours, pathology & genetics. Tumours of haematopoietic and lymphoid tissues. IARC Press, Lyon, pp 291–302
2. Horny H-P, Metcalfe DD, Bennett JM, Bain BJ, Akin C, Escribano L et al (2008) Mastocytosis (Mast cell disease). In: Swerdlow SH, Campo E, Harris NL, Jaffe ES, Pileri SA, Stein H, Thiele J, Vardiman JW (eds) WHO classification of tumours of haematopoietic and lymphoid tissues. IARC Press, Geneva, Switzerland, pp 54–63
3. Stein DH (1986) Mastocytosis: a review. Pediatr Dermatol 3:365–375
4. Lennert K, Parwaresch MR (1979) Mast cells and mast cell neoplasia: a review. Histopathology 3:349–365
5. Yarden Y, Kuang WJ, Yang-Feng T, Coussens L, Munemitsu S, Dull TJ et al (1987) Human proto-oncogene c-kit: a new cell surface receptor tyrosine kinase for an unidentified ligand. EMBO J 6:3341–3351
6. Qiu FH, Ray P, Brown K, Barker PE, Jhanwar S, Ruddle FH et al (1988) Primary structure of c-kit: relationship with the CSF-1/PDGF receptor kinase family–oncogenic activation of v-kit involves deletion of extracellular domain and C terminus. EMBO J 7:1003–1011
7. Ashman LK, Cambareri AC, To LB, Levinsky RJ, Juttner CA (1991) Expression of the YB5. B8 antigen (c-kit proto-oncogene product) in normal human bone marrow. Blood 78: 30–37
8. Papayannopoulou T, Brice M, Broudy VC, Zsebo KM (1991) Isolation of c-kit receptor-expressing cells from bone marrow, peripheral blood, and fetal liver: functional properties and composite antigenic profile. Blood 78: 1403–1412
9. Reisbach G, Bartke I, Kempkes B, Kostka G, Ellwart J, Birner A et al (1993) Characterization of hemopoietic cell populations from human cord blood expressing c-kit. Exp Hematol 21:74–79
10. Ogawa M, Matsuzaki Y, Nishikawa S, Hayashi S, Kunisada T, Sudo T et al (1991) Expression and function of c-kit in hemopoietic progenitor cells. J Exp Med 174:63–71
11. Orr-Urtreger A, Avivi A, Zimmer Y, Givol D, Yarden Y, Lonai P (1990) Developmental expression of c-kit, a proto-oncogene encoded by the W locus. Development 109:911–923
12. Manova K, Nocka K, Besmer P, Bachvarova RF (1990) Gonadal expression of c-kit encoded at the W locus of the mouse. Development 110:1057–1069
13. Koch CA, Anderson D, Moran MF, Ellis C, Pawson T (1991) SH2 and SH3 domains: elements that control interactions of cytoplasmic signaling proteins. Science 3:668–674
14. Pawson T (1995) Protein-tyrosine kinases. Getting down to specifics [news; comment]. Nature 373:477–478
15. Furitsu T, Tsujimura T, Tono T, Ikeda H, Kitayama H, Koshimizu U et al (1993) Identification of mutations in the coding sequence of the proto-oncogene c-kit in a human mast cell leukemia cell line causing ligand-independent activation of c-kit product. J Clin Invest 92:1736–1744
16. Kitayama H, Kanakura Y, Furitsu T, Tsujimura T, Oritani K, Ikeda H et al (1995) Constitutively activating mutations of c-kit receptor tyrosine kinase confer factor-independent growth and tumorigenicity of factor-dependent hematopoietic cell lines. Blood 85:790–798

17. Kemmer K, Corless CL, Fletcher JA, McGreevey L, Haley A, Griffith D et al (2004) KIT mutations are common in testicular seminomas. Am J Pathol 164:305–313
18. Gari M, Goodeve A, Wilson G, Winship P, Langabeer S, Linch D et al (1999) c-kit proto-oncogene exon 8 in-frame deletion plus insertion mutations in acute myeloid leukaemia. Br J Haematol 105:894–900
19. Andersson J, Sjogren H, Meis-Kindblom JM, Stenman G, Aman P, Kindblom LG (2002) The complexity of KIT gene mutations and chromosome rearrangements and their clinical correlation in gastrointestinal stromal (pacemaker cell) tumors. Am J Pathol 160:15–22
20. Hongyo T, Li T, Syaifudin M, Baskar R, Ikeda H, Kanakura Y et al (2000) Specific c-kit mutations in sinonasal natural killer/T-cell lymphoma in China and Japan. Cancer Res 1:2345–2347
21. Kong Y, Si L, Zhu Y, Xu X, Corless CL, Flaherty KT, Li L, Li H, Sheng X, Cui C, Chi Z, Li S, Han M, Mao L, Lu A, Guo J (2011) Large-scale analysis of KIT aberrations in Chinese patients with melanoma. Clin Cancer Res 17:1684–1691
22. Orum H, Nielsen PE, Egholm M, Berg RH, Buchardt O, Stanley C (1993) Single base pair mutation analysis by PNA directed PCR clamping. Nucleic Acids Res 21:5332–5336
23. Thiede C, Bayerdorffer E, Blasczyk R, Wittig B, Neubauer A (1996) Simple and sensitive detection of mutations in the ras proto-oncogenes using PNA-mediated PCR clamping. Nucleic Acids Res 24:983–984
24. Behn M, Thiede C, Neubauer A, Pankow W, Schuermann M (2000) Facilitated detection of oncogene mutations from exfoliated tissue material by a PNA-mediated 'enriched PCR' protocol. J Pathol 190:69–75
25. Wittwer CT, Ririe KM, Andrew RV, David DA, Gundry RA, Balis UJ (1997) The LightCycler: a microvolume multisample fluorimeter with rapid temperature control. Biotechniques 22:176–181
26. Mangasser-Stephan K, Tag C, Reiser A, Gressner AM (1999) Rapid genotyping of hemochromatosis gene mutations on the LightCycler with fluorescent hybridization probes. Clin Chem 45:1875–1878
27. Elenitoba-Johnson KS, Bohling SD, Wittwer CT, King TC (2001) Multiplex PCR by multicolor fluorimetry and fluorescence melting curve analysis. Nat Med 7:249–253
28. Sotlar K, Escribano L, Landt O, Möhrle S, Herrero S, Torrelo A et al (2003) One-step detection of c-kit point mutations using peptide nucleic acid-mediated polymerase chain reaction clamping and hybridization probes. Am J Pathol 162:737–746
29. Horny HP, Sotlar K, Sperr WR, Valent P (2004) Systemic mastocytosis with associated clonal haematological non-mast cell lineage diseases: a histopathological challenge. J Clin Pathol 57:604–608
30. Sotlar K, Bache A, Stellmacher F, Bültmann B, Valent P, Horny HP (2008) Systemic mastocytosis associated with chronic idiopathic myelofibrosis: a distinct subtype of systemic mastocytosis associated with a clonal hematological non-mast cell lineage disorder carrying the activating point mutations KITD816V and JAK2V617F. J Mol Diagn 10:58–66
31. Sotlar K, Colak S, Bache A, Berezowska S, Krokowski M, Bültmann B et al (2010) Variable presence of KITD816V in clonal haematological non-mast cell lineage diseases associated with systemic mastocytosis (SM-AHNMD). J Pathol 220:586–595

Chapter 5

Detection of Recurrent Cytogenetic Abnormalities in Acute Lymphoblastic and Myeloid Leukemias Using Fluorescence In Situ Hybridization

Gail H. Vance

Abstract

Cytogenetic identification of clonal abnormalities present in leukemia is critical for accurate diagnosis of the disease and determination of specific therapeutic interventions for the patient. Fluorescence in situ hybridization (FISH) studies complement the diagnostic karyotype by providing a higher resolution of analysis with clarification of rearrangements observed by G-banding and identification of cryptic abnormalities not observed by the light microscope. This chapter will discuss FISH methodology as practiced in the cancer cytogenetic laboratory.

Key words Cytogenetics, Chromosomes, Molecular cytogenetics, Fluorescence in situ hybridization

1 Introduction

Cancer cytogenetics is a field built upon the identification of nonrandom chromosome abnormalities in cancer. Identification of recurring numerical and structural cytogenetic abnormalities by G-banded chromosome analysis and fluorescence in situ hybridization (FISH) studies is critical for the diagnosis, prognosis, and assessment of effectiveness of treatment in patients with hematological malignancies (1). Since the first determination of a structural abnormality associated with chronic myeloid leukemia by Nowell in 1960 (2), the field has progressed to include both banded chromosomes and molecular cytogenetic methods. The emergence of the discipline of molecular cytogenetics in 1986 advanced the power of resolution beyond the G-banded chromosome and dramatically increased the yield of detected chromosomal aberrations (3, 4). Recent years have seen further development of molecular cytogenetic methods with increasing resolution and sensitivity of detection promoting the important discovery of previously cryptic abnormalities (5, 6).

Magdalena Czader (ed.), *Hematological Malignancies*, Methods in Molecular Biology, vol. 999,
DOI 10.1007/978-1-62703-357-2_5, © Springer Science+Business Media New York 2013

Table 1
2001 World Health Organization (WHO) classification for AML recurrent genetic abnormalities

AML with t(8;21)(q22;q22) (*AML1/ETO*)
AML with inv(16)(p13.1q22) (*CBFB/MYH11*)
APL with t(15;17)(q22;q21.1) (*PML/RARA*)
AML with 11q23 (*MLL*) abnormalities

The World Health Organization (WHO) Classification of Tumours of Haematopoietic and Lymphoid Tissues published in 2001 reflected for the first time a myeloid neoplasm classification scheme with integrated cytogenetic information (7). The category, "Acute myeloid leukemia with recurrent cytogenetic abnormalities" listed four entries (Table 1). Thus, a cytogenetic diagnosis was required to report a case of acute myeloid leukemia (AML) in this category. The fourth edition of the WHO text published in 2008 expanded the category to include nine subclassifications of AML with recurrent genetic abnormalities (8). These abnormalities spanned recognized recurring cytogenetic translocations in AML but also included molecularly detected DNA mutations observed in specimens with normal chromosomes (Table 2). This chapter discusses methods for performing fluorescence in situ (FISH) on cell suspensions and uncultured cells from a bone marrow smear (or tissue touch prep). FISH studies can be performed rapidly and complement G-banded analyses to enhance the detection of cytogenetic abnormalities in hematological malignancies and lymphomas.

Conventional cytogenetic and FISH studies for leukemia are routinely performed on bone marrow, unstimulated peripheral blood, and bone marrow clot specimens. Dividing cells are required for conventional cytogenetics (9). FISH, however, is performed on both dividing and interphase cells in suspension as well as uncultured cells from smears, touch preps, and paraffin-embedded tissue.

Probes utilized in FISH are typically prepared from nucleic acid sequences and include the following:

- Repetitive DNA sequences.
  - Centromere (alpha satellite) probes.
- Specific DNA loci or single copy probes.
  - Gene(s) of interest.
  - Subtelomere probe.

Table 2
2008 World Health Organization (WHO) classification for AML with recurrent genetic abnormalities

AML with t(8;21)(q22;q22)(*RUNX1/RUNX1T1*)
AML with inv(16)(p13.1q22)(*CBFB/MYH11*) or t(16;16)(p13.1;q22)
AML with t(15;17)(q22;q21.1)(*PML/RARA*)
AML with t(9;11)(p22;q23)(*MLLT3/MLL*)
AML with t(6;9)(p23;q34)(*DEK/NUP214*)
AML with inv(3)(q21q26.2)(*RPN1/EVI1*) or t(3;3)(q21;q26.2)
AML with t(1;22)(p13;q13)(*RBM15/MKL1*)
AML with mutated *NPM1*
AML with mutated *CEBPA*

- Whole chromosome painting probe.
  - Multiple DNA sequences that span the entire chromosome of interest.

Probes may be prepared in the laboratory or purchased commercially following good manufacturing practices (GMP). Most cytogenetic labs purchase labeled probes from a vendor. If preparing the probe in the laboratory, the DNA must be isolated and labeled. Typically bacterial artificial chromosome (BAC) clones are utilized in probe development. Once isolated, the DNA must be labeled with a fluorophore either by nick translation or polymerase chain reaction (PCR) labeling (10, 11).

Performing the FISH procedure is similar to a Southern blot in that both the probe and the cells need to be denatured (conversion of double-stranded DNA to single-stranded DNA) prior to hybridization and excess probe washed off prior to detection. The complete FISH procedure is outlined in Fig. 1.

FISH probes used in hematological malignancies have been developed into various schemes depending on the specific abnormality to be detected. Translocation probes, such as the t(9;22)(q34;q11.2) utilized for detecting a rearrangement of *BCR* and *ABL1*, are usually developed as dual-color, dual-fusion probes. In this scheme, each locus of interest is labeled in a specific color (red or green) and probes flank the breakpoints of the translocation, such that the derivative chromosomes are identified with fused (yellow) signals due to the juxtaposition of the red fluor next to the green or vice versa (Fig. 2a, b).

A breakapart probe is structured to identify the rearrangement of a specific gene such as *MLL*. For these probes a fluor (red or green) labels the 5′ end of the gene and a different color (red or green)

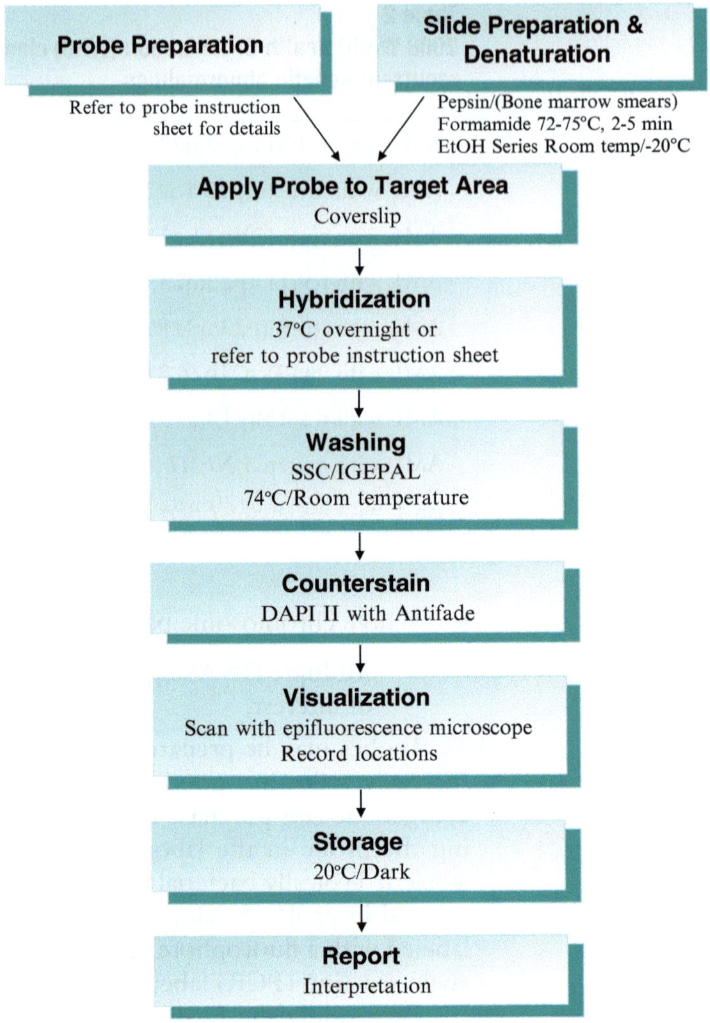

Fig. 1 Diagram of the FISH procedure

identifies the 3′ end of the gene. When the gene of interest is intact, the two colors lie juxtaposed and typically appear yellow. With a rearrangement of the gene the two colors are separated and single red and green colors are observed (Fig. 2c).

A third probe scheme for translocations, such as the t(12;21)(p13;q22), is a dual-color, single-fusion, extra signal probe which utilizes two colors (red for *AML1/RUNX1* on chromosome 21 and green for *ETV6* located on chromosome 12) that hybridize to these genes on each chromosome. However, in this arrangement, one probe spans the breakpoint at the *AML1RUNX1* locus (red fluor) but not the *ETV6* locus (green). So, the signal pattern for a translocation includes one fusion signal (green and red together on the derivative chromosome21) and one extra (residual) signal (red) residing on the derivative chromosome 12 (Fig. 2d, e) (12).

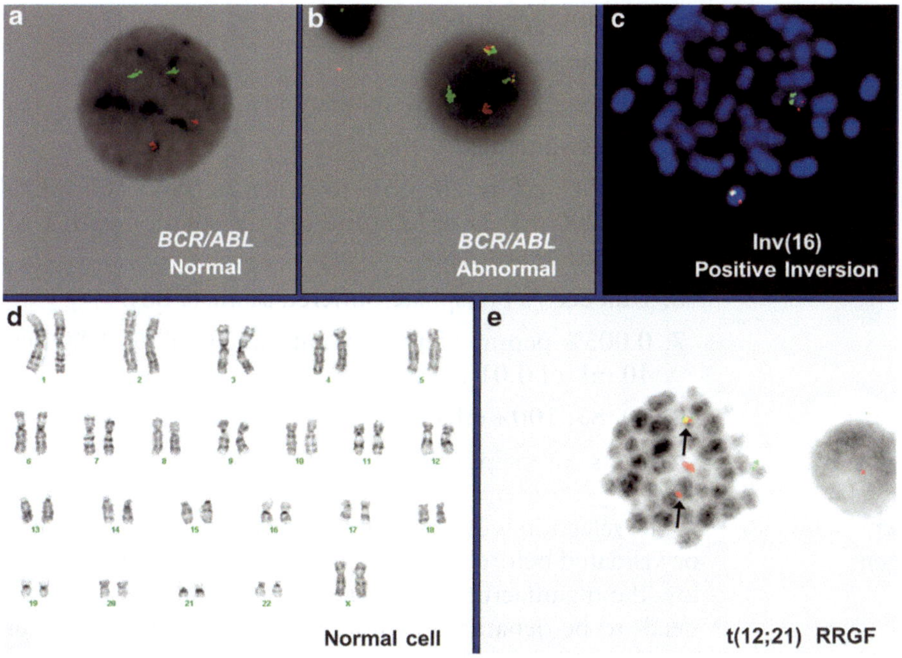

Fig. 2 (**a**) Normal interphase cells hybridized with probes for *BCR* (*green*) and *ABL1* (*red*). (**b**) Abnormal nucleus demonstrating dual-color, dual-fusion (*yellow*) patterns representative of a t(9;22). (**c**) Metaphase cells with a breakapart pattern demonstrating a normal chromosome 16 (*yellow signals*) and rearranged chromosome 16 (separate *red* and *green signals*). (**d**) Normal G-banded image of a bone marrow cell with a t(12;21) detected by FISH in (**e**). *Top arrow* indicates the fusion of *AML1* and *ETV6*. The *lower arrow* demonstrates the residual (*red*) signal on the derivative chromosome 21

This chapter presents detailed step-by-step FISH methodology used in our cancer cytogenetic laboratory for the determination of recurrent genetic abnormalities in acute leukemias.

2 Materials

2.1 Slide Preparation for FISH Performed on Cell Suspensions

1. Absolute methanol (ACS grade).
2. Glacial acetic acid.
3. Fixative: 3:1 absolute methanol to acetic acid.
4. Pasteur pipettes.
5. Cleaned microscope slides (Gold Seal Ultra Frost Rite-on Micro Slides, Fisher Scientific, Pittsburg, PA) (see Note 1).
6. 2× SSC: dilute 20× SSC to make 2× SSC (100 mL 20× SSC and 900 mL 3× dH_2O) and pH the solution with 1 N HCl to desired pH of 7.0.
7. Ethanol series of 70, 85, 100% ethanol solutions.
8. Glass coverslips (12 mm circle, 18×18 mm, or 22×22 mm).

2.2 Slide Preparation for FISH on Bone Marrow Smears

1. Absolute methanol.
2. Glacial acetic acid.
3. Fixative: 3:1 absolute methanol to acetic acid.
4. Pasteur pipettes.
5. 2× SSC: dilute 20× SSC to make 2× SSC (100 mL 20× SSC and 900 mL 3× dH_2O) and pH the solution with 1 N HCl to desired pH of 7.0.
6. Dulbecco's phosphate buffered saline (PBS).
7. 0.005% pepsin working solution: 20 μl of 10% pepsin and 40 mL of 0.01 N HCl.
8. 70, 85, 100% ethanol series.
9. Glass coverslips (12 mm circle, 18 × 18 mm, or 22 × 22 mm).

2.3 Probe Preparation

Probe selection is dependent on the target. All FISH probes should be validated before use (see Note 2). Probe preparation should follow the manufacturer's protocol noting whether or not the probe needs to be denatured or not. Some probes do not require denaturation prior to hybridization.

1. Remove the probe from the freezer and aliquot the volume required into an Eppendorf tube.
2. Then return the probe vial to the freezer.
3. Keep aliquoted probe on ice.
4. Remove probe hybridization buffer from freezer and warm to room temperature.

2.4 Denaturation

1. 70% formamide/2× SSC: in a plastic Coplin jar, combine 5 mL 20× SSC, 10 mL of 3× H_2O, and 35 mL of formamide (Hi-Di Formamide, Applied Biosystems, Foster City, CA). Adjust the solution a pH of 7.0 adding drops of 1 N HCl (see Note 3).
2. Prepare a Coplin jar with 50 mL 2× SSC at 37°C.
3. Cold (−20°C) ethanol series of 70% (make two 50 mL Coplin jars with 70% ethanol), 85%, and 100% ethanol in 50 mL plastic Coplin jars.

2.5 Post-hybridization Wash Solutions

1. Post-hybridization wash solution 1: 0.4× SSC/0.3% IGEPAL. Make 1,000 mL of the solution by mixing 977 mL 3× H_2O, 20 mL 20× SSC, and 3 mL IGEPAL. Adjust pH to 7.0.
2. Post-hybridization wash solution 2: 2× SSC/0.1% IGEPAL. Make 1,000 mL of the solution with 899 mL 3× H_2O, 100 mL 20× SSC, and 1 mL IGEPAL. Adjust pH to 7.0.
3. 2× SSC: prepare 500 mL of the solution by adding 450 mL 3× dH_2O and 50 mL 20× SSC. Adjust pH to 7.0.

4. DAPI (4,6,-diamidino-2-phenylindole-dihydrochloride) II counterstain (Abbott Molecular/Vysis, Abbott Park, IL). Store at −20°C. Store in the dark as the solution is light sensitive. Also, do not leave at room temperature for extended periods of time.

2.6 Instrumentation

1. Fluorescence microscope equipped with 100 W mercury lamp and filters appropriate for FITC/Texas Red/DAPI (triple filter), FITC/Texas Red (dual filter), FITC, Texas Red, Aqua, and DAPI (single filters) fluorescence detection.
2. FISH imaging system (Applied Imaging, Santa Clara, CA).
3. Phase contrast microscope.
4. Slide warmer (65°C).

3 Methods

A normal control slide should be run with each batch of patient samples.

3.1 Slide Preparation from Cell Suspensions

1. Suspend the cells in a freshly prepared fixative of 3:1 methanol:acetic acid. The best results are obtained with bone marrow and unstimulated peripheral blood cells that have been cultured and harvested according to standard cytogenetic procedures for hematological malignancies.
2. Remove a cold slide from the carrier and wipe off excess water (see Note 1 for preparation of clean slides).
3. Aspirate and fill a Pasteur pipette with cell suspension.
4. Allow 2–3 drops per 1/2 of the slide to fall from an approximate distance of 2–3 ft onto cold, clean, wet slides. Dropping height varies by technologist. The goal is to obtain chromosomes/nuclei that lie flat on the slide with a gray (not black) hue.
5. Place the slide on the 65°C slide warmer.
6. Leave on the hot plate until all the liquid has evaporated and the slide is dry.
7. Check the cells with phase microscopy to see that they are flat with a gray hue.
8. Label and store in a desiccator until use. Slides may be stored up to 3 months in a desiccator at room temperature or in a slide box at −20°C.
9. When ready to use, immerse slide in 2× SSC for 10 min at 37°C. The Coplin jar with 50 mL of 2× SSC should be warmed to 37°C in a water bath for approximately 30 min prior to use.
10. Dehydrate in room temperature ethanol series (70, 85, 100%) for 2 min each. Air dry.

3.2 Slide Preparation for Bone Marrow Smears

1. Place the slide in a Coplin jar containing 50 mL of 3:1 methanol:acetic glacial acid fixative for 5 min. Repeat in fresh fixative and then air dry.
2. Place the slide in a second Coplin jar containing 50 mL 2× SSC in a 37°C water bath for 15 min.
3. Remove from 2× SSC and place in the 0.005% pepsin solution for 20 min at 37°C.
4. Rinse slide in PBS at room temperature for 5 min.
5. Dehydrate in 70, 85, and 100% ethanol series for 2 min each at room temperature.

3.3 Slide Denaturation

1. Place the slide into the Coplin jar containing 70% formamide/2× SSC at 72–75°C for 3 min (see Note 4). More time may be required for thick bone marrow smears.
2. Remove the slide and place immediately into a wash solution of 70% cold (−20°C) ethanol for 2 min to remove formamide.
3. Run the slide through an alcohol series of cold 70, 85, and 100% ethanol for 2 min each.
4. Air dry or place on 42°C slide warmer to dry.
5. Cells may also be denatured (and hybridized) utilizing a bench-top denaturation/hybridization system.

3.4 Hybridization

1. Place 3–5 μl of probe mixture (probe, H_2O, and buffer) or 10 μl of probe for FDA-cleared or -approved probes onto the slide (see Notes 5 and 6).
2. Cover with a coverslip. The size of the coverslip to be used depends on the volume of probe placed on a slide. Usually a 22×22 mm slide is used for 10 μl of probe.
3. Seal the coverslip with rubber cement by applying sealant along the perimeter of the coverslip. A 5 mL syringe or Pasteur pipette can be used to disperse air bubbles.
4. Place in a humidified chamber and incubate at 37°C for 4–16 h (usually overnight) (see Note 7).

3.5 Post-hybridization Washes

1. Using forceps, remove the rubber cement from the slide. Gently slide the coverslip over the edge of the slide.
2. Preheat 40 mL 0.4× SSC/0.3% IGEPAL in a Coplin jar to 74°C. Immerse slide and wash for 2 min agitating gently.
3. Immediately transfer to 40 mL of 2× SSC/0.1% IGEPAL at room temperature. Wash for 1 min.
4. Allow the slide to dry protected from light.
5. Apply 10 μl of DAPI II counterstain to the target area of the slide (see Note 8). Place a coverslip over the counterstain and allow it to spread evenly.

6. Seal the edges of the slide with nail polish. Do not expose the slide to light. Store the slide in the dark at −20°C. The slide is ready to view when the nail polish is dry.

3.6 Analysis

1. Allow the fluorescence microscope to warm up. Place the slide on the microscope stage and view with the filter appropriate for the fluorophore. Dual pass filters will allow for both green and red signals to be observed simultaneously.
2. Scan the slide to identify the target area with probe and assess the hybridization efficiency of the probe in the target area by determining that at least one copy of the probe fluors (red, green, and/or aqua) is present.
3. Score per laboratory scoring criteria, marking the locations of cells for photography (see Notes 9 and 10).
4. Photograph two images for normal results and two images of a clonal abnormality as well as one image of a normal cell.
5. Interpret results and utilize current ISCN to write the nomenclature (13) (see Notes 11 and 12).

4 Notes

1. The following is one procedure for cleaning glass slides (Gold Seal Ultra Frost Rite-on Micro Slides) for use in both conventional cytogenetics and FISH analyses:
   (a) Place slides in a slide carrier with frosted label facing forward.
   (b) When the slide carrier is full, place in a container containing 100% acetone for 8 min.
   (c) Next place the slide carrier in a container with 10 mL HCL mixed with 100 mL EtOH (12.1 N HCl/100% ethanol) mixture. Let it sit in this solution for 8 min.
   (d) Rinse slide carrier in tap-distilled water 8 min.
   (e) Fill carrier with 3× dH_2O. Label lid with date and initials. Store at 2–8°C.
2. All FISH probes should be validated in the laboratory prior to offering them for clinical testing. Recommended is a validation process that incorporates three steps, including (1) familiarization, (2) pilot study, and (3) clinical study (14). The validation of FISH tests is designed to assess probe performance, determine the probe signal pattern in normal and abnormal specimens, establish scoring criteria, set normal and abnormal reference ranges, and establish the ability of laboratory personnel to perform the test consistently. Documentation of test or analytic validation is required under CLIA '88 for any new test being placed into clinical service after September 1992. Regulations require

that proper validation of the performance of FISH tests be completed. Guidelines have been produced by the American College of Medical Genetics (ACMG) (15) and the Clinical Laboratory Standards Institute (CLSI, formerly NCCLS) (16).

(a) *Familiarization Study*: The familiarization study is intended to gain initial experience (become familiar) with the performance of each FISH probe and determine the analytical specificity and sensitivity of the assay utilizing metaphase and interphase nuclei from the peripheral blood specimen of five normal male controls. Each probe is hybridized to metaphase and interphase cells from five karyotypically normal male controls. Ten metaphase spreads are analyzed per observer and 25 interphase cells are analyzed per observer for a total of 20 metaphase and 50 interphase cells per control. Chromosomal localization must be confirmed by one of the following methods: Inverted DAPI staining or use of a cell line or patient specimen containing the chromosomal region of interest as an independent and identifiable target (e.g., structural rearrangement, trisomy). Sequential staining may be performed to confirm FISH hybridization to locus/region of interest (i.e., destaining of G-banded slide, followed by FISH). An image of at least one metaphase and one interphase cell is taken for each normal control demonstrating the most consistently observed signal pattern.

(b) *Pilot Study*: The purpose of the pilot study is to gain experience with the FISH assay for both normal and abnormal specimens using the tissue for which the test is intended and to revise scoring criteria, establish the normal cutoff, analytical sensitivity, and performance of the test. Validation for each type of tissue that is intended to be tested in clinical practice should be performed. A minimum of at least five patients should be analyzed (three abnormal and two normal are recommended). Metaphase FISH: Ten metaphase spreads and at least one interphase cell each are analyzed by two observers (total of 20 metaphases and two interphase cells). All signal patterns observed should be recorded. At least one image is recorded and labeled of one metaphase spread and one interphase cell. An image should also be captured of an unexpected cross-hybridization pattern observed in 5% or more of cells. Interphase FISH: 500 interphase cells are analyzed by two observers (250 cells per observer) and images captured of at least two interphase cells with the common pattern. All signal patterns observed should be recorded. An image should also be captured of a frequently observed unexpected signal pattern. The standard operating procedure (SOP) for the probe/FISH test methodology should be established following the conclusion of the pilot study.

(c) *Clinical Study*: The clinical study tests predictable parameters encountered in clinical practice, refines the normal cut-off and abnormal reference range, and validates the standard operating procedure. It is recommended that in the clinical study at least ten patients (five normal and five abnormal patients) are analyzed using either metaphase or interphase cells depending upon the type of probe used.

Biannual (twice per year) calibration or continuous quality monitoring verification is required under CLIA '88 (see 42 CFR §493.1217) in the use of all FISH probes (17). This requirement may be satisfied by enrollment in a commercially available proficiency testing or laboratory-initiated alternative assessment (18).

3. Formamide is toxic. Do not pour formamide down the sink. After use discard formamide solutions into a container marked "formamide waste" and dispose with the institutional or company hazardous waste division.
4. The denaturation solution must be pre-warmed to 72 + 1 °C for each additional slide to be added to the Coplin jar. So for example, if three slides were denatured simultaneously, the temperature of the denaturation solution would be 74°C. The temperature and time of exposure of the denaturation solution are critical for satisfactory hybridization and cell morphology. Denature slides by immersing in the pre-warmed solution and agitating periodically. Denature metaphase chromosomes for approximately 2 min and 20 s and interphase nuclei for 3–4 min. For best results, denature no more than three slides at a time.
5. Many reagents contain azide. Wear gloves and a lab coat when handling. Use proper disposal procedures.
6. The chromosome probes are sensitive to enzymes that degrade DNA (DNAses). Wear gloves and do not handle pipette tips with fingers as this could result in degradation of the probe.
7. A humidified chamber may be created using a Rubbermaid or Tupperware (plastic) rectangular container. Moisten towels in 2× SSC and line the bottom of the chamber. Lay two plastic pipettes (cut to the length of the container) parallel to one another. Preheat the chamber in a 37°C incubator prior to use. When slides are ready for hybridization, lay each slide across the pipettes so they are elevated in the chamber and not touching the bottom. Close tightly with the lid and place again in a 37°C incubator for the duration of the hybridization time.
8. The DAPI II antifade reagent contains light-sensitive reagents. Keep caps tightly closed and limit exposure to light.
9. Probe signals (red, green, aqua, gold) are observed against a background of blue DAPI. For interphase analysis, typically 200–500 cells are analyzed for each probe by two observers. Each observer is blinded to the results of the other. Once the

case is completed, the assessment of normal or abnormal results is made based upon (1) the laboratory data for the normal range established during the validation procedure, (2) FDA-approved interpretation, and/or (3) guidelines established by professional organizations (19).

10. Scoring criteria for technologist analysis should be defined for each probe. Such criteria may include:
    (a) Selecting only singular cells and not scoring cells which are overlapped.
    (b) Determining if the signal is a diffuse single signal or more than one signal.
    (c) Determining the minimum number of signals that must be present for a cell to be scored.

    The above criteria will help the technologists with uniform selection of cells and alignment of their scoring results. However, it is also important for the technologist to recognize cells with an unexpected and unusual signal patterns that may represent a clone with uncommon numerical and structural abnormalities. Each technologist should photograph cells representative of the clones observed. Additionally, in an abnormal case, a cell with a normal karyotype or signal pattern should be taken and filed with the patient's record.

11. The nomenclature for conventional cytogenetics and FISH is written according to the most recent version of the International Standards of Cytogenetic Nomenclature (13).

12. Discrepancies between G-banded chromosomes and FISH are not unexpected. Sometimes the morphology of the G-banded chromosomes is poor, and abnormalities cannot be fully discerned by conventional cytogenetics. However, FISH can detect cryptic abnormalities not observable by G-banded chromosomes even with acceptable chromosomal morphology. For example, masked or cryptic variants of the Philadelphia chromosome involve a submicroscopic translocation that is not evident by conventional cytogenetics but is detectable by FISH with probes for the *BCR* and *ABL1* genes (20). The subtle translocation between *ETV6* (*TEL*) and *RUNX1* (*AML1*) representing 25% of childhood ALL was ignore not fully recognized until the advent of FISH (21).

Acknowledgments

The author would like to acknowledge the IU Cytogenetics Laboratory personnel and especially the FISH team members: Haki Choi, Ryan Stohler, Ryanne Berger, Lisa Wright, Matthew Sweckor, and Virginia Thurston. Thanks also to Shani Stiles for her talented clerical assistance.

References

1. Byrd JC, Mrozek K, Dodge RK, Carroll AJ, Edwards CG, Artheru DC et al (2002) Pretreatment cytogenetic abnormalities are predictive of induction success, cumulative incidence of relapse, and overall survival in adult patients with de novo acute myeloid leukemia: results from Cancer and Leukemia Group B (CALGB 8461). Blood 100:4325–4336
2. Nowell P, Hungerford D (1960) A minute chromosome in human chronic granulocytic leukemia. Science 132:1497
3. Pinkel D, Straume T, Gray JW (1986) Cytogenetic analysis using quantitative, high sensitivity, fluorescence hybridization. Proc Natl Acad Sci USA 83:2934–2938
4. Heerema NA, Maben KD, Bernstein J, Breitfeld PP, Neiman RS, Vance GH (1996) Dicentric (9;20)(p11;q11) identified by fluorescence in situ hybridization in four pediatric acute lymphoblastic leukemia patients. Cancer Genet Cytogenet 92:111–115
5. Brown J, Jawad M, Twigg SRF, Saracoglu K, Sauerbrey A, Thomas AD et al (2002) A cryptic t(5;11)(q35;p15.5) in 2 children with acute myeloid leukemia with apparently normal karyotypes, identified by multiplex fluorescence in situ hybridization telomere assay. Blood 99:2526–2531
6. Dierlamm J, Stul M, Vranckx H, Michaux L, Weghuis DE, Speleman F et al (1998) FISH identifies inv(16)(p13q22) masked by translocations in three cases of acute myeloid leukemia. Genes Chromosomes Cancer 22: 87–94
7. Jaffe ES, Harris NL, Stein H, Vardiman JW (eds) (2001) World Health Organization classification of tumours, pathology and genetics of tumours of haematopoietic and lymphoid tissues. IARC, Lyon
8. Swerdlow SH, Campo E, Harris NL, Jaffe ES, Pileri SA, Stein H et al (eds) (2008) WHO classification of tumours of haematopoietic and lymphoid tissues. IARC, Lyon
9. Spurkbeck JL, Adams SA, Stupca PJ, Dewald GW (2004) Primer on medical genomics, part XI: visualizing human chromosomes. Mayo Clin Proc 79:58–75
10. Telenius H, Carter NP, Bebb C, Nordenskjold M, Ponder BJ, Tunnacliffe A (1992) Degenerate oligonucleotide-primed PCR: general amplification of target DNA by a single degenerate primer. Genomics 13:718–725
11. Cushman LJ, Torres-Martinez W, Cherry AM, Manning MA, Abdul-Rahman O, Anderson CE et al (2005) A report of three patients with an interstitial deletion of chromosome 15q24. Am J Med Genet 137A:65–71
12. http://www.abbottmolecular.com/LSITELAML1ESDualColorTranslocationProbe_5397.aspx
13. Shaffer LG, Slovak ML, Campbell LJ (eds) (2009) ISCN (2009): an international system for human cytogenetic nomenclature. S. Karger, Basel
14. Wiktor AE, Van Dyke DL, Stupca PJ, Ketterling RP, Thorland EC, Shearer BM et al (2006) Preclinical validation of fluorescence in situ hybridization assays for clinical practice. Genet Med 8:16–23
15. American College of Medical Genetics (2006) Standards and guidelines for clinical genetics laboratory. Section E. www.acmg.net/Pages/ACMG_Activities/Stds-2002/e.htm
16. Clinical Laboratory Standards Institute (2004) Fluorescence in situ hybridization (FISH) methods for medical genetics; Approved guidelines, vol MM7-A. 24. Wayne, PA, pp 1–46
17. Clinical Laboratory Improvement Amendments, 1988. http://www.access.gpo.gov/nara/cfr/waisidx_04/42cfr493_04.html
18. Proficiency Testing. http://www.cap.org/
19. Wolff AC, Hammond E, Schwartz JN, Hagerty K, Allred DC, Cote R et al (2007) American Society of Clinical Oncology/College of American Pathologists Guideline recommendations for HER2 testing in breast cancer. J Clin Oncol 25:118–143
20. Dewald GW, Schad CR, Christensen ER, Tiede AL, Zinsmeister AR, Spurbeck JL et al (1993) The application of fluorescent in situ hybridization to detect *Mbcr/abl* fusion in variant Ph chromosomes in CML and ALL. Cancer Genet Cytogenet 71:7–14
21. Romana SP, Mauchauffe M, Le Coniat M, Chumakov I, Le Paslier D, Berger R et al (1995) The t(12;21) of acute lymphoblastic leukemia results in a tel-AML1 gene fusion. Blood 85:3662–3670

Chapter 6

Liquid Bead Array Technology in the Detection of Common Translocations in Acute and Chronic Leukemias

Rodney E. Shackelford, Keith D. Jackson, Michael J. Hafez, and Christopher D. Gocke

Abstract

Hematologic malignancies often have specific chromosomal translocations that promote cancer initiation and progression. Translocation identification is often vital in the diagnosis, prognosis, and treatment of malignancies. A variety of methods including metaphase cytogenetics, in situ hybridization, microarray techniques, Southern blotting, and many variations of PCR are used to identify translocations. While all these techniques have utility, many have drawbacks limiting their clinical usefulness: high cost, slow turnaround time, low density, large sample requirements, high complexity, and difficult validation and standardization. Multiplexed RT-PCR combined with liquid bead array detection overcomes many of these limitations, allowing simultaneous amplification and detection of multiple translocations within one patient sample. This system has high reliability, reproducibility, and flexibility; low cost and low complexity; rapid turnaround time; and appropriate analyte density. Recently, Asuragen Inc. has developed a multiplexed RT-PCR liquid bead array panel that simultaneously analyzes 12 fusion transcripts found in four major types of hematologic malignancies, allowing rapid and efficient diagnosis. In this chapter, we review liquid bead array technology in relation to the specific hematologic translocations analyzed in the Signature LTx panel.

Key words Hematologic malignancy, Translocation, Liquid bead array, PCR, Acute myeloid leukemia, Chronic myelogenous leukemia, Acute lymphoblastic leukemia, Acute promyelocytic leukemia

1 Introduction

Although disturbances in chromosomal structure were hypothesized to play a role in malignancy as early as 1914, it was not until 1960 that an association between cancer and chromosomal rearrangements was established owing to the identification of the Philadelphia chromosome in chronic myelogenous leukemia (CML) (1, 2). Since then over 500 recurrent chromosomal translocations have been identified in hematologic malignancies, far more than found in solid tumors (3, 4). Typically, translocations result in either the production of a chimeric protein unique for a specific entity,

Magdalena Czader (ed.), *Hematological Malignancies*, Methods in Molecular Biology, vol. 999,
DOI 10.1007/978-1-62703-357-2_6,

and the placement of novel regulatory elements in front of proto-oncogenes may result in gene product over-expression with malignancy-promoting effects (3, 4).

There are many techniques employed to detect translocations. The more common ones include classical karyotypic and fluorescence in situ hybridization analyses, oligonucleotide and cDNA microarrays, and variations on polymerase chain reaction (PCR). Standard DNA PCR, reverse transcriptase PCR (RT-PCR), and real-time quantitative RT-PCR may be used and may be nested and/or multiplexed to increase specificity and sensitivity, allowing multiple target sequence analysis. Combined with clinical data, histology, and immunohistochemical studies, each of these molecular techniques is useful in diagnosing hematologic malignancies (5). However, each technique has significant limitations lowering its clinical usefulness, including slow turnaround time, low density, the need for a large amount of patient sample (50–200 μg RNA or 10^7 cells for microarray), and high cost. High-density microarray in particular, while useful in research applications, often lacks standardization and reproducibility; is complex to implement, analyze, and validate; has high redundancy; and results in a large amount of clinically irrelevant data, reducing assay cost-effectiveness and efficiency (6, 7).

Recently a molecular testing technology has been developed that combines multiplexed PCR with a microarray, employing translocation-specific DNA probes covalently conjugated to different internally dyed microspheres (or beads). The microspheres have two or more fluorophores in different ratios, allowing the spectral identification of different bead subsets, each carrying a specific DNA capture probe. Additionally, the multiplexed PCR products have an incorporated fluorophore. Thus, following transcript-microsphere hybridization, spectral analysis can identify and quantify a given analyte (6). The beads are suspended in a solution and analyzed by a modified flow cytometer. The advantages of this system are high throughput (the assay can be done in 5–7 h), high density (up to 100 different analytes/single sample), low cost (approximately $8.00/assay), efficient hybridization (approaching that of solution hybridization kinetics), easy reproducibility, and high flexibility (6–8).

The Signature LTx liquid bead microarray translocation analysis platform from Asuragen Inc. uses reverse transcription, multiplexed PCR, and liquid bead array hybridization in a clinical assay analyzing 12 different translocation transcripts, associated with chronic myelogenous leukemia (CML), acute lymphoblastic leukemia (ALL), and acute myeloid leukemia (AML). Each of these translocations results in a malignancy-unique chimeric transcript (3). The clinical significance of each of these translocations in specific hematologic malignancies is briefly summarized in the following paragraphs.

CML by definition carries a t(9;22)(q34;q11) translocation, resulting in *BCR-ABL1* chimeric transcript and protein expression

(9–12). Combined with appropriate morphologic and clinical findings, the *BCR-ABL1* fusion protein is necessary and sufficient for CML diagnosis. Individuals with similar clinical presentation and/or laboratory features, but without detectable *BCR-ABL1* fusion products, are diagnosed with other subtypes of chronic myeloid neoplasms (9, 13, 14). Several different breakpoints can occur in *BCR* gene, such as the "major breakpoint cluster region" and "minor breakpoint region" (9–12). The Signature LTx liquid bead microarray translocation panel detects the vast majority of the CML t(9;22) translocations and those occurring in a subset of acute lymphoblastic leukemia.

ALL is a heterogeneous group of precursor stage lymphoblastic leukemias, which diagnosis depends mostly on immunophenotyping by flow cytometry combined with translocation identification (5). The Signature LTx panel detects and quantifies the major translocations seen in ALL, all of which have therapeutic or prognostic implications (15). B lymphoblastic leukemia/lymphoma with MLL gene rearrangement is considered a separate entity in WHO classification of hematolymphoid neoplasms. The *t(4;11)(q21;q23), MLL-AF4 (e9e5)* is the most common of more than 40 chromosomal translocations involving the *MLL* gene that have been identified in ALL. The *MLL-AF4* fusion protein causes aberrant histone methylation, resulting in an increased expression of numerous genes that promote transformation to ALL (16, 17). t(4;11)(q21;q23) carries a poor prognosis, with poor chemotherapy response, lineage heterogeneity, *FLT3* deregulation/mutation, and hyperleukocytosis, conferring a median survival of 7 months in adults and 9 months in children (15, 18–22). Another ALL translocation detected by the Signature LTx liquid bead assay is t(12;21)(p12,q22) TEL/AML-1 fusion. This translocation carries an excellent prognosis with standard chemotherapy (16). This fusion causes disruption of normal *TEL* and *AML* functions, repressing gene expression needed for normal cell differentiation (23). Some data indicates that MRD testing may be useful for this translocation, giving the Signature LTx panel an additional potential clinical use (24, 25). The t(1;19)(q23;p13); *PBX/E2A* fusion carries a poor prognosis, with high leukocyte count at presentation. However, intensified chemotherapy improves the prognosis and may nullify the adverse prognostic impact of this translocation (15, 25, 26). The identification of t(9;22)(q34;q11); ABL/BCR fusion (e1a2) in ALL allows for the upfront identification of poor prognosis disease and indicates that imatinib mesylate therapy is warranted. Unfortunately, ALL with t(9;22)(q34;q11) often develops imatinib mesylate resistance quickly (15, 24, 27).

Similar to ALL, AML classification requires cytogenetic/molecular data. The 2008 WHO classification divides AML into four major categories: (1) AML with recurrent genetic abnormalities; (2) AML with multilineage dysplasia; (3) AML, therapy related;

and (4) AML not otherwise specified (5, 28). The Signature LTx panel detects two AML translocations and three fusion gene transcripts relevant to diagnosis, prognosis, and treatment in AML. The AML with t(8;21)(q22;q22); AML1/ETO is a separate disease entity with a favorable prognosis, a good response to chemotherapy, and long median survival (5, 17, 28). The *AML1/ETO* fusion protein functions by blocking normal AML1 protein activity, AML1 target gene expression, and hematopoietic differentiation (5, 28–30). Another separate AML subtype defined by inv(16)(p13;q22); *CBFB/MYH11 fusion* can be diagnosed by Signature LTx liquid bead array. *CBFB/MYH11* fusion exerts its oncogenic effects by blocking the expression of genes involved in hematopoietic differentiation (31). The inv(16)(p13;q22) is heterogeneous with different breakpoints in the *CBFB* and *MYH11* genes generating at least ten different fusion transcripts, all preserving the *CBFB* and *MYH11* reading frames. Roughly 85% of patients have an "A-type" transcript and about 10% have the "D-type" transcript (31, 32). The Signature LTx panel detects types A and D, covering the majority of the AML fusion transcripts. The Signature LTx liquid bead microarray translocation panel includes t(15;17)(q22;q21), PML-RARA defining acute promyelocytic leukemia. The t(15;17)(q22;q21) has breakpoints in the retinoic acid receptor α (*RAR*α) gene on chromosome 17 and the *PML* locus on chromosome 15 (33–35). The chimeric PML-RARα protein binds all-*trans* retinoic acid (ATRA), inducing dramatic APL promyelocyte differentiation. Combined with chemotherapeutic agents, ATRA has markedly improved the prognosis of APL from extremely poor to a 5-year disease-free survival of roughly 74% (36). Multiple t(15;17)(q22;q21) exist, and the Signature LTx liquid bead microarray translocation panel detects the three most common types, allowing the identification of the majority of APL translocations. The 2008 WHO classification introduced an entity of AML with mutated *NPM1*. Nucleophosmin (*NPM1*) is a nucleolar protein regulating both proliferative and growth suppression pathways, with overexpression correlating with uncontrolled cell growth and transformation (37, 38). Fifty to sixty percent of AML with a normal karyotype carry these mutations (38). In AML, 26 different insertions have been identified in the *NPM1* exon 12, nucleotides 956–971, all causing frame-shift mutations ablating nucleolar localization motifs. As a result, the *NPM1* dimer aberrantly localizes to the cytoplasm (38). The type A insertion mutation occurs in 80% of AML cases. Types B and D are seen in 9.1% and 3.1% cases, respectively. Interestingly, these AML mutations confer an improved prognosis, with a lower relapse incidence and better disease-free survival (39, 40). Asuragen offers tests for mutations types A, B, and D, thus covering all but very rare *NPM1* mutations. Presently, this test (Signature NPM1 Mutations [RUO]) is separate from the translocation panel described above, but may be run in parallel in the laboratory.

Last, recent applications of liquid bead array technology have included such diverse analyses as the detection of biothreat agents such as *B. anthracis*, *Y. pestis*, *F. tularensis*, and *B. melitensis*, and the detection of male infertility (41, 42).

In the following sections, we describe the Signature LTx liquid bead microarray translocation analysis platform and outline the major steps of the method including reverse transcription, multiplexed PCR, and liquid bead array hybridization.

2 Materials

2.1 Sample Requirements and Sample Preparation

1. The assay requires a minimum of 6 ml whole blood or 3 ml bone marrow, with 1 ml of either sample being the bare minimum required. The samples must be received in an EDTA tube within 24 h from collection. Bone marrow collected in heparin should be transferred to EDTA.
2. Qiagen QIAamp RNA Blood Mini Kit (Qiagen, Valencia, CA).

2.2 Signature LTx Liquid Bead Microarray Translocation Assay

1. RT amplification reagent package (Asuragen, Austin, TX).
2. Amp reagent package (Asuragen, Austin, TX).
3. Hybridization reagent package (Asuragen, Austin, TX).
4. Control package from Asuragen.
5. Appropriate ASR Primers from Asuragen.
6. Appropriate ASR Probes from Asuragen.
7. 96-well plate (USA Scientific, Orlando, FL).
8. Strip caps (USA Scientific, Orlando, FL).
9. *Taq* Gold (5 U/μl) (Applied Biosystems, Carlsbad, CA).
10. Microseal "A" film (BioRad, Hercules, CA).
11. Thermowell 96 well plate (Corning Life Sciences, Lowell, MA).
12. Luminex Instrument (Asuragen, Austin, TX).

3 Methods

3.1 RNA Extraction

RNA extraction is performed with a commercial kit, such as the Qiagen QIAamp RNA Blood Mini Kit, and can be completed within 1.5 h. This is the specific protocol we employ. All buffers are from the Qiagen QIAamp RNA Blood Mini Kit (see Note 1).

1. Mix 1 volume of blood with 5 volumes of RL buffer in an appropriate tube.
2. Incubate for 10–15 min on ice. Mix periodically by vortexing twice during the incubation. The cloudy solution will become translucent, indicating red blood cell lysis.

3. Centrifuge at 400 × *g* for 10 min at 4°C and completely remove and discard the supernatant. This should remove all or nearly all lysed red blood cells.
4. Add 2 volumes buffer EL to the cell pellet for every volume of blood in the original sample. Resuspend cells by vortexing briefly.
5. Centrifuge at 400 × *g* for 10 min and discard the supernatant.
6. Add buffer RLT to pelleted leukocytes, 350 μl for 0.5 ml starting blood volume and 600 μl for 0.5–1.5 ml starting blood volume.
7. Pipette lysate directly into a QIAshredder spin column sitting in a 2 ml collection tube and centrifuge at maximum rotor speed for 2 min.
8. Add 1 volume (350 or 600 μl) of 70% ethanol to the homogenized lysate and mix by pipetting.
9. Pipette the sample into a new QIAamp spin column sitting in a 2 ml collection tube and centrifuge for 15 s at ≥8,000 × *g*. Use a maximal loading volume of 700 μl. If the sample volume is greater than 700 μl, the sample is spilt into 2 columns and centrifuged.
10. Transfer the QIAamp spin column to a new 2 ml collection tube.
11. Apply 700 μl buffer RPE into the QIAamp spin column and centrifuge for 15 s at 8,000 × *g* to wash.
12. Place the QIAamp spin column into a new 2 ml collection tube.
13. Pipette 500 μl buffer RPE into the QIAamp spin column and centrifuge for 15 s at ≥8,000 × *g*.
14. Open the QIAamp spin column and add 500 μl of buffer RPE. Close the cap and centrifuge at full centrifuge speed (20,000 × *g*) for 3 min.
15. Transfer QIAamp spin column into a 1.5 ml microcentrifuge tube and pipette 30–50 μl of RNase-free water onto the QIAamp membrane. Centrifuge for 1 min at ≥8,000 × *g* to elute.
16. The total RNA sample may now be put directly onto the MagNA Pure for mRNA isolation, or may be frozen at −70°C for mRNA isolation at a later time.

3.2 Reverse Transcription of mRNA

3 μl of RNA is reverse transcribed using the Signature® RT Reagents Kit which employs the Moloney murine leukemia virus reverse transcriptase. The procedure takes approximately 30 min of hands-on setup and 55 min in a thermocycler:

1. Quick-thaw frozen RNA samples, controls, and general purpose RT reagents; immediately place them on ice.

Table 1
Master mix for the reverse transcription of mRNA

1× RT master mix	Component
5.0 μl	Annealing buffer
4.0 μl	RT buffer I
4.0 μl	RT buffer II
1.0 μl	RNase inhibitor
1.0 μl	MMLV
2.0 μl	Diluent
17.0 μl	Total mix volume
3.0 μl	RNA sample
20.0 μl	Grand total

2. Aliquot the appropriate amount of RT reagents into a 1.5 ml Eppendorf tube (see Asuragen worksheet).
3. Pipette 17 μl of the master mix as shown in Table 1 into the appropriate wells.
4. Aliquot 3 μl of the RNA samples/controls into the appropriate wells. The total reaction volume is 20 μl. Note: If RNA concentration is low (<50 ng/μl), you may add up to 5 μl RNA (adjust amount of H_2O in master mix).
5. Cover each column used, as well as the columns to be used for amplification reaction, with strip caps to seal.
6. Spin plate briefly to collect fluid in the bottom of the wells.
7. Place the tubes in the thermal cycler and run the LTX RT-PCR amplification program:
   (a) 42°C for 45 min.
   (b) 93°C for 10 min.
   (c) 4°C indefinitely.
8. Proceed to next step or freeze cDNA at −20°C.

3.3 Amplification of cDNA

1. The resulting fusion transcript cDNAs are amplified with PCR utilizing biotinylated probes specific for each translocation (cDNA from a housekeeping gene such as unmutated *NPM1* or *GAPDH* is analyzed in parallel to ensure adequate sample preparation). As this PCR step is multiplexed, the presence or absence of 12 different fusion transcripts can be simultaneously examined with one patient sample in one reaction volume (see Note 2). Sample preparation time for this step is 30 min,

Table 2
LTX DNA AMP master mix/NPM1 DNA AMP master mix

LTX		NPM1	
1×	Component	1×	Component
9.5 μl	Diluent	8.5 μl	Diluent
5.0 μl	DNA Amp buffer	5.0 μl	AMP buffer I
5.0 μl	DNA primer mix	5.0 μl	AMP buffer II
0.5 μl	AmpliTaq gold	1.0 μl	NPM1 primer
20.0 μl	Total	0.5 μl	AmpliTaq gold
5.0 μl	cDNA product	20.0 μl	Total
		5.0 μl	cDNA product

while the PCR reaction requires 150 min. The LTX DNA AMP master mix/NPM1 DNA AMP master mix is prepared as shown in Table 2.

2. Typical PCR employs the following amplification cycles:

(a)	37°C	15 min
(b)	95°C	10 min
(c)	94°C	30 s
(d)	55°C	30 s ×45 cycles
(e)	72°C	30 s
(f)	4°C	indefinitely

3.4 Hybridization

1. Using a multichannel micropipettor, add 5 μl of each amplified patient sample to internally dyed microspheres with covalently conjugated DNA probes (Table 3).
2. Denature the samples via heating for 5 min at 95°C.
3. Hybridize the sample by incubating for 25 min at 52°C. The protocol allows the sample to remain at 52°C for up to an additional 10 min before continuing (see Note 3).
4. Add a 25 μl of reporter mix to each well to bind the biotinylated amplified fusion transcripts and incubate at RT for 10 min. The reporter is streptavidin with a conjugated fluorophore, such as phycoerythrin.

3.5 Detection and Interpretation

Spectral analysis employing a Luminex 100 IS or 200 system allows the final identification and quantification of the amplified fusion transcript and is completed in approximately 30 min. The readout

Table 3
Hybridization mixes

LTX		NPM1	
1×	**Component**	**1×**	**Component**
45 μl	Bead mix	40 μl	Hyb buffer
5.0 μl	PCR product	5.0 μl	NPM1 probe
		45 μl	Total mix
		5.0 μl	PCR product

from the Luminex system is numeric, indicating transcript-specific fluorescence units (see Note 4).

During validation, each laboratory will set its own thresholds and demonstrate linearity, but in general the assays are linear over at least four logs of target concentration, and the sensitivities are in the range of hundreds of molecules, or the presumed equivalent of tens of cells.

4 Notes

1. RNA is easily degraded by ubiquitous RNase present in the environment and on most surfaces and liquids. Extreme care must be used when working with RNA to avoid sample degradation. All water used to isolate and store RNA should be pretreated with diethylpyrocarbonate (DEPC) to inactivate any RNAs present.
2. Mixing of probe sets is very important. Thoroughly vortex and sonicate probe sets before use.
3. It is very important to add reporter solution to the hybridization plate (*step 8*) as soon as the hybridization reaction is complete (not longer than 10 min after hybridization reaction completes). Assay quality will be greatly reduced if the 10 min period at step 8 is lengthened.
4. Avoid bubbles when adding reporter solution to hybridization plate that will be run on Luminex instrument. Bubbles will interfere with the instrument readout.

Acknowledgment

We would like to thank Lisa M. LaChance, B.A. for her help in the preparation of this manuscript.

References

1. Boveri T (1914) Zur frage der entstehung maligner tumoren. Gustav Fischer, Jena
2. Nowell PC, Hungerford DA (1960) A minute chromosome in human chronic granulocytic leukemia. Science 132:1497–1501
3. Namibia M, Kari V, Raghavan SC (2008) Chromosomal translocations in cancer. Biochim Biophys Acta 1786:139–152
4. Mitelman F, Johansson B, Mertens F (2007) The impact of translocations and gene fusions on cancer causation. Nat Rev Cancer 7: 233–245
5. Swerdlow SH, Campo E, Harris NL, Jaffe ES, Pileri SA, Stein H et al (eds) (2008) WHO classification of tumours of haematopoietic and lymphoid tissues. IARC, Lyon
6. Hadd AG, Brown JT, Andruss BF, Ye F, WalkerPeach CR (2005) Adoption of array technologies into the clinical laboratory. Expert Rev Mol Diagn 5:409–420
7. Vercoutere W, Akeson M (2002) Biosensors for DNA sequence detection. Curr Opin Chem Biol 6:816–822
8. Wallace J, Zhou Y, Usmani GN, Reardon M, Newburger P, Woda B et al (2003) BARCODE-ALL: accelerated and cost-effective genetic risk stratification in acute leukemia using spectrally addressable liquid bead microarrays. Leukemia 7:1404–1410
9. Goldman JM, Melo JV (2008) BCR-ABL in chronic myelogenous leukemia—how does it work? Acta Haematol 119:212–217
10. Elefanty AG, Hariharan IK, Cory S (1990) Bcr-abl, the hallmark of chronic myeloid leukaemia in man, induces multiple haemopoietic neoplasms in mice. EMBO J 9:1069–1078
11. Kelliher MA, McLaughlin J, Witte ON, Rosenberg N (1990) Induction of a chronic myelogenous leukemia-like syndrome in mice with v-abl and BCR/ABL. Proc Natl Acad Sci USA 87:6649–6653
12. Pear WS, Miller JP, Xu L, Pui JC, Soffer B, Quackenbush RC et al (1998) Efficient and rapid induction of a chronic myelogenous leukemia-like myeloproliferative disease in mice receiving P210 bcr/abl-transduced bone marrow. Blood 92:3780–3792
13. Hehlmann R, Hochhaus A, Baccarani M (2007) Chronic myeloid leukemia. Lancet 370: 342–350
14. Pasternak G, Hochhaus A, Schultheis B, Hehlmann R (1998) Chronic myelogenous leukemia: molecular and cellular aspects. J Cancer Res Clin Oncol 124:643–660
15. Teitell MA, Pandolfi PP (2009) Molecular genetics of acute lymphoblastic leukemia. Annu Rev Pathol 4:175–198
16. Gleissner B, Gökbuget N, Bartram CR, Janssen B, Rieder H, Janssen J et. al. German Multicenter Trials of Adult Acute Lymphoblastic Leukemia Study Group (2002) Leading prognostic relevance of the BCR-ABL translocation in adult acute B-lineage lymphoblastic leukemia: a prospective study of the German Multicenter Trial Group and confirmed polymerase chain reaction analysis. Blood 99: 1536–1543
17. Ribeirok RC, Abromowitch M, Raimondi SC, Murphy SB, Behm F, Williams DL (1987) Clinical and biologic hallmarks of the Philadelphia chromosome in childhood acute lymphoblastic leukemia. Blood 70:948–953
18. Zeisig BB, Cheung N, Yeung J, So CW (2008) Reconstructing the disease model and epigenetic networks for MLL-AF4 leukemia. Cancer Cell 14:345–347
19. Krivtsov AV, Feng Z, Lemieux ME, Faber J, Vempati S, Sinha AU et al (2008) H3K79 methylation profiles define murine and human MLL-AF4 leukemias. Cancer Cell 14: 355–368
20. van Dongen JJ, Macintyre EA, Gabert JA, Delabesse E, Rossi V, Saglio G et al (1999) Standardized RT-PCR analysis of fusion gene transcripts from chromosome aberrations in acute leukemia for detection of minimal residual disease. Report of the BIOMED-1 Concerted Action: investigation of minimal residual disease in acute leukemia. Leukemia 13:1901–1928
21. Biondi A, Cimino G, Pieters R, Pui CH (2000) Biological and therapeutic aspects of infant leukemia. Blood 96:24–33
22. Poi CH, Frankel LS, Carroll AJ, Raimondi SC, Shuster JJ, Head DR et al (1991) Clinical characteristics and treatment outcome of childhood acute lymphoblastic leukemia with the t(4;11)(q21;q23): a collaborative study of 40 cases. Blood 78:2471–2473
23. Fischer M, Schwieger M, Horn S, Niebuhr B, Ford A, Roscher S et al (2005) Defining the oncogenic function of the TEL/AML1 (ETV6/RUNX1) fusion protein in a mouse model. Oncogene 24:7579–7591
24. Borowitz MJ, Pullen DJ, Shuster JJ, Viswanatha D, Montgomery K, Willman CL, et. al. Children's Oncology Group study (2003) Minimal residual disease detection in childhood precursor-B-cell acute lymphoblastic leukemia: relation to other risk factors. A Children's Oncology Group study. Leukemia 17: 1566–1572
25. Pui CH, Raimondi SC, Hancock ML, Rivera GK, Ribeiro RC, Mahmoud HH et al (1994)

Immunologic, cytogenetic, and clinical characterization of childhood acute lymphoblastic leukemia with the t(1;19) (q23; p13) or its derivative. J Clin Oncol 12:2601–2606
26. Raimondi SC, Behm FG, Roberson PK, Williams DL, Pui CH, Crist WM et al (1990) Cytogenetics of pre-B-cell acute lymphoblastic leukemia with emphasis on prognostic implications of the t(1;19). J Clin Oncol 8:1380–1388
27. Willemse MJ, Seriu T, Hettinger K, d'Aniello E, Hop WC, Panzer-Grümayer ER et al (2002) Detection of minimal residual disease identifies differences in treatment response between T-ALL and precursor B-ALL. Blood 99:4386–4393
28. Buzzai M, Licht JD (2008) New molecular concepts and targets in acute myeloid leukemia. Curr Opin Hematol 15:82–87
29. Ohki M (1993) Molecular basis of the t(8;21) translocation in acute myeloid leukaemia. Semin Cancer Biol 4:369–375
30. Yuan Y, Zhou L, Miyamoto T, Iwasaki H, Harakawa N, Hetherington CJ et al (2001) AML1-ETO expression is directly involved in the development of acute myeloid leukemia in the presence of additional mutations. Proc Natl Acad Sci USA 98:10398–10403
31. Schnittger S, Bacher U, Haferlach C, Kern W, Haferlach T (2007) Rare CBFB-MYH11 fusion transcripts in AML with inv(16)/t(16;16) are associated with therapy-related AML M4eo, atypical cytomorphology, atypical immunophenotype, atypical additional chromosomal rearrangements and low white blood cell count: a study on 162 patients. Leukemia 21:725–731
32. Reilly JT (2005) Pathogenesis of acute myeloid leukaemia and inv(16)(p13;q22): a paradigm for understanding leukaemogenesis? Br J Haematol 128:18–34
33. Rowley JD, Golomb HM, Dougherty C (1977) 15/17 translocation, a consistent chromosomal change in acute promyelocytic leukemia. Lancet 1:549–550
34. de Thé H, Chomienne C, Lanotte M, Degos L, Dejean A (1990) The t(15;17) of acute promyelocytic leukemia fuses the retinoic acid receptor alpha gene to a novel transcribed locus. Nature 347:558–561
35. Kakizuka A, Miller WH Jr, Umesono K, Warrell RP Jr, Frankel SR, Murty VV et al (1991) Chromosomal translocation t(15;17) in human acute promyelocytic leukemia fuses RAR alpha with a novel putative transcription factor, PML. Cell 66:663–674
36. Wang ZY, Chen Z (2008) Acute promyelocytic leukemia: from highly fatal to highly curable. Blood 111:2505–2515
37. Okuwaki M (2008) The structure and functions of NPM1/Nucleophsmin/B23, a multifunctional nucleolar acidic protein. J Biochem 143:441–448
38. Grisendi S, Mecucci C, Falini B, Pandolfi PP (2006) Nucleophosmin and cancer. Nat Rev Cancer 6:493–505
39. Chen W, Rassidakis GZ, Medeiros LJ (2006) Nucleophosmin gene mutations in acute myeloid leukemia. Arch Pathol Lab Med 130: 1687–1692
40. Thiede C, Koch S, Creutzig E, Steudel C, Illmer T, Schaich M et al (2006) Prevalence and prognostic impact of NPM1 mutations in 1485 adult patients with acute myeloid leukemia (AML). Blood 107:4011–4020
41. Gallagher RE, Li YP, Rao S, Paietta E, Andersen J, Etkind P et al (1995) Characterization of acute promyelocytic leukemia cases with PML-RAR alpha break/fusion sites in PML exon 6: identification of a subgroup with decreased in vitro responsiveness to all-trans retinoic acid. Blood 86:1540–1547
42. Wilson WJ, Erler AM, Nasarabadi SL, Skowronski EW, Imbro PM (2005) A multiplexed PCR-coupled liquid bead array for the simultaneous detection of four biothreat agents. Mol Cell Probes 19:137–144

Chapter 7

Molecular Genetic Tests for *FLT3*, *NPM1*, and *CEBPA* in Acute Myeloid Leukemia

Qing Zhang, Shaochun Bai, and Gail H. Vance

Abstract

Patients with acute myeloid leukemia (AML) and a normal karyotype constitute the single largest cytogenetic group of AML. It is important to identify prognostic markers that predict patients' outcome more precisely. The presence of mutations in *FLT3* (FMS-like tyrosine kinase 3), *NPM1* (Nucleophosmin), and *CEBPA* (CCAAT/enhancer-binding protein alpha) genes hold prognostic significance in patients with AML and normal cytogenetics. Therefore, mutation identification may help to optimize therapeutic approaches in this group of patients. Polymerase chain reaction (PCR)-based fragment length analysis for mutations in *FLT3* and *NPM1* has been shown to be a fast and sensitive method, while nucleotide sequencing represents a gold standard for *CEBPA* heterogeneous mutational screening. We describe both fragment length assay and sequencing methods for mutational analysis of these three genes.

Key words Acute myeloid leukemia (AML), *FLT3*, *NPM1*, *CEBPA*, PCR, Capillary electrophoresis, DNA sequencing, Mutational detection

1 Introduction

Acute myeloid leukemia (AML) is a clinically and genetically heterogeneous disease. Cytogenetic identification of recurring abnormalities at diagnosis classifies patients into favorable, adverse, or intermediate risk groups with implications for risk-adapted therapy (1, 2). However, 40–50% of AML patients will have a normal karyotype (AML-NK) at diagnosis (1–3). The genetic events leading to AML-NK have been more difficult to decipher as individual patients may have considerably different clinical courses. Recently, molecular diagnostics have identified novel markers that define new prognostic subgroups and provide important clinical implications (4, 5). The 2008 edition of the World Health Organization classification of AML integrates both *NPM1* and *CEBPA* mutations as entities under "AML with recurrent genetic abnormalities" (6). At present, the most common independent prognostic

Magdalena Czader (ed.), *Hematological Malignancies*, Methods in Molecular Biology, vol. 999,
DOI 10.1007/978-1-62703-357-2_7, © Springer Science+Business Media New York 2013

factors for AML-NK include mutations in the FMS-like tyrosine kinase 3 (*FLT3*), Nucleophosmin (*NPM1*), and CCAAT/enhancer-binding protein alpha (*CEBPA*) genes (5, 7).

FLT3 is a member of the class III receptor tyrosine kinase family mapped on chromosome 13q12 (8). The FLT3 protein is normally expressed on hematopoietic stem progenitor cells and appears to play an important role in the regulation of stem cell proliferation and differentiation (9). Two specific *FLT3* mutations have important implications for AML prognosis. An in-frame internal tandem duplication (ITD) mutation arises from duplications of the juxtamembrane domain of the gene (exons 11 and 12) to produce activation of the FLT3 protein identified in approximately 40% of AML-NK patients (3). The second type is a missense mutation at aspartic acid residue 835 (D835) within the second tyrosine kinase domain (exon 20) occurring in about 7% of AML-NK cases (3, 10). Both mutations activate the FLT3 protein and associated signaling pathways and appear to be associated with a poor prognosis in patients with AML. *FLT3*-ITD testing is recommended in all cytogenetically normal AML patients who are candidates for allogeneic transplantation or investigational therapies (5, 11).

The *NPM1* gene is mapped to chromosome 5q35 and contains 12 exons (12). NPM1 protein shuttles between the nucleus and cytoplasm and is involved in ribosomal regulation, centrosome duplication, and regulation of apoptosis (13). Heterozygous mutations of *NPM1* have been identified in about 35% of all AML patients and 50–60% of AML-NK (13). The most common alterations are insertions of short nucleotide stretches (4–11 bp) in *NPM1* exon 12 (13, 14). These mutations result in mislocalization of the mutant protein to the cytoplasm (NPMc+) in the leukemic blasts. Immunohistochemical detection of NPMc+ in AML is predictive of *NPM1* mutations (15). A *NPM1* mutation, in the absence of FLT3 mutations, confers a more favorable prognosis and an intermediate prognosis if *FLT3*-ITD is present (13).

CEBPA localizes to 19q13.1 and is an intronless gene (16). It encodes the transcription factor CCAAT/enhancer-binding protein alpha which is crucial for normal granulocyte differentiation (16). *CEBPA* mutations are identified in approximately 15% of AML-NK patients (16). The mutations can be largely divided into two common types: N-terminal frameshift mutations resulting in a truncated 30-kDa protein, whereas C-terminal in-frame mutations affect DNA binding as well as homo- and heterodimerization with other C/EBP family members (17). The majority of AML-NK patients with *CEBPA* mutations have biallelic mutations involving the N-terminal mutation and typically a C-terminal mutation (17). Mutated patients preferentially belong to M1 or M2 French–American–British morphological subtypes associated with lower relapse rate and improved survival (17–19). Besides genetic mutations, *CEBPA* can be also silenced by aberrant DNA methylation.

Thus, DNA methylation analysis of the promoter region of *CEBPA* is recommended to capture all of the relevant dysfunctional changes of CEBPA (20).

Molecular tests for mutations in *FLT3, NPM1*, and *CEBPA* genes can be performed using genomic polymerase chain reaction (PCR), followed by capillary gel electrophoresis (fragment sizing) for *FLT3*-ITD mutations and *NPM1* exon 12 insertions; restriction enzyme digestion with EcoRV for identification of the *FLT3* D835 mutation; and PCR followed by sequencing analysis of the entire coding region for *CEBPA*.

Note: Clinical testing for FLT3 mutations by PCR is patent-protected by in- vivoscribe company. Therefore, all diagnostic testing for FLT3 in the U.S. is restricted to Lab PMM in San Diego, CA.

2 Materials

2.1 Control Samples

1. FLT3-ITD and D835 negative control: Polyclonal control DNA from IVS-0000 (InVivoScribe Technologies, San Diego, CA) and DNA from MOLT-4 cells (Abcam Inc, Cambridge, MA).
2. FLT3-ITD positive control: Clonal control DNA from IVS-0017 (InVivoScribe Technologies, San Diego, CA) and DNA from MV-4–11 cells (ATCC, Manassas, Virginia).
3. FLT3-D835 positive control: Clonal control DNA from IVS-P001 (InVivoScribe Technologies, San Diego, CA). A positive patient sample may also be implemented as an additional or alternative D835 positive control.
4. NPMl negative control: Cell line OCI-AML2 cells (DMSZ, Germany).
5. NPMl positive control (exon 12 insertion): Cell line OCI-AML3 cells (DMSZ, Germany).

2.2 Cell Lysis/DNA Extraction

1. Red Blood Cell (RBC) Lysis Solution (QIAGEN Sciences, Germantown, MD).
2. Cell Lysis Solution (QIAGEN Sciences, Germantown, MD).
3. Protein Precipitation Solution (QIAGEN Sciences, Germantown, MD).
4. Hydration Solution (QIAGEN Sciences, Germantown, MD).
5. Isopropanol, 100%.
6. Ethanol, 70%.
7. Ethanol, 95–100%.

2.3 PCR Reagents

1. AmpliTaq gold® with GeneAmp® DNA polymerase pack (Applied Biosystems, Foster City, CA): 5 U/μl AmpliTaq;

Table 1
Primers used to amplify *FLT3*-ITD, *FLT3*-D835, *NPM1* exon 12, and *CEBPA* coding region from genomic DNA

FLT3-ITD	
Forward—FLT3-ITD-E14F-fluo	5′-5FAM-CAATTTAGGTATGAAAGCCAGC-3′
Reverse—FLT3-ITD-E15R	5′-CTTTCAGCATTTTGACGGCAACC-3′
FLT3-D835	
Forward—FLT3-835-E20-F-fluo	5′-TET-CCGCCAGGAACGTGCTTG-3′
Reverse—FLT3-835-E20R	5′-CAGGAAACAGCTATGACCgatat[a]CAGCCTCACATT GCCCC-3′
NPM1	
Forward—NPM1-E12F-fluo	5′-HEX-GATGTCTATGAAGTGTTGTGGTTCC-3′
Reverse—NPM1-E12R	5′-ACCATTTCCATGTCTGAg[b]CAC-3′
CEBPA	
Forward 1 CEBPA_ex_1_1_-91F	CGAGCAGGGTCTCCGGGTG
Reverse 1 CEBPA_ex_1_1_250R	GCTGGAACAGGTCGGCCAGG
Forward 2 CEBPA_ex_1_2_179F	CGTCCATCGACATCAGCGCCTA
Reverse 2 CEBPA_ex_1_2_521R	GCCAGCTGCTTGGCTTCATCCT
Forward 3 CEBPA_ex_1_3_469F	CCGCTGGTGATCAAGCAGGAGC
Reverse 3 CEBPA_ex_1_3_840R	TGTCCACCGACTTCTTGGCCTTG
Forward 4 CEBPA_ex_1_4_651F	CATGCACCTG CAGCCCGGT
Reverse 4 CEBPA_ex_1_4_1140R	CCCCAAACCACTCCCTGGGTC

[a]Enzyme cut site introduced
[b]Primer designed as a mismatch in the 3′ end to enhance specificity

gold® DNA polymerase, 10× PCR gold buffer w/o $MgCl_2$, 25 mM $MgCl_2$.

2. 10 mM dNTP mix (10 mM each dATP, dTTP, dCTP, and dGTP) (Invitrogen, Carlsbad, CA) diluted to 2 mM with nuclease-free H_2O.
3. FailSafe™ PCR 2× PreMix K (Epicentre, Madison, WI). FailSafe™ PCR enzyme mix, 2 U/µl (Epicentre, Madison, WI).

2.4 Primers

Primers are ordered with standard desalting purification (Integrated DNA Technologies, Coralville, IA) and reconstituted to a 100 µM stock and stored at −20°C (Table 1). Working solutions are prepared by dilution in nuclease-free H_2O to 10 µM and are stored at −20°C (see Note 1).

2.5 Post-PCR Purification

1. ExoSAP-IT (Affymetrix, Santa Clara, CA).

2.6 Sequencing/ BigDye® Reaction Purification

1. BigDye® terminator v3.1 cycle sequencing kit (Applied Biosystems, Foster City, CA): Ready reaction mix, 5× sequencing buffer.
2. Ethanol, 70%.

2.7 Electrophoresis Reagents

1. Agarose (Sigma, St. Louis, MO).
2. Ethidium bromide, prepared to 10 mg/ml working solution. Store in a light-proof container (Sigma, St. Louis, MO).
3. TBE Buffer (10×): 0.89 M Tris–HCl, 0.89 M boric acid, 0.02 M EDTA, pH 8.3. Store at room temperature. Prepare working buffer by diluting to 1× with dH_2O.
4. 10× Gel Loading Buffer: 24.0 ml nuclease-free H_2O, 65.0 ml glycerol, 270 mg bromophenol blue, 1.0 g SDS, 10.0 ml 10× TE buffer. Store at room temperature. The stock is diluted to 3× working concentration with nuclease-free H_2O.
5. 100 bp DNA ladder (New England Biolabs, Ipswich, MA).
6. 10× genetic analyzer buffer with EDTA (Applied Biosystems, Foster City, CA).
7. Hi-Di formamide (Applied Biosystems, Foster City, CA).
8. POP-7 performance optimized polymer (Applied Biosystems, Foster City, CA).
9. GeneScan 500 TAMRA sizing standard (Applied Biosystems, Foster City, CA).
10. Fluorescent amidite matrix standards for filter set C (Applied Biosystems, Foster City, CA).

2.8 Equipment and Supplies

1. Mikro 200 microcentrifuge (Hettich, Beverly, MA).
2. TJ-6 centrifuge (Beckman Coulter, Brea, CA) with rotor to support 15 ml conical tubes.
3. Vortex machine.
4. Pipettes (10, 20, 100, 200 μl, 1 ml) and aerosol-resistant pipette tips.
5. 15 ml centrifuge tubes.
6. 0.2 ml PCR tubes.
7. 1.5 ml microcentrifuge tubes.
8. Nanodrop ND-2000 spectrophotometer (ThermoScientific, Waltham, MA).
9. Thermal Cyclers: GeneAmp® PCR System 9700 (Applied Biosystems, Foster City CA); Mastercycler® epgradient (Eppendorf, Hauppauge, NY).
10. Gel cast, box, and power supply.

11. ABI PRISM® 3130*xl* Genetic Analyzer and related components including: Buffer reservoirs and Septa Mats, gel block assembly, anode buffer jar, 36 cm 16 capillary array, 96-well sample tray assembly, 96-well MicroAmp® reaction plate, 96-well plate septa (Applied Biosystems, Foster City, CA).
12. 3130xl Data Collection v3.0; Sequencing Analysis Software v5.3.1; GeneMapperID v3.2 (Applied Biosystems, Foster City, CA). Mutation Surveyor 4.0 (Softgenetics, State College, PA).

3 Methods

3.1 FLT3-ITD, D835, and NPM1 Mutational Analysis by PCR (See Note 2)

Patient DNA is isolated, purified, and subjected to PCR amplification using specific oligonucleotide primers directed at exons 14, 15, and 20 of the *FLT3* gene (Table 1). Each assay includes a positive control reaction using DNA from a specimen or cell line known to contain an *FLT3*-ITD mutation or exon 20 point mutation and a negative control reaction using DNA from a specimen or cell line containing the wild-type *FLT3* sequence. Amplicons for exon 20 are digested with EcoRV. PCR products are separated by capillary gel electrophoresis detected by fluorescence.

3.2 CEBPA Mutational Screening by Sequencing

The entire coding region of the CEBPA gene was amplified using four overlapping PCR primer pairs as shown in Table 1. PCR products were sequenced in both directions using BigDye Terminator-Mix Version3.1 (see Note 1).

3.3 DNA Extraction Using QIAGEN DNA Isolation Kit

This is a conventional DNA isolation method for large volumes of blood (3–5 ml). It will yield ~50–100 μg amount of DNA. The procedure consists of cell lysis (steps 1–7), protein precipitation (steps 8–11), and DNA precipitation (steps 12–23).

1. Pipette 9 ml of RBC Lysis Solution into a 15 ml centrifuge tube.
2. Add 3 ml of whole blood.
3. Mix by inversion and incubate 10 min at room temperature. Invert at least once again during the incubation.
4. Centrifuge in Beckman TJ-6 at approximately 816×*g* for 10 min.
5. Remove the supernatant solution. Leave behind the white cell pellet and about 100 μl of the residual liquid.
6. Vortex the tube vigorously to suspend the cells in the residual liquid.
7. Add 3 ml of Cell Lysis Solution to the suspended cells and pipette up and down to lyse the cells. Usually, no incubation is required. If, however, cell clumps are visible, incubate at 37°C until the solution is homogeneous. Samples are stable

in cell lysis solution for at least 18 months at room temperature.

8. Cool samples to room temperature, if necessary.
9. Add 1 ml of Protein Precipitation Solution to the cell lysate.
10. Vortex vigorously for 20 s to mix the Protein Precipitation Solution and cell lysate uniformly.
11. Centrifuge in Beckman TJ-6 at approximately 816×*g* for 10 min. The precipitated protein should form a tight, dark-brown pellet. If the precipitated protein pellet is not tight, repeat steps 9 and 10, followed by incubation on ice for 5 min. Repeat the centrifugation for 10 min.
12. Pipette 3 ml of 100% isopropanol into a clean 15-ml centrifuge tube.
13. Pour the supernatant solution containing the DNA into the isopropanol. Leave pellet behind.
14. Mix by inverting gently at least 50 times, until the white threads of DNA form a visible clump.
15. Centrifuge in TJ-6 at approximately 816×*g* for 3 min. The DNA will be visible as a small white pellet.
16. Pour off the supernatant solution and drain the tube briefly on clean absorbent paper.
17. Add 3 ml of 70% ethanol and invert the tube several times to wash the DNA pellet.
18. Centrifuge for 3 min to precipitate the pellet.
19. The pellet may still be loose, so pour alcohol off slowly and watch the pellet!
20. Invert and drain the tube on clean absorbent paper and allow to air-dry for 10–15 min.
21. Add the proper amount (250–1,000 μl) of DNA hydration solution or 1× TE buffer according to the size of the pellet. Mix by pipetting up and down several times and transfer to a 2 ml tube for use or storage (250 μl of DNA Hydration Solution will give a concentration of 400 ng/μl if the total yield is 100 μg of DNA).
22. Rehydrate DNA by incubating at 65°C for 1 h and overnight at room temperature. Or, place on rotator at room temperature overnight. Tap tube periodically to aid in dispersing the DNA.
23. For storage, centrifuge briefly and transfer to 1.5-ml microfuge tube. For short-term storage, store DNA at 4°C or −20°C. Store long term at −80°C.

3.4 PCR

1. *FLT3*-ITD, *FLT3*-D835, and *NPM1* PCRs are composed of 3.0 μl of 10× PCR buffer without $MgCl_2$ (1× final concentration),

2.4 μl of 25 mM $MgCl_2$ (2 mM final concentration), 3.0 μl of 2 mM dNTP mix (200 μM each dNTP final concentration), 1.0 μl of each 10 μM primer (0.33 μM final concentration, each), 0.2 μl 5 U/μl AmpliTaq® Gold DNA polymerase, 1 μl of 100 ng/μl DNA, and 18.4 μl of nuclease-free H_2O for a 30 μl of total reaction volume.

2. *CEBPA* PCRs are composed of 12.5 μl of 2.5× FailSafe PCR Mix K (1.25× final concentration), 0.5 μl of each 10 μM primer (0.2 μM final concentration, each), 0.25 μl of 2 U/μl Fail Safe enzyme mix (0.5 U total), 1 μl of 100 ng/μl DNA, and 6.25 μl nuclease-free H_2O for a 25 μl total reaction volume (see Note 3).
3. Controls should be amplified with each PCR batch (see Subheading 2.1). A non-template blank control (H_2O) should also be run simultaneously.
4. Amplify samples using the following thermal cycling conditions for *FLT3*-ITD, *FLT*-D835, and *NPM1*: 94°C for 5 min followed by 35 cycles of 94°C for 45 s, 58°C for 45 s, 72°C for 1 min, with a final extension at 72°C for 10 min, followed by a 4°C hold.
5. *CEBPA* amplification conditions are as follows: 95°C for 5 min followed by 35 cycles of 94°C for 45 s, 65°C for 45 s, 72°C for 1 min, with a final extension at 72°C for 10 min, followed by a 4°C hold.

3.5 PCR Product Assessment Using Agarose Gel Electrophoresis

1. Prior to further analysis, PCR products should be assessed by electrophoresis on a 1% agarose gel, containing EtBr: 1.0 g agarose, 100 ml 1× TBE buffer, 5 μl EtBr (10 mg/ml).
2. Add 5 μl of PCR product to 5 μl of 3× loading buffer. Add 2 μl of 100 bp DNA ladder to 5 μl 3× loading buffer. Load samples onto gel and run electrophoresis for 30 min at 100 V.
3. Visualize PCR product on UV gel box and save electronic image.
4. PCR products that have been successfully amplified can be carried into subsequent analysis steps. If PCR has failed, or if PCR products have nonspecific band(s), repeat amplification should be performed. If the non-template blank control exhibits visible bands, repeat amplification should be performed (see Note 4).

3.6 EcoRV Digestion of D835 PCR Products

1. Prepare the enzyme master mix in a sterile 1.5 ml Eppendorf tube: 1.0 μl of EcoRV enzyme (20 U/μl), 1.5 μl of 10× NE buffer 3, 4.5 μl of nuclease-free water, 8.0 μl of D835 PCR products for a total volume of 15.0 μl.
2. Incubate in a 37°C water bath for 1 h.

3.7 Purification of PCR Product for CEBPA Sequencing Analysis

1. Add 2 μl of ExoSAP-IT to a new PCR tube for each sample. Add 5 μl of PCR product to each tube.
2. Quick spin the tube and place on a thermal cycler using the following conditions: 37°C for 15 min, 80°C for 15 min, followed by a 4°C hold.

3.8 BigDye® Terminator v3.1 Cycle Sequencing Kit Protocol

1. Prepare a master mix of the sequencing reagents using the following volumes per sample: 1.0 μl Big Dye v3.1 ready reaction premix, 1.5 μl 5× sequencing buffer, 4.5 μl nuclease-free H_2O.
2. Add 7.0 μl of the master mix to a 96-well plate for each sample to be sequenced. Add 2.0 μl of 2.5 μM sequencing primer to the master mix in the plate and then add 1.0 μl of purified PCR product to the master mix/primer (see Note 6).
3. Quick spin the plate to pull down the reaction components and run the sequencing program on a thermal cycler using the following parameters: 96°C for 1 min followed by 25 cycles of 96°C for 10 s, 50°C for 5 s, 60°C for 4 min, followed by a 4°C hold.

3.9 Ethanol Precipitation

1. Briefly spin the plate down in a centrifuge. Add 90 μL of 70% EtOH to the desired wells.
2. Securely place new caps on the samples and invert the tray a few times to mix.
3. Allow to incubate in the dark at room temperature for 20 min.
4. Spin the plate down in the centrifuge on 4500 rpm (or 2050 rcf) for 45 min.
5. Remove caps, invert tray onto a paper towel, and spin again for 1 min at 1000 rpm.
6. Let stand to completely evaporate EtOH.
7. Add 10 μL of Hi-Di Formamide to each well (including non-sample wells). Seal tubes with caps and Run denature on thermal cycler (95°C for 10 min then 4°C hold).
8. Keep at 4°C until needed for loading.

3.10 Sequencing Protocol for CEBPA in ABI 3130xl

1. Assemble the 96-well plate and place the plate assembly on the autosampler as described in the maintenance section of the 3130 User's Guide.
2. Run plate using a Sequencing Analysis Plate Record in the Data Collection software using the ABI RapidSeq36_POP7 Instrument Protocol and "3130POP7_BDTv3-KB-Denovo_5.2" Analysis Method.

3.11 Sequencing Alignment Analysis Using Mutation Surveyor v4.0

1. Mutation Surveyor v4.0 is used to align sample sequences against a reference sequence. The software creates a consensus sequence of all the overlapping sample sequences and can detect the presence of sequence variations as compared to the reference. Summary reports of software identified mutations can also be generated.
2. Mutation Summary Reports can be generated and exported in .txt format and formatted using Microsoft Excel.

3.12 ABI Fluorescence Detection with an ABI 3130xl Instrument

PCR products from *FLT3*-ITD, D835, and *NPM1* are electrophoresed in the capillary-based ABI 3130xl genetic analyzer. The samples are analyzed with the ABI GeneScan software and the sizes of the fragments are calculated.

1. Prepare a sample loading master mix with the following volumes per sample: 12.0 μl of Hi-Di formamide, 0.5 μl of GeneScan-500 TAMRA. Aliquot 12.5 μl of the master mix into each sample tube.
2. Transfer 1 μl of diluted PCR product to each tube (see Note 7). Mix gently and spin down briefly.
3. Denature samples 5 min at 95°C and cool to 4°C until ready to use.
4. ABI Data Collection software is used to prepare a 96-well sample sheet. Samples are run using the ABI "FragmentAnalysis36_POP7" module.

3.13 GeneMapperID v.3.2 Fragment Analysis

1. Samples are added to a new project and analyzed using the following settings: FLT3 analysis method, FLT3 Panel, TAMRA size standard (include 35–400 bp fragment for FLT3-D835 and 75–500 bp fragment for FLT3-ITD and NPM1).
2. Data can be visualized in the green, blue, yellow, and red channels for FLT3-D835, FLT3-ITD, NPM1, and TAMRA sizing standard, respectively.

3.14 Acceptable Assay Performance Criteria for FLT3-ITD

1. The "no template" control (water) must be blank and without a signal corresponding to a base pair size of 328 bp for the ITD PCR.
2. ITD negative control (MOLT-4) must show a visible signal corresponding to a base pair size of 328 bp for the ITD PCR.
3. ITD positive control must show a visible signal corresponding to a base pair size larger than 328 bp for the ITD PCR (Fig. 1).
4. Failure to achieve these criteria requires repeating this portion of the procedure.

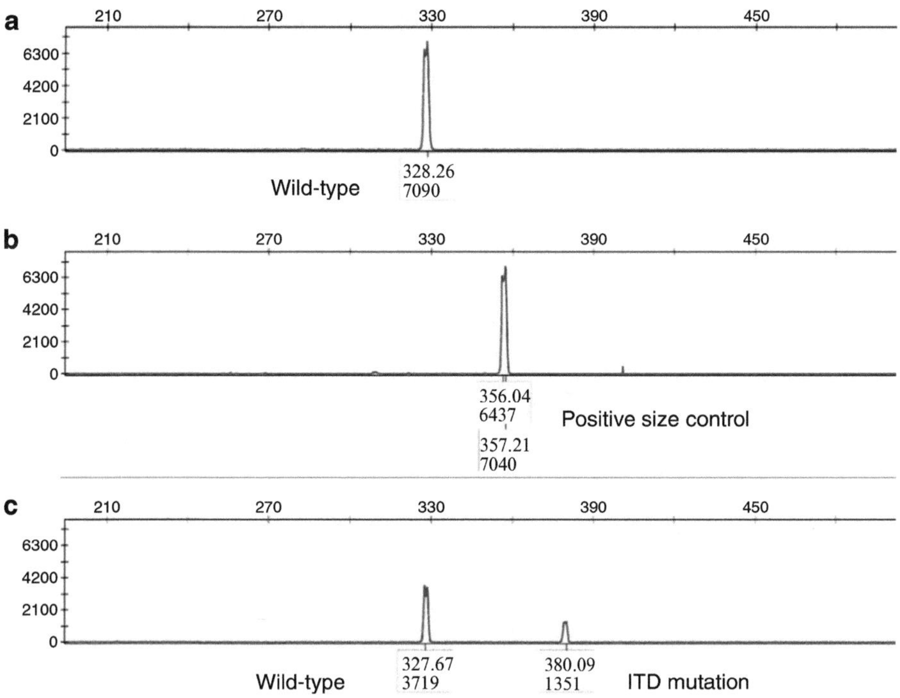

Fig. 1 FLT3-ITD mutation detection. FLT-3 was amplified using PCR followed by capillary electrophoresis. (**a**) Approximately 328 bp amplicon represents the wild-type allele. A larger than 328 bp amplicon represents the internal tandem duplication. (**a**) Normal control. (**b**) Positive control. (**c**) Patient sample harboring both normal and ITD alleles

3.15 Acceptable Assay Performance Criteria for FLT3-D835

1. The "no template" control (water) must be blank without signal corresponding to a base pair size of 134 bp for the D835 PCR.
2. All samples except the "no template" control must show a visible signal corresponding to a base pair size of 134 bp for the D835 PCR *before* restriction enzyme digestion.
3. D835 positive control (IVS-P001) must show a signal corresponding to the size of 111 bp *after* the restriction enzyme digestion. The reverse primer FLT3-835-E20R is designed to introduce an EcoRV cut site in order to monitor a partial digestion.
4. D835 negative control (MOLT-4) must show visible signals corresponding to base pair sizes of 65, 46, and 23 bp fragments on the gel, but only a 65 bp fragment on ABI after digestion with EcoRV (Fig. 2).

3.16 Acceptable Assay Performance Criteria for NPM1

1. The "no template" control (water) must be blank without a signal corresponding to a base pair size of 362 bp for the *NPM1* exon12 PCR.

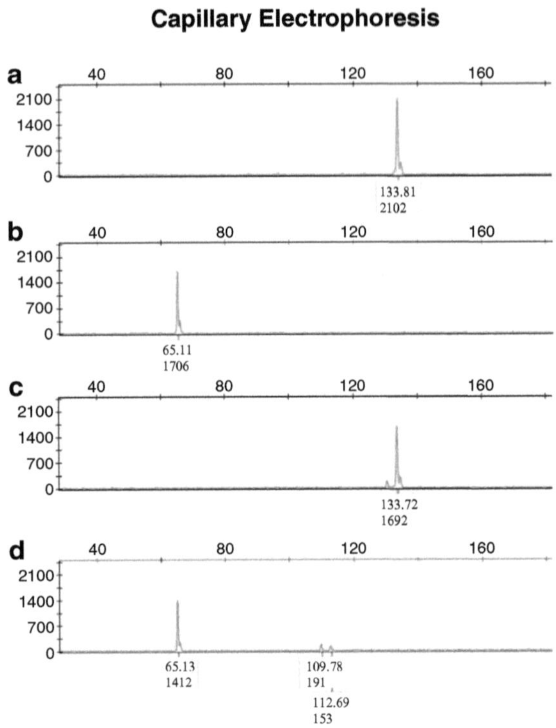

Fig. 2 FLT3-D835 mutation detection by capillary electrophoresis (CE). The amplicon is 134 bp. EcoRV digestion of wild-type product generates fragments of 65, 46, and 23 bp. The D835 mutation results in a ~110 bp fragment. (**a**) Normal undigested; (**b**) normal digested; (**c**) D835 mutation undigested; (**d**) D835 mutation digested

2. *NPM1* negative control (OCI-AML2) must show a visible signal corresponding to a base pair size of 362 bp as a PCR product.
3. *NPM1* positive control (OCI-AML3) must show a visible signal corresponding to a base pair size larger than 362 bp for the NPM1 exon12 PCR (see Fig. 3 and Note 8).
4. Failure to achieve these criteria requires repeating this portion of the procedure.

3.17 Acceptable Assay Performance Criteria for CEBPA

1. Sequencing data should cover the entire coding region of the gene.
2. Sequencing data should be aligned with reference sequencing from GenBank (NC_000019.8) using ABI GeneScan software.
3. Determine the type of alteration (missense, nonsense, silent, etc.).
4. Perform evaluation of variants with unknown clinical significance found in the coding region of the gene (see Note 11).

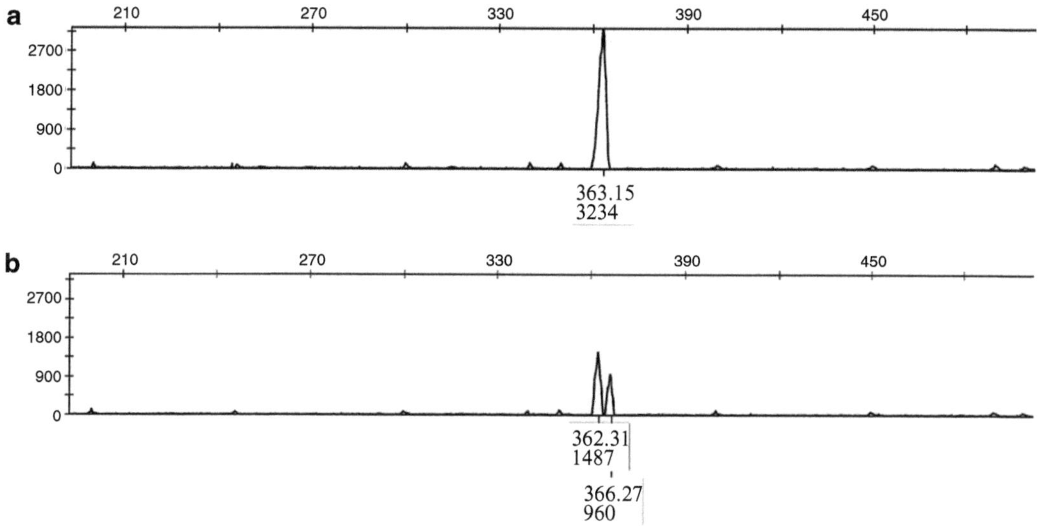

Fig. 3 NPM1 exon 12 mutation detection. PCR followed by capillary electrophoresis. (**a**) Normal allele (362 ± 1 bp). (**b**) Exon 12 heterozygote with normal (~362 bp) and mutant (4 bp larger, ~366 bp) alleles

3.18 Assay Sensitivity

In order to detect *FLT3* and *NPM1* mutations, acceptable specimens of blood or bone marrow must have a minimum of 10% blast cells (5% mutation). The sequencing assay is expected to detect >99% of germline and/or somatic variants within the *CEBPA* coding and regions, if the mutation is present at a level of 20% (equivalent to 40% of blast cells) or greater (see Fig. 4).

4 Notes

1. *NPM1* mutations and *FLT3*-ITD mutations frequently occur together; therefore, molecular testing of *NPM1* is usually done in conjunction with *FLT3* testing. *CEBPA* mutation analysis can be ordered separately or as a reflex test when both *FLT3* and *NPM1* tests are negative.
2. Some tips on primer design: primers should be 17–28 bases in length, have a base composition of 50–60% GC, and a Tm between 55 and 80°C. Primers should end (3′) in a G or C, or CG, or GC to increase efficiency; Avoid runs of three or more Cs or Gs at the 3′-ends of primers that may promote mispriming at G- or C-rich sequences (because of stability of annealing); Avoid complimentary 3′-ends of primers as primer dimers will form preferentially; Avoid primer self-complementarity (ability to form 2° structures such as hairpins); and of course, avoid SNPs in the primers that may fail PCR.
3. *CEBPA* gene has a GC-rich (more than 70%) coding region that is contained within a single exon. Therefore, a GC-rich

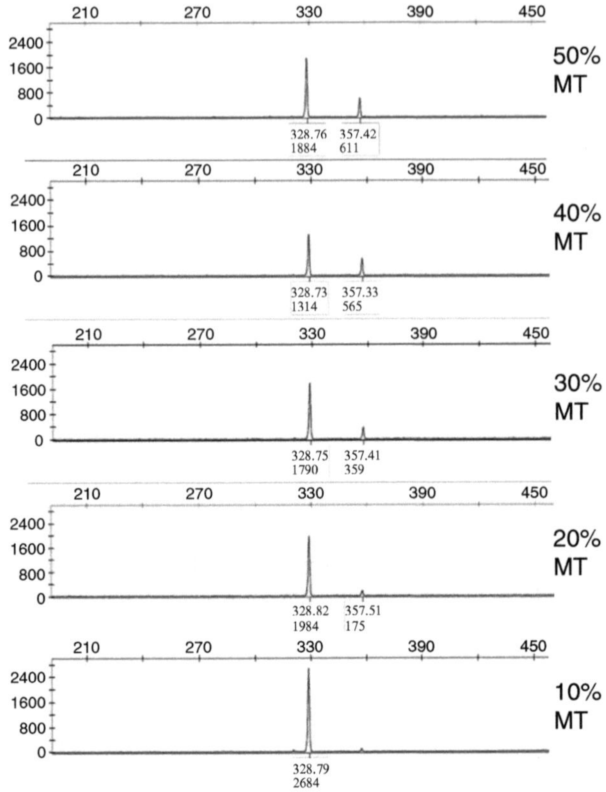

Fig. 4 Sensitivity of FLT3-ITD assay. A cloned plasmid DNA harboring FLT-ITD mutant allele was serially diluted with wild-type plasmid DNA. The mixed plasmid template were PCR amplified and followed by capillary electrophoresis. Percentages on the figures show the expected amount of mutant DNA in the mixture

PCR kit (FailSafe PCR Mix K Kit, Roche GC-rich PCR System) may be needed to facilitate amplification of GC-rich templates. Several reagents also have been used to disrupt base paring or isostabilize DNA like DMSO, formamide, glycerol, TMAC, Betaine, and 7-deaza dGTP.

4. Presence of a PCR product in the blank indicates contamination. To prevent carry-over contamination, separated working stations of pre-PCR and post-PCR and separate sets of pipettes and tips are necessary. A one-way work flow, where nothing from post-PCR goes back into pre-PCR (including gloves, gown, pens, paper, tube racks), is important.

5. *FLT3*-ITD PCR products and *FLT3*-D835 undigested and digested PCR products are separated by capillary electrophoresis. In our lab, the sensitivity of mutant detection is approximately 10% of mutant in a wild-type and mutant-type mixture.

6. The software allows for data to be viewed in several ways including raw data format, mobility corrected electropherogram format, and sequence format. Information useful for troubleshooting, such as injection parameters, electrophoretic history, and general sample information, can also be viewed.
7. PCR products should be diluted with nuclease-free H_2O prior to addition to the TAMRA master mix. We typically dilute the PCR products approximately 50–100-fold. Excessive DNA template will cause saturation of the fluorescent signal and increased background.
8. The human genome contains multiple *NPM1*-like elements (pseudogenes) that lack intron sequences. To avoid amplifying pseudogene fragments, the forward primer for *NPM1* exon 12 was designed within intron 11. Additionally, the poly-T track in intron 11 may cause +1 or −1 length variation in samples.
9. To evaluate variants of unknown clinical significance identified by sequencing, the following online tools/databases can be utilized:

   Search dbSNP to see if listed as SNP:

   http://www.ensembl.org (gives exact location of SNP with dbSNP number)

   Search mutation database (if exist) to see if reported as mutation:

   http://www.hgmd.cf.ac.uk; or check disease-specific database if available

   Search PubMed to see if reported in literature

   Check conservation of amino acid across species

   Check conservation of amino acid across related proteins

   Use Polyphen and Panther programs to predict effect of the variants

   http://www.bork.embl-heidelberg.de/ployphen

   http://www.pantherdb.org/tools/csnpscoreform.isp

   Use sorting intolerant from Tolerant program to predict effect

   http://blocks.fhcrc.org/sift/sift.html

   Check for effects on splicing, cryptic splice sites, alternative splice sites, transcription factor binding sites depending on the type of variant

   http://www.fruitfly.org

   http://bioweb.uwlax.edu/Genweb/molecular/seq_anal/splice_sites/splice_sites.html

   Alterative splice site predictor

   http://es.embnet.org/~mwang/assp.html

   Transcription factor binding sites

http://mordor.cgb.ki.se/cgi-bin/consite/consite

Predict effect on protein (alters binding site, conformation, etc.)

http://swissmodel.expasy.org//swiss-model.html

Acknowledgment

The authors wish to thank Dr. Stephen Dlouhy for his review of the manuscript.

References

1. Grimwade D, Walker H, Oliver F, Wheatley K, Harrison C, Harrison G et al (1998) The importance of diagnostic cytogenetics on outcome in AML: analysis of 1612 patients entered into the MRC AML 10 trail: the medical research council adult and children's leukaemia working parties. Blood 92:2322–2333
2. Grimwade D, Hills RK, Moorman AV, Walker H, Chatters S, Goldstone AH et al (2010) Refinement of cytogenetic classification in acute myeloid leukemia: determination of prognostic significance of rare recurring chromosomal abnormalities among 5876 younger adult patients treated in the United Kingdom Medical Research Council trials. Blood 116:354–365
3. Gulley ML, Shea TC, Fedoriw Y (2010) Genetic tests to evaluate prognosis and predict therapeutic response in acute myeloid leukemia. J Mol Diagn 12:3–16
4. Rau R, Brown P (2009) Nucleophosmin (NPM1) mutations in adult and childhood acute myeloid leukaemia: towards definition of a new leukaemia entity. Hematol Oncol 27:171–181
5. Marcucci G, Haferlach T, Dohner H (2011) Molecular genetics of adult acute myeloid leukemia: prognostic and therapeutic implications. J Clin Oncol 29(5):475–486
6. Swerdlow SH, Campo E, Harris NL, Jaffe ES, Pileri SA, Stein H et al (eds) (2008) WHO classification of tumours of haematopoietic and lymphoid tissues. Lyon, IARC, pp 120–122
7. Dohner H, Estey EH, Amadori S, Applebaum FR, Buchner T, Burnett AK et al (2010) Diagnosis and management of acute myeloid leukemia in adults. Recommendations from an international expert panel, on behalf of the European Leukemia Net. Blood 115: 453–474
8. Rosnet O, Mattei M-G, Marchetto S, Birnbaum D (1991) Isolation and chromosomal localization of a novel FMS-like tyrosine kinase gene. Genomics 9:380–385
9. Turner AM, Lin NL, Issarachai S, Lyman SD, Broudy VC (1996) FLT3 receptor expression on the surface of normal and malignant hematopoietic cells. Blood 88:3383–3390
10. Whitman SP, Ruppert AS, Radmacher MD, Mrózek K, Paschka P, Langer C et al (2008) FLT3 D835/I836 mutations are associated with poor disease-free survival and a distinct gene-expression signature among younger adults with de novo cytogenetically normal acute myeloid leukemia lacking FLT3 internal tandem duplications. Blood 111:1552–1559
11. Bacher U, Haferlach C, Schnittger S, Kern W, Kroeger N, Zander AR et al (2009) Interactive diagnostics in the indication to allogeneic SCT in AML. Bone Marrow Transplant 43: 745–756
12. Chang JH, Olson MO (1990) Structure of the gene for rat nucleolar protein 23. J Biol Chem 265:18227–18233
13. Falini B, Nicoletti I, Martelli MF, Mecucci C (2007) Acute myeloid leukemia carrying cytoplasmic/mutated nucleophosmin (NPMc+AML): biologic and clinical features. Blood 109: 874–885
14. Szankasi P, Jama M, Bahler DW (2008) A new DNA-based test for detection of nucleophosmin exon 12 mutations by capillary electrophoresis. J Mol Diagn 10:236–241
15. Falini B, Martelli MF, Bolli N, Bonasso R, Ghia E, Pallotta MT et al (2006) Immuohistochemistry predicts nucleophosmin (NPM) mutations in acute myeloid leukemia. Blood 108:1999–2005
16. Hendricks-Taylor L, Bachinski LL, Siciliano MJ, Fertitta A, Trask B, de Jone P et al (1992) The CCAAT/enhancer binding protein (C/EBP alpha) gene (CEBPA) maps to human chromosome 19q13 and related nuclear factor NF-IL6 (C/EBP beta) gene (CEBPB) maps to human chromosome 20q13.1. Genomics 14:12–17
17. Koschmieder S, Halmos B, Levantini E, Tenen DG (2009) Dysregulation of the C/EBPα differentiation pathway in human cancer. J Clin Oncol 27:619–628
18. Renneville A, Roumier C, Biggio V, Nibourel O, Boissel N, Fensux P et al (2008) Cooperating

gene mutations in acute myeloid Leukemia: a review of the literature. Leukemia 22: 915–931

19. Pabst T, Eyholzer M, Fos J, Mueller BU (2009) Heterogeneity within AML with CEBPA mutatons; only CEBPA double mutations, but not single CEBPA mutations are associated with favorable prognosis. Br J Cancer 100:1343–1346
20. Hackanson B, Bennett KL, Brena RM, Jiang J, Claus R, Chen SS et al (2008) Epigenetic modification of CCAAT/enhancer binding protein a expression in acute myeloid leukemia. Cancer Res 68:3142–3151

Chapter 8

Flow Cytometric Monitoring of Residual Disease in Acute Leukemia

Brent L. Wood

Abstract

Multiparameter flow cytometry offers the unique ability to simultaneously assess and correlate multiple cellular properties at the single cell level in a timely and efficient manner. Application of this technique to the detection of residual acute leukemia after therapy has been shown to be of singular importance to monitor response to therapy and provide prognostic information. Principles and methods that allow for the sensitive detection of acute leukemia following therapy are presented. The basic protocol outlines a simple and efficient method for the labeling of white cells with monoclonal antibodies directed against cell surface antigens. A second method describes a general method for the simultaneous assessment of surface and cytoplasmic antigens using a combination of fixation followed by membrane permeabilization. An illustrative panel of validated reagents currently in use for residual disease detection for acute lymphoblastic leukemia of B or T cell lineage as well as acute myeloid leukemia is provided. Principles of data analysis that allow for the reproducible detection of small populations of abnormal hematopoietic cells in peripheral blood and bone marrow are presented.

Key words Immunophenotyping, Minimal residual disease, Flow cytometry, Acute lymphoblastic leukemia, Acute myeloid leukemia

1 Introduction

Flow cytometry offers the unique ability to simultaneously assess and correlate multiple cellular properties at the single cell level in a timely and efficient manner and so is ideally suited for the evaluation of complex mixtures of hematopoietic cells obtained from peripheral blood and bone marrow (1). As a result, multiparametric flow cytometry is widely used in the clinical laboratory for the identification of abnormal hematopoietic populations and the determination of lineage and maturational stage for diagnosis and classification, particularly for acute leukemia (2). More recently, multiparametric flow cytometry has been applied to the detection of leukemic populations following induction and consolidation

Magdalena Czader (ed.), *Hematological Malignancies*, Methods in Molecular Biology, vol. 999,
DOI 10.1007/978-1-62703-357-2_8,

therapy for acute leukemia in an attempt to identify patients who have responded successfully to therapy and to identify those in whom therapy has been suboptimal and may be at increased risk of relapse. If therapy has been at least partially successful, the residual neoplastic population will be small in number, generally present at sub-morphologic levels. Consequently, minimal residual disease (MRD) analysis represents an example of rare event detection where identification and enumeration of the neoplastic population and discrimination from normal hematopoiesis is the primary objective and may represent a significant technical challenge compared with diagnostic assessment.

The ability to detect MRD by flow cytometry for patients with acute leukemia is well described in the literature (3–5). The basic method relies on the discovery of antigens that are differentially expressed between leukemic populations and their normal counterparts in bone marrow, i.e., informative antigens. The use of combinations of monoclonal antibodies against these antigens, in concert with reagents that allow recognition of specific hematopoietic cell lineages and maturational stages, allows for the detection of immunophenotypic abnormalities on discrete subpopulations and is key to the success of the method. Many of the antigens that show differential expression suitable for MRD assessment are the same antigens commonly used diagnostically for assignment of lineage and maturational stage, allowing for efficient antibody combinations and emphasizing similarities between diagnostic and post-therapeutic monitoring applications. Given the multiparametric nature of these assays, the use of more simultaneous parameters allows for more precise definition of lineage, maturational stage, and assessment of abnormality, provided the antigens are informative. While much of the published MRD literature to date has assessed three or four simultaneous antigens, the current generation of assays utilizes up to ten simultaneous fluorochromes (6) and this approach is the focus of this chapter.

The detection and enumeration of residual acute leukemia after therapy is an important prognostic factor that has been correlated with outcome in a large number of studies. The best studied is acute lymphoblastic leukemia of B cell lineage (B-ALL), particularly in the pediatric population (7–14). Multiple investigators have shown that detection of MRD at levels greater than 0.01% of mononuclear cells at end of induction or end of consolidation is associated with an increased risk of both long and short term relapse as well as decreased event-free survival. MRD significance is also seen in good cytogenetic risk groups, suggesting that the assay is not simply detecting patients with less favorable cytogenetics. Similar data exists for T cell lineage acute leukemia (T-ALL), but is less robust, in part due to the relatively low frequency of disease and consequently fewer patients evaluated. In acute myeloid leukemia (AML), multiple studies demonstrate the significance of MRD detection for survival and relapse, with levels of detection between 0.01 and 0.1% of white cells at either end of induction or consolidation being associated with poorer outcome (15–18). Taken together, the data compellingly demonstrate that the identification of MRD after therapy is associated with a poor outcome for acute leukemia; however, whether the natural history of the disease can be influenced by additional therapeutic maneuvers is unknown and is the subject of the current generation of ongoing clinical trials.

2 Materials

2.1 Reagents

1. *PBS/BSA/azide (Phosphate buffered saline with 0.3% BSA (w/v) and 0.1% sodium azide)*: Add one packet of PBS mix (Gibco), 10 ml of 30% bovine serum albumin (BSA) and 1 g of sodium azide to a 1 L volumetric flask and fill to 1 L with reagent grade deionized water. Mix thoroughly and filter through a 45 μm Millipore filter. Store up to 2 months at 4°C.
2. Buffered NH_4Cl lysing solution containing 0.25% formaldehyde (w/v): add 80.2 g ammonium chloride (NH_4Cl), 8.4 g sodium bicarbonate ($NaHCO_3$) and 3.7 g disodium EDTA to a 1 L volumetric flask and fill flask to 1 L with reagent grade deionized water. Mix thoroughly and filter through a 45 μm Millipore filter. This results in a 10× stock that can be stored at 4°C for 3 months. Add 50 ml of 10× stock and 11.25 ml of 10% formaldehyde (Polysciences methanol-free ultrapure) to 500 ml volumetric flask. Fill flask to 500 ml and mix thoroughly. Prepare lysing solution fresh every day of use.

2.2 Monoclonal Antibody Panels

Panels of monoclonal antibodies that are suitable for the detection of residual acute leukemia of B cell, T cell, and myeloid lineages are presented in Tables 1, 2, 3, and 4. Each of these reagents should be carefully titered to optimize signal to noise ratio in the volume of total reagents to be delivered (see Note 1). IgG1 reagents are preferred to minimize the potential for complement mediated antibody interactions (19).

3 Methods

These methods assume appropriate and standardized instrument setup including correct compensation settings, topics beyond the scope of this chapter, but critical to the success of these methods.

3.1 Simultaneous Labeling of White Cells with Monoclonal Antibodies Against Surface Antigens

The following method is intended to minimize sample manipulation and maximize recovery for all white blood cell populations while providing low fluorescence background and the preservation of spectral characteristics of tandem fluorochromes (see Note 2). The addition of a low-level fixative to the lysing solution allows for

Table 1
Immunophenotyping panel for the detection of residual acute lymphoblastic leukemia of B cell lineage

	FITC	PE	PCP5.5	PC7	APC	APC7
Tube 1	CD20	CD10	CD38	CD19	CD58	CD45
Tube 2	CD9	CD13+33	CD34	CD19	CD10	CD45

These combinations require a 2-laser flow cytometer having excitation at 488 nm (FITC, PE, PCP5.5, PC7), and 635 nm (APC, APC7). The numbers indicate cluster designations, i.e., CD antigens
FITC, fluorescein isothiocyanate; *PE*, phycoerythrin; *PCP5.5*, PerCP-Cy5.5; *PC7*, PE-Cy7; *APC*, allophycocyanin; *APC7*, APC-Cy7

Table 2
Immunophenotyping panel for the detection of residual acute lymphoblastic leukemia of B cell lineage (alternate single combination)

	PB	FITC	PE	PCP5.5	PC7	A594	APC	APC7
Tube 1	CD20	Syto16	CD10	CD34	CD19	CD38	CD58	CD45

These combinations require a 4-laser flow cytometer having excitation at 488 nm (FITC, PE, PCP5.5, PC7), 635 nm (APC, APC7), 407 nm (PB or V450), and 594 nm (A594). Syto16 is a permeant nucleic acid binding dye that may be used for nucleated cell identification. The numbers indicate cluster designations, i.e., CD antigens
PB, Pacific Blue or V450; *FITC*, fluorescein isothiocyanatel; *PE*, phycoerythrin; *PCP5.5*, PerCP-Cy5.5; *PC7*, PE-Cy7; *APC*, allophycocyanin; *APC7*, APC-Cy7; *A594*, Alexa 594

Table 3
Immunophenotyping panel for the detection of residual acute lymphoblastic leukemia of T cell lineage

	PB	FITC	PE	PE-TR	PC5	PC7	A594	APC	APC7
Tube 1	CD16	cCD3	CD7	–	CD56	CD5	CD38	sCD3	CD45
Tube 2	CD8	CD2	CD5	CD34	CD56+16	CD3	CD4	CD7	CD45

These combinations require a 4-laser flow cytometer having excitation at 407 nm (PB), 488 nm (FITC, PE, PE-TR, PCX, PC7), 594 nm (A594), and 635 nm (APC, A700, APC7). The numbers indicate cluster designations, i.e., CD antigens
cCD3, cytoplasmic CD3; *sCD3,* surface CD3; *PB*, Pacific Blue; *FITC*, fluorescein isothiocyanate; *PE*, phycoerythrin; *PE-TR,* PE-Texas Red, *PC5*, PE-Cy5; *PC7*, PE-Cy7; *A594*, Alexa 594; *APC*, allophycocyanin; *APC7*, APC-Cy7

Table 4
Immunophenotyping panel for the detection of residual acute myeloid leukemia

	PB	FITC	PE	PE-TR	PCX	PC7	A594	APC	APC-A700	APC7
Tube 1	HLA-DR	CD15	CD33	CD19	CD117	CD13	CD38	CD34	CD71	CD45
Tube 2	HLA-DR	CD64	CD123	CD4	CD14	CD13	CD38	CD34	CD16	CD45
Tube 3	HLA-DR	CD56	CD7	–	CD5	CD33	CD38	CD34	–	CD45

These combinations require a 4-laser flow cytometer having excitation at 407 nm (PB), 488 nm (FITC, PE, PE-TR, PCX, PC7), 594 nm (A594), and 635 nm (APC, A700, APC7). The numbers indicate cluster designations, i.e., CD antigens
PB, Pacific Blue; *FITC*, fluorescein isothiocyanate; *PE*, phycoerythrin; *PE-TR*, PE-Texas Red; *PCX*, PE-Cy5 or PE-Cy5.5 or PerCP-Cy5.5; *PC7*, PE-Cy7; *A594*, Alexa 594; *APC*, allophycocyanin; *APC-A700*, APC-alexa 700; *APC7*, APC-Cy7

the simultaneous lysing and fixing of the sample, preservation of the light scatter properties of the sample, and provides improved separation of compromised from viable cells. Addition of a subsequent wash step reduces background fluorescence due to unbound fluorochrome and provides more controlled timing for fixation that enhances the stability of certain tandem fluorochromes. The procedure outlined is generic and will allow for the use of a variety of different panels of monoclonal antibodies.

1. Add 100 μl of cell suspension (white cell concentration equal to or less than 10,000 cells/μl) to tube (see Note 3).
2. Add 100 μl of antibody cocktail (see Tables 1, 2, 3, and 4) to a 12 × 75 mm polystyrene tube and gently vortex to mix.
3. Incubate in the dark for 15 min at room temperature.
4. Add 1.5 ml of NH_4Cl lysing solution containing 0.25% formaldehyde and gently vortex to mix.
5. Incubate in the dark for 15 min at room temperature.
6. Centrifuge at 550 × *g* for 5 min and decant supernatant.
7. Add 3 ml of PBS/BSA/azide and vortex gently to mix.
8. Centrifuge at 550 × *g* for 5 min and decant supernatant.
9. Add 100 μl of PBS/BSA/azide and gently resuspend.
10. Run sample on flow cytometer optimized for the simultaneous detection of the fluorochromes used.

3.2 Simultaneous Labeling of White Cells with Monoclonal Antibodies Against Surface and Cytoplasmic Antigens

The following method allows the detection of cytoplasmic antigens, as well as assessment of abnormalities in the expression of surface antigens. Although the method works for many cytoplasmic antigens, it uses a cross-linking fixative to stabilize cellular contents prior to labeling with antibodies against cytoplasmic antigens and may not be suitable for intracellular antibodies directed against fixation-sensitive epitopes or which require protein denaturation to expose epitopes. Antibodies against cytoplasmic antigens, in particular, require careful titration to optimize the signal-to-noise ratio and often must be used at sub-saturating concentrations to minimize background (see Note 4). The outlined procedure utilizes the "Fix and Perm" kit from Invitrogen, but other manufacturer's products may be used in a similar manner with equivalent results after appropriate validation.

1. Add 100 μl of cell suspension to a 12 × 75 mm polystyrene tube.
2. Add appropriate amount (e.g., 100 μl) of titered surface antibody cocktail to tube and gently vortex to mix.

   Use antibody cocktail lacking reagents directed against cytoplasmic antigens, e.g., *Tube 1 from Table 3 without cytoplasmic CD3.*

3. Incubate in the dark for 15 min at room temperature.
4. Add 3 ml of PBS/BSA/azide to tube and gently vortex to mix.
5. Centrifuge at 550 × *g* for 5 min and decant supernatant.
6. Repeat addition of PBS/BSA/azide, centrifugation and decantation of supernatant.
7. Add 100 μl Reagent A (fixation) and gently vortex to mix.
8. Incubate for 15 min at room temperature.
9. Add 3 ml of PBS/BSA/azide to tube and gently vortex to mix.
10. Centrifuge at 550 × *g* for 5 min and decant supernatant.
11. Repeat addition of PBS/BSA/azide, centrifugation and decantation of supernatant.
12. Add 100 μl Reagent B (permeabilization).
13. Add appropriate amount of titered cytoplasmic antibody cocktail to tube and gently vortex to mix.

    Use cocktail containing only reagents directed against cytoplasmic antigens, e.g., *cytoplasmic CD3.*
14. Incubate in the dark for 30 min at room temperature.
15. Add 3 ml of PBS/BSA/azide to tube and gently vortex to mix.
16. Centrifuge at 550 × *g* for 5 min and decant supernatant.
17. Repeat addition of PBS/BSA/azide, centrifugation and decantation of supernatant (optional).
18. Add 100 μl of PBS/BSA/azide and gently resuspend.
19. Run sample on flow cytometer optimized for the simultaneous detection of the fluorochromes used (see Note 5).

3.3 Sample Acquisition

The number of total cellular events to acquire will depend on the desired sensitivity for the assay. For acceptable reproducibility, the population of interest should consist of a minimum of 100 cells to give a theoretical coefficient of variation (CV) of 10%. For an assay where a detection sensitivity of 0.01% of white cells is desired, this will require the acquisition of 1,000,000 total white cell events (see Note 6). Populations consisting of smaller numbers of events can be enumerated, e.g., 0.001%, but with a corresponding increase in CV. For samples where 1,000,000 events cannot be obtained, the sensitivity and/or CV of the assay will be proportionately decreased and/or increased, respectively.

To minimize data file size, gated acquisition may be performed using parameters believed to be consistently able to include the population of interest, e.g., CD19 positivity for B-ALL. However, this assumes that the parameter used for gating is invariably present,

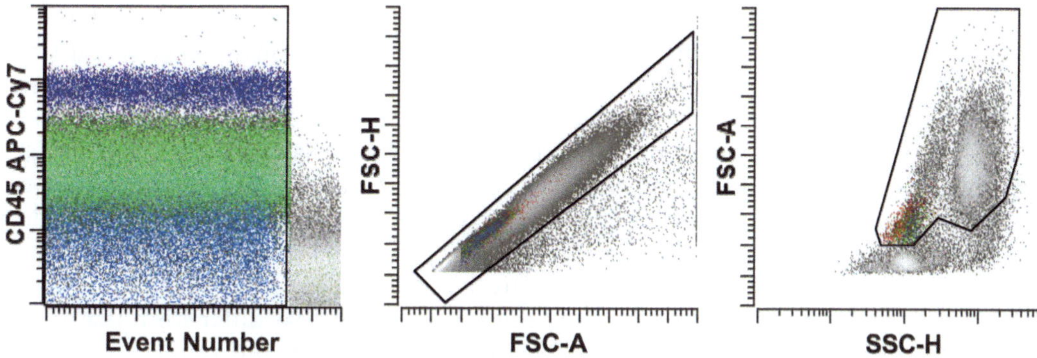

Fig. 1 Basic analysis strategies to minimize artifact. (*Left*) Evaluation of data over time or event number to exclude air aspirated following exhaustion of sample. (*Center*) Exclusion of doublets and aggregates by gating on singlets using forward scatter area and height. (*Right*) Exclusion of nonviable cells and debris for white blood cell evaluation using forward and side scatter gating

which will undoubtedly be false for some subset of cases, in which case the acquired data will be unable to detect the population of interest. This is particularly a problem after therapy where antigenic changes may occur, for instance the loss of CD19 in B-ALL. Given that data storage is now relatively abundant and cheap, it is probably more prudent to simply acquire all events for a more comprehensive analysis.

3.4 Data Analysis

3.4.1 Data Quality

Initial evaluation of flow cytometric data should focus on assessing the quality of the data by identifying artifact or other problems within the data, and noting or correcting problems where possible. One useful strategy is to observe the data over event number (time), as this allows assessment of the quality and consistency of the data that has been acquired. In particular, on multi-laser instruments one should monitor one parameter from each of the lasers used versus time to identify fluidic instabilities that might have result in changes in apparent antigen intensity (see Fig. 1). The same strategy will allow identification of samples that were exhausted during acquisition, resulting in signals from air bubbles being acquired. In both circumstances, spurious data may be generated that can significantly compromise identification of residual disease, but which can be easily corrected by excluding data via gating during the time periods where artifact was present.

Whenever a sample is evaluated by flow cytometry it is assumed that the instrument measures a single cell at a time. However, this is rarely true due the combined effects of the statistical likelihood that two cells in solution are near each other at the time of aspiration into the instrument, a phenomenon that increases with high cell concentration or high sample aspiration rates, or the direct association of cells due to sample processing as may be induced by centrifugation or antibody binding. The consequence is that some events consist of two or more cells with the measured properties being a composite of the cells in the aggregate. This artifact can be a significant problem for rare event assays, like MRD detection, and measures should be taken to minimize this problem at the time of sample preparation and acquisition. In addition, during data analysis one may use doublet discrimination techniques where a combination of peak area, width and/or height for one or more parameters are used to exclude events that differ from that of the singlet population (see Fig. 1). However, this requires that these parameters be collected at the time of acquisition.

Loss of cell viability can result in significant artifact through changes in light scatter properties, particularly loss of forward scatter, and progressive loss of antigen as the cell degenerate. Use of a viability gate to exclude low forward scatter events, usually in conjunction with side scatter, can significantly minimize artifact of this type (see Fig. 1). However, care must be used that such a gate does not entirely exclude the population of interest, as can happen rarely in highly proliferative neoplasms where cell degeneration is rapid, and the consequences for enumeration should be carefully assessed to ensure that degeneration of all cell populations is roughly proportional. Highly correlated relationships between antigens should raise concern for nonspecific antibody binding on those events, and is commonly seen with certain reagents on degenerating cell populations.

3.4.2 Identification of Target Population

Once artifact is recognized and eliminated, where possible, attention turns to identification of populations within the sample. The populations that may be recognized are highly dependent on the reagent combination used, but each discrete cluster of events (population) that is identified should be accounted for as a normal population, an abnormal population, or artifact. Neoplastic or leukemic populations are recognized by an immunophenotype that is different or deviates from that seen on normal populations (see Note 7). It is the immunophenotype of the normal populations that remain relatively constant and serve as reference points for population identification and assessment. Use of color to define normal stages of maturation within a lineage can greatly facilitate recognition of normal and abnormal populations during data analysis. Description of the immunophenotypes of normal populations is well outside of the scope of this manuscript, and readers are referred to other resources on the topic (1). However, it is the understanding of the immunophenotypic features at specific maturational stages for each cell lineage that allows one to identify when a population may be normal or potentially neoplastic. Examples are provided for B lineage ALL, T lineage ALL and AML MRD detection in Figs. 2, 3, and 4.

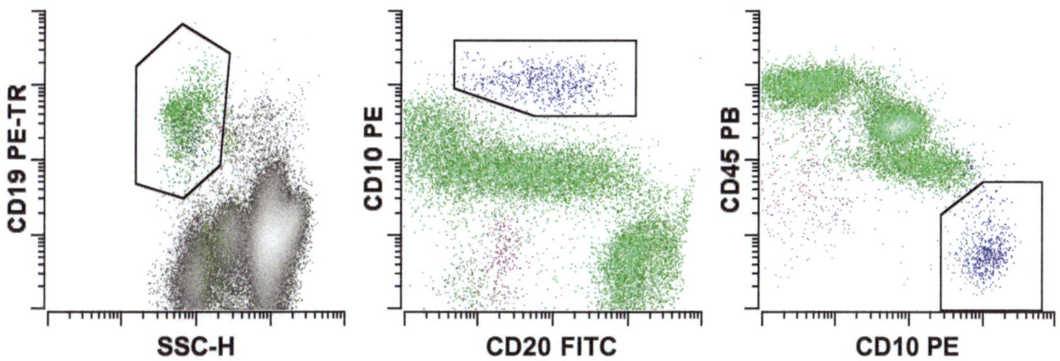

Fig. 2 Identification of minimal residual disease for Precursor B-cell lymphoblastic leukemia/lymphoma (ALL). The identification of the B cell population is achieved using CD19 and Side scatter gating (*left*). Only B cells are displayed in the remaining *dot plots* and the abnormal residual population identified by its abnormal expression of increased CD10 with variable CD20 (*center*) or abnormal loss of CD45 with increased CD10 (*right*) in comparison with the remaining mature and immature B cells. The abnormal population represents 0.1% of the white cells

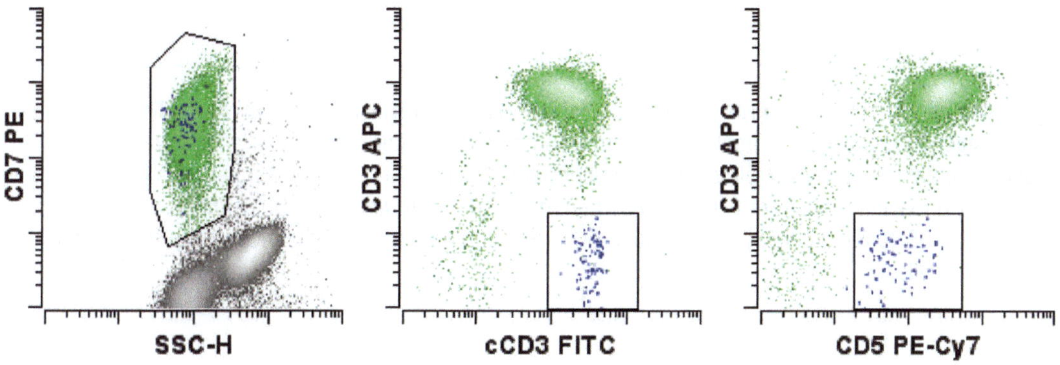

Fig. 3 Identification of minimal residual disease for Precursor T-cell lymphoblastic leukemia/lymphoma (ALL). The identification of the T/NK cell population is achieved using CD7 and Side scatter gating (*left*). Only T cells are displayed in the remaining *dot plots* and the abnormal residual population identified by its abnormal expression of absent surface CD3 with presence of cytoplasmic CD3 (*center*) in combination with abnormal loss of CD3 with decreased CD5 (*right*) compared to the remaining mature and immature T and NK cells. The abnormal population represents 0.1% of the white cells

One basic strategy used as a starting point for identifying cell populations is the use of lineage-associated antigens in combination with side scatter. B cells of all types may be well identified by the use of CD19 in combination with side scatter and the maturational expression of other antigens such as CD10, CD20, CD38, and CD45 used to define normal maturational subpopulations. Similarly, CD7 in combination with side scatter is a reliable way to

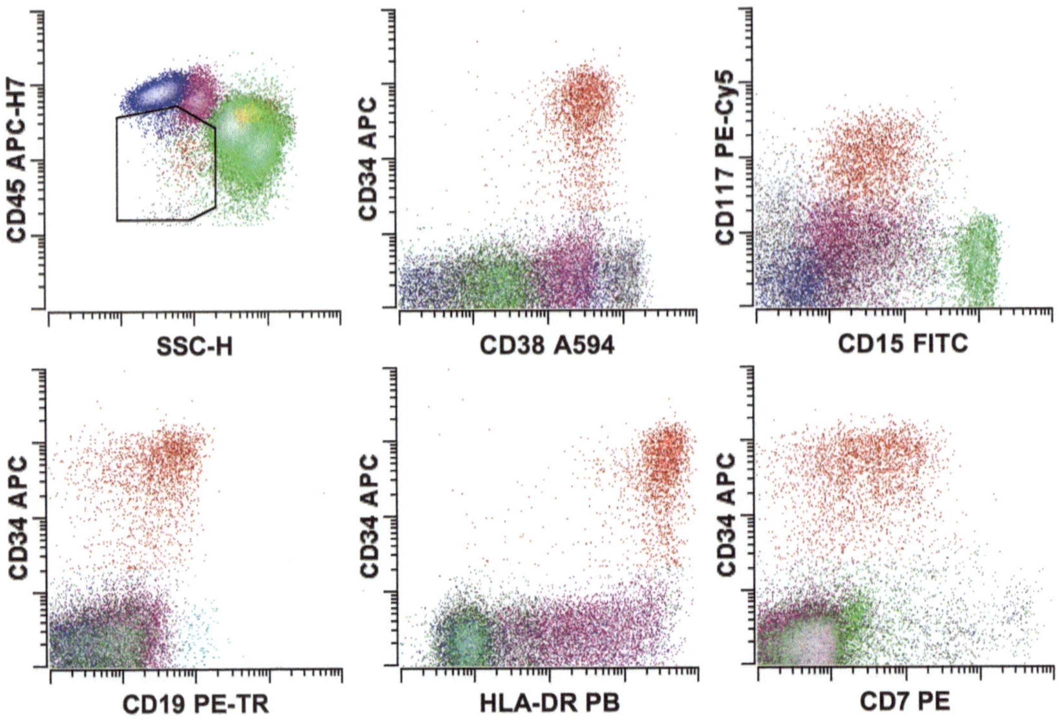

Fig. 4 Identification of minimal residual disease for t(8;21) acute myeloid leukemia (AML). The identification of the progenitor population is achieved using CD45 and Side scatter gating (*top left*). Only progenitors are displayed in the remaining dot plots and the abnormal CD34-positive residual population is identified by its abnormal expression of uniform CD38 (*top center*), dim CD15 (*top right*), dim CD19 (*bottom left*), increased uniform HLA-DR (*bottom center*), and variable CD7 (*bottom left*). The abnormal population represents 1.4% of the white cells

identify immature T cells and will also encompass most mature T cells and NK cells which can be further subdivided using CD2, CD3, CD4, CD5, CD7, CD8, CD45, and CD16/56. For immature populations in general, the use of CD45 versus side scatter is a good starting point to allow the identification of progenitors characteristically having lower CD45 and/or side scatter than mature cells with specificity for lineage and maturational stage provided by other antigens in the reagent combination.

With any analysis strategy, the exclusion of events assumes that the population of interest remains within the events retained, but this is an assumption that must be consistently checked to ensure that events of interest are not excluded. For instance, reliance on CD19 to identify B cells will fail in a small subset of cases of B lineage ALL where CD19 is absent, so routine use of a second method is advised, such as evaluation of events with lymphocyte light scatter characteristics for expression of CD10 or CD20 without CD19. In general, the reliance on population identification by expression of a single antigen is to be avoided. Rather it is a multiparameteric assessment that provides the sensitivity and specificity for population identification.

Changes in immunophenotype on populations in acute leukemia are common after therapy (20–23). Consequently, the use of fixed methods of population identification based on the immunophenotype of the leukemic population as determined at the time of initial diagnosis will fail in a subset of cases, particularly if reduced or limited reagent combinations are used at post-therapeutic time points. A population based approach where each relevant population is identified and compared with normal maturational patterns of antigen expression will allow more consistent identification of residual leukemia, even in the presence of significant post-therapeutic changes in immunophenotype. While this type of analysis may be successfully performed on samples where the diagnostic immunophenotype is not known, knowledge of the diagnostic immunophenotype can simplify data analysis by providing a starting point for analysis and will improve sensitivity and consistency by focusing attention on populations with similar immunophenotypes. Consequently, it is recommended that diagnostic material be assessed prior to therapy by the same panel of reagents that is to be used for residual disease detection whenever possible.

4 Notes

1. If the reagent combinations are to be used frequently, cocktailing of the reagents allows efficient laboratory practice and minimizes error. Of importance is the accurate titering of each monoclonal antibody to be used in the larger incubation volume that inevitably results from the addition of large numbers of antibodies to a sample. The selection of a target total reagent volume to be delivered, e.g., 100 μl, provides a standardized way to determine reagent performance under the conditions that are to be used. The resulting data is then inspected to select the titer having the optimal signal-to-noise ratio, i.e., greatest separation between positive and negative populations without an associated significant increase in intensity for the negative population. In many instances, the amount of reagent used can be reduced from that recommended by the manufacturer. Once the appropriate titers for each reagent have been determined, a recipe for the cocktail can be constructed using a diluent such as PBS containing protein to achieve the desired final delivery volume, e.g., 100 μl per sample. The amount of each cocktail to prepare should be based on the anticipated rate of utilization in the laboratory, and each new cocktail should be evaluated on a test sample prior to being put into use. The stability of the cocktail should be determined by the

repeated staining of samples over time, the usual limiting factor being the stability of the tandem fluorochromes.

2. Prolonged fixation and exposure to fluorescent light may degrade Cy7-containing tandem fluorochromes. Labeling prior to lysis, decreased light exposure, and limited fixation as outlined above, minimizes fluorochrome degradation.
3. The target number of cells to add to the assay is 1,000,000 white cells delivered in 100 μl sample volume or 10,000 cells/μl. For cell suspensions having lower cell concentrations, the volume of cell suspension may generally be increased up to 200 μl to allow the addition of one million white blood cells without increasing the amount of antibody cocktail used. For samples where this still will not provide adequate numbers of cells, the sample may be centrifuged and the supernatant aspirated to yield a more concentrated sample that may then be used in the usual protocol. For old samples, this may result in some incomplete erythrocytes lysis, which a second round of lyse-fixing will correct. If more events are still desired, more than one aliquot of sample may be prepared and pooled prior to acquisition. An alternative is to lyse a larger volume of sample with NH_4Cl lacking fixative, wash and then prepare as per protocol without the lysing step. While this works, it can result in some increased cell loss due to large volume washing, as well as activate some cell types, monocytes in particular with changes in antigen expression.
4. Each of the cytoplasmic antigens used should be carefully titered to optimize signal-to-noise ratio rather than to achieve antibody saturation as is routinely done for surface antigens. Use of excessive antibody will result in a disproportionate increase in background and compromise the ability to detect the antigen of interest. The permeabilization required for cytoplasmic antigen expression results in a decrease in forward light scatter and requires an increase in gain on the forward scatter detector to adjust for this loss.
5. For this type of analysis, the focus is on population identification rather than determination of absolute levels of antigen expression. Consequently, negative controls are of little use for this type of analysis and are not recommended.
6. Populations of interest are invariably reported as a percentage of an aggregate population, but the denominator used varies in the literature. Since most assays contain CD45 as a gating reagent and the lysing reagents used for specimen preparation are designed for preservation of white cells, total CD45-positive white cells is probably the most common denominator used for enumeration. Historically, density gradient centrifugation was used for sample preparation, which depletes samples of neutrophils and retains nucleated erythrocytes, so total mononuclear cells (all cells except maturing neutrophils) were used as a

denominator. Another option is to use total nucleated cells. Both total mononuclear or nucleated cells require the use of a DNA binding dye to exclude contaminating non-nucleated erythrocytes, which may require an additional aliquot of sample to be prepared and the percentage calculated as the product of cell proportions using data from two aliquots of sample. None of these methods takes into account the extent of peripheral blood dilution present in bone marrow aspirate samples, a major source of error in enumeration for some samples.

7. The identification of small populations in assays of this type is determined by two basic factors: (1) the degree to which the neoplastic population deviates from normal maturation, and (2) the relative number of normal cells with a similar immunophenotype present in the sample. The former is in large part related to the particular antibody combinations utilized and the extent to which those particular antigens are differentially modulated by neoplasia. The latter is influenced by the time at which residual disease assessment is performed and the type of therapy utilized. For example in acute leukemia of B cell lineage, commonly used therapies result is near complete annihilation of the normal B cell progenitors which persists for the first 1–2 months of therapy before active B cell regeneration occurs. As a result, determination of residual disease at early time points, such as day 15 or day 29 after induction therapy, is relatively sensitive while samples from later time points will often contain larger numbers of normal immature B cells (hematogones) which reduce the sensitivity of these assays, particularly in children. The opposite is true for AML, since active marrow regeneration occurs between day 17 and day 28 following induction therapy, resulting in increased normal regenerating myeloid progenitors with an attendant reduction in sensitivity, while at later time points the marrow has reached a steady state with a relatively lower number of myeloid progenitors.

References

1. Wood BL (2004) Multicolor immunophenotyping: human immune system hematopoiesis. Methods Cell Biol 75:559–576
2. Craig FE, Foon KA (2008) Flow cytometry immunophentoyping for hematopoietic neoplasms. Blood 111:3941–3967
3. Vidriales MB, San-Miguel JF, Orfao A, Coustan-Smith E, Campana D (2003) Minimal residual disease monitoring by flow cytometry. Best Pract Res Clin Haematol 16:599–612
4. Weir EG, Cowan K, LeBeau P, Borowitz MJ (1999) A limited antibody panel can distinguish B-precursor acute lymphoblastic leukemia from normal B precursors with four color flow cytometry: implications for residual disease detection. Leukemia 13:558–567
5. Al-Mawali A, Gillis D, Hissaria P, Lewis I (2008) Incidence, sensitivity, and specificity of leukemia-associated phenotypes in acute myeloid leukemia using specific five-color multiparameter flow cytometry. Am J Clin Pathol 129:934–945
6. Wood B (2006) 9 and 10 color flow cytometry in the clinical laboratory. Arch Pathol Lab Med 130:680–690
7. Coustan-Smith E, Song G, Clark C, Key L, Liu P, Mehrpooya M et al (2011) New markers for minimal residual disease detection in

acute lymphoblastic leukemia. Blood 117: 6267–6276

8. Borowitz MJ, Devidas M, Hunger SP, Bowman WP, Carroll AJ, Carroll WL et al (2008) Clinical significance of minimal residual disease in childhood acute lymphoblastic leukemia and its relationship to other prognostic factors: a Children's Oncology Group study. Blood 111:5477–5485
9. Bruggemann M, Raff T, Flohr T, Gökbuget N, Nakao M, Droese J et al German Multicenter Study Group for Adult Acute Lymphoblastic Leukemia (2006) Clinical significance of minimal residual disease quantification in adult patients with standard-risk acute lymphoblastic leukemia. Blood 107:1116–1123
10. Krampera M, Vitale A, Vincenzi C, Perbellini O, Guarini A, Annino L et al (2003) Outcome prediction by immunophenotypic minimal residual disease detection in adult T-cell acute lymphoblastic leukaemia. Br J Haematol 120: 74–79
11. Borowitz MJ, Pullen DJ, Shuster JJ, Viswanatha D, Montgomery K, Willman CL et al Children's Oncology Group study (2003) Minimal residual disease detection in childhood precursor-B-cell acute lymphoblastic leukemia: relation to other risk factors. A Children's Oncology Group study. Leukemia 17:1566–1572
12. Bjorklund E, Mazur J, Soderhall S, Porwit-MacDonald A (2003) Flow cytometric follow-up of minimal residual disease in bone marrow gives prognostic information in children with acute lymphoblastic leukemia. Leukemia 17:138–148
13. Dworzak MN, Froschl G, Printz D, Mann G, Pötschger U, Mühlegger N et al Austrian Berlin-Frankfurt-Münster Study Group (2002) Prognostic significance and modalities of flow cytometric minimal residual disease detection in childhood acute lymphoblastic leukemia. Blood 99:1952–1958
14. Coustan-Smith E, Sancho J, Hancock ML, Boyett JM, Behm FG, Raimondi SC et al (2000) Clinical importance of minimal residual disease in childhood acute lymphoblastic leukemia. Blood 96:2691–2696
15. Al-Mawali A, Gillis D, Lewis I (2009) The use of receiver operating characteristic analysis for detection of minimal residual disease using five-color multiparameter flow cytometry in acute myeloid leukemia identifies patients with high risk of relapse. Cytometry B Clin Cytom 76:91–101
16. Kern W, Voskova D, Schoch C, Hiddemann W, Schnittger S, Haferlach T (2004) Determination of relapse risk based on assessment of minimal residual disease during complete remission by multiparameter flow cytometry in unselected patients with acute myeloid leukemia. Blood 104:3078–3085
17. Buccisano F, Maurillo L, Gattei V, Del Poeta G, Del Principe MI, Cox MC et al (2006) The kinetics of reduction of minimal residual disease impacts on duration of response and survival of patients with acute myeloid leukemia. Leukemia 20:1783–1789
18. San Miguel JF, Vidriales MB, López-Berges C, Díaz-Mediavilla J, Gutiérrez N, Cañizo C et al (2001) Early immunophenotypical evaluation of minimal residual disease in acute myeloid leukemia identifies different patient risk groups and may contribute to postinduction treatment stratification. Blood 98:1746–1751
19. Wood BL, Levin GR (2006) Interactions between mouse IgG2 antibodies are common and mediated by plasma C1q. Cytometry B Clin Cytom 70:321–328
20. Gaipa G, Basso G, Aliprandi S, Migliavacca M, Vallinoto C, Maglia O et al I-BFM-ALL-FCM-MRD-Study Group (2008) Prednisone induces immunophenotypic modulation of CD10 and CD34 in nonapoptotic B-cell precursor acute lymphoblastic leukemia cells. Cytometry B Clin Cytom. 74:150–5
21. Borowitz MJ, Pullen DJ, Winick N, Martin PL, Bowman WP, Camitta B (2005) Comparison of diagnostic and relapse flow cytometry phenotypes in childhood acute lymphoblastic leukemia: implications for residual disease detection: a report from the Children's Oncology Group. Cytometry B Clin Cytom 68: 18–24
22. Baer MR, Stewart CC, Dodge RK, Leget G, Sulé N, Mrózek K et al (2001) High frequency of immunophenotype changes in acute myeloid leukemia at relapse: implications for residual disease detection (Cancer and Leukemia Group B Study 8361). Blood 97:3574–3580
23. Langebrake C, Brinkmann I, Teigler-Schlegel A, Creutzig U, Griesinger F, Puhlmann U et al (2005) Immunophenotypic differences between diagnosis and relapse in childhood AML: implications for MRD monitoring. Cytometry B Clin Cytom 63:1–9

Chapter 9

Chimerism Analysis Following Hematopoietic Stem Cell Transplantation

Kathleen M. Murphy

Abstract

Allogeneic hematopoietic stem cell transplantation (HSCT) is an effective therapeutic approach for several hematological diseases. Chimerism studies can be helpful to assess donor engraftment, detect early signs of graft rejection, and monitor minimal residual disease. Currently the most common method for monitoring chimerism following HSCT is by PCR amplification of STR loci followed by capillary electrophoresis. Prior to transplantation, multiple STR loci in both the donor and recipient are analyzed in order to identify loci that differentiate the two individuals. Informative loci are selected to calculate the percent donor and recipient present in post-transplant specimens. This is a rapid, sensitive, and cost-effective method for monitoring chimerism in patients following HSCT.

Key words Hematopoietic stem cell transplantation, Engraftment, Short tandem repeat (STR), Capillary electrophoresis

1 Introduction

Allogeneic hematopoietic stem cell transplantation (HSCT) is an effective therapeutic approach for several hematological diseases. Engraftment of donor cells in the recipient results in chimerism, a term used to refer to the presence of lymphohematopoietic cells of non-host origin. Complete or full chimerism generally refers to the presence of only cells of donor origin, while mixed chimerism indicates the presence of both donor and recipient cells. Chimerism studies can be helpful to assess donor engraftment, detect early signs of graft rejection, and monitor minimal residual disease. Peripheral blood and bone marrow specimens are both suitable for chimerism studies; however peripheral blood studies may be more useful (1). In addition, it may be desirable to analyze specific leukocyte subsets, particularly in the setting of nonmyeloablative and reduced-intensity conditioning (1–3).

Detection and quantification of donor and recipient cells are most effectively achieved by genetic analysis of the cells present.

Magdalena Czader (ed.), *Hematological Malignancies*, Methods in Molecular Biology, vol. 999,
DOI 10.1007/978-1-62703-357-2_9, © Springer Science+Business Media New York 2013

There are several DNA technologies that can be used to differentiate donor and recipient cells. For sex-mismatched transplants, fluorescent in situ hybridization (FISH) analysis of the X and Y chromosomes can be performed using commercially available probes and standardized procedures. This procedure is limited however to transplants involving a donor and recipient of opposite gender. More universally applicable methods for monitoring engraftment involve analysis of noncoding repeat polymorphisms, either variable number tandem repeats (VNTRs) or short tandem repeats (STRs). VNTR loci provide excellent discrimination between individuals, such that only a few loci (approximately four) need to be analyzed to differentiate the donor from the recipient. The primary limitation of VNTR loci is that they are composed of relatively large repeat elements that are generally not amenable to PCR amplification. These loci are generally analyzed by Southern blot, which has several limitations including the need for large (microgram) quantities of high-quality DNA, a long and laborious procedure, and potentially the need for radioactivity.

Currently the most common method for monitoring chimerism following HSCT is by PCR amplification of STR loci followed by capillary electrophoresis (4–8). STR loci are smaller than VNTR loci, allowing them to be analyzed by PCR amplification. The advantages of this method over VNTR Southern blot include the ability to use small (nanogram) amounts of DNA, a shorter turnaround time, and elimination of radioactivity. The accurate sizing achieved with capillary electrophoresis allows for multiple STR loci to be analyzed in a single reaction, increasing the speed and throughput capacity of the assay. Multiple STR loci must be analyzed in order to identify loci that differentiate the donor and recipient. This is especially true since the donor and recipients are often related and thus often share multiple genetic determinants. Loci that can be used to differentiate the individuals are said to be "informative," while loci that do not are "not informative."

More recently described methods for monitoring bone marrow engraftment include pyrosequencing (9), allele-specific real-time PCR of SNP markers (10, 11), allele-specific real-time PCR of insertion/deletion (indel) markers (12–15), and TaqMan real-time PCR of SNP markers (16, 17). The advantage of the real-time PCR format is that no post-amplification manipulations are necessary, which significantly reduces the time required for the assay. This method also reduces the potential for contamination in the laboratory because the PCR tubes are never opened following amplification. The disadvantage of the real-time format is that it is limited to SNP and indel markers. Each of these markers has a relatively low discrimination power. In general, an SNP locus has two or three possible alleles, while STR loci can have greater than 50 alleles. Thus, a relatively large number of SNP loci would have to be evaluated in order to achieve the same discrimination power of relatively few STR loci. Development of commercially available reagents that evaluate multiple high frequency SNP and/or indel markers may make this technology a cost-effective alternative in the future.

This chapter describes a multiplex STR chimerism assay that is rapid and cost-effective. This assay is one of several commercially available STR assays that analyze multiple (approximately 4–15) STR loci in single PCR reactions. Many of these assays have been created for forensics, criminal, and paternity purposes, and thus are very robust and have very high discrimination power. Regardless of which STR loci are used for chimerism analysis, validation of the assay, including linearity, reproducibility, and limit-of-detection studies, is required if the results are to be reported for clinical use.

2 Materials

2.1 DNA Isolation and Quantification

1. QIAamp DNA Mini spin columns (Qiagen, Valencia, CA) (see Note 1).
2. Microcentrifuge (minimum 8,000 rpm, 6,000 × *g*).
3. 100% EtOH.
4. 1.5 ml microcentrifuge tubes.
5. NanoDrop ND-1000 Spectrophotometer (Thermo Scientific, Houston, TX) (see Note 2).
6. Sterile dH_2O (Sigma, St. Louis, MO).

2.2 PCR Amplification

1. AmpF*l*STR® Profiler™ kit (Applied Biosystems, Foster City, CA).
2. *Taq*Gold (5 U/μl) (Applied Biosystems).
3. Sterile dH_2O (Sigma).
4. Thermal cycler ABI 9700 (Applied Biosystems) (see Note 3).

2.3 Capillary Electrophoresis

1. Hi-Di Formamide (Applied Biosystems).
2. GeneScan 500 [ROX] size standard (Applied Biosystems).
3. ABI3100 capillary electrophoresis instrument (Applied Biosystems) (see Note 3).
4. Reagents for the ABI3100 including POP4 polymer, 36 cm capillary array, and running buffer (Applied Biosystems).

3 Methods

3.1 DNA Isolation Using QIAamp Reagents

Specimens suitable for isolation and downstream analysis include peripheral blood, bone marrow, and sorted cell fractions (see Note 4).

1. Pipette 20 μl of Qiagen Protease into the bottom of a 1.5 ml microcentrifuge tube.

2. Add 200 μl of blood, bone marrow, or cells (up to 5×10^6 cells total).
3. Add 200 μl Buffer AL. Mix by pulse-vortexing for 15 s.
4. Incubate at 56°C for 15 min.
5. Add 200 μl EtOH (96–100%). Mix by pulse-vortexing for 15 s.
6. Apply the sample to a labeled QIAamp spin column without wetting the rim. Close the cap and microfuge at room temperature (RT) for 1 min at a minimum of 8,000 rpm (6,000 × *g*). Discard the collection tube containing the filtrate and place column on a new collection tube.
7. Add 500 μl Buffer AW1 without wetting the rim. Close the cap and microfuge at RT for 1 min at a minimum of 8,000 rpm (6,000 × *g*). Discard the collection tube containing the filtrate and place the column on a new collection tube.
8. Add 500 μl Buffer AW2 without wetting the rim. Close the cap and microfuge at RT for 3 min at a minimum of 8,000 rpm (6,000 × *g*). Discard the collection tube containing the filtrate and place the column on a new collection tube.
9. Microfuge the column at RT for an additional 1 min at a minimum of 8,000 rpm (6,000 × *g*) to ensure that all Buffer AW2 is removed. Discard the collection tube containing the filtrate.
10. Place the column in a clean, labeled 1.5 ml microcentrifuge tube. Add 75 μl Buffer AE. Incubate at RT for 5 min and then microfuge at RT for 1 min at 8,000 rpm (6,000 × *g*).
11. Store DNA at 4°C ± 3°C for up to 1 week or at −20°C for long-term storage.

3.2 DNA Quantification and Dilution

1. Turn on computer and open the NanoDrop software program.
2. Select the "Nucleic Acid" icon.
3. With the sampling arm open, pipette 2 μl of dH_2O onto the center of the lower measurement pedestal.
4. Carefully close the upper sampling arm and click "OK" to first initialize the instrument.
5. With the sample arm still closed, click the "Blank" button at the top of the screen.
6. With the sample arm still closed, type "dH_2O" into the sample ID Box and click on the green arrow labeled "Measure". If the reading for the dH_2O is >1 ng/μl repeat steps 3–6 using a fresh sample of dH_2O.
7. Raise the sampling arm and wipe the sample from both the upper and lower pedestals using a Kimwipe.
8. Pipette 2 μl of DNA specimen onto the center of the lower measurement pedestal.

Table 1
PCR master mix

Component	Amount (μl) per reaction
AmpFlSTR PCR reaction mix	9.55
AmpFlSTR Profiler primer mix	5.00
AmpliTaq Gold DNA polymerase	0.45
dH_2O	9.00
Total volume	24.00

9. Close the upper sampling arm and click "OK."
10. Type the sample ID into the sample ID Box and click on the green arrow labeled "Measure."
11. Raise the sampling arm and wipe the sample from both the upper and lower pedestals using a Kimwipe.
12. Repeat steps 8–11 for each sample to be measured.
13. Choose "Show Report." This will display all the readings and concentrations for each sample.
14. Make a dilution of each specimen to a final concentration of 2 ng/μl using sterile dH_2O.

3.3 PCR Amplification

1. Prepare a master mix of PCR reagents as indicated in Table 1 (see Note 5). Multiply each amount by the total number of reactions plus 1.
2. Aliquot 1 μl of diluted DNA into each PCR tube (see Note 6).
3. Aliquot 24 μl of the reaction mixture into each of the sample tubes.
4. Pipette gently up and down to mix.
5. Cap all tubes tightly.
6. Place the tubes in the thermal cycler and run the following program:

   95°C for 11 min.

   28 cycles of (see Note 7):

   94°C for 1 min.

   59°C for 1 min.

   72°C for 1 min.

   60°C for 45 min.
7. Store reactions at 4°C ± 3°C in the dark until capillary electrophoresis is performed.

3.4 Capillary Electrophoresis

1. Prepare a size standard reaction pool by combining 8.5 μl of Hi-Di Formamide and 0.5 μl of ROX GS500 size standard for each sample.
2. Pipette 1.0 μl of PCR product into a well of a 96-well plate.
3. Pipette 9.0 μl of the Hi-Di Formamide/ROX reaction mixture to each well containing PCR product and place a gray septa over the plate.
4. Denature samples at 95°C for 2 min in the thermal cycler.
5. Place the reaction on ice for at least 1 min.
6. Place the 96-well plate in a black 3100 base plate and cover with the white 3100 plate retainer.
7. Set the following parameters on the ABI3100 (see Note 8):

   Project name: 3100 Project1.

   Dye set: F.

   Run module: GeneScan36_POP4 45 s.

   Analysis module: GS500 Profiler.gsp.
8. After capillary electrophoresis is complete, analyze the samples using the GeneScan software.

3.5 Comprehensive (Pre-transplant) Analysis: Selection of Informative Loci and Calculations for Posttransplant Analysis

1. After electrophoresis, the genetic pattern of the pre-transplant recipient and the donor is determined. At each locus a single peak (homozygous) or two peaks (heterozygous) are identified. In addition to the allele peaks, one may notice small "stutter" peaks that occur four bases smaller than the allele peaks (see Note 9).
2. The donor and recipient alleles at each locus are compared. Loci must be identified that are informative for low amounts of donor and for low amounts of recipient. The following describes the identification of loci that are informative for low amounts of recipient. The same process can be used for identifying loci that are informative for low amounts of donor.
3. Loci that are NOT informative occur when all of the recipient alleles are either shared with the donor or are located in stutter down positions from donor alleles.
4. Informative loci occur when a recipient allele is longer than all donor alleles, or is eight or more bases shorter than donor alleles.
5. Calculations for informative alleles are shown in Fig. 1. Note that the calculation can be performed using either peak height or peak area (see Note 10). In these examples, the informative recipient allele is always the longest allele. The same calculation can be performed if the informative recipient allele is eight or more bases shorter than donor alleles.

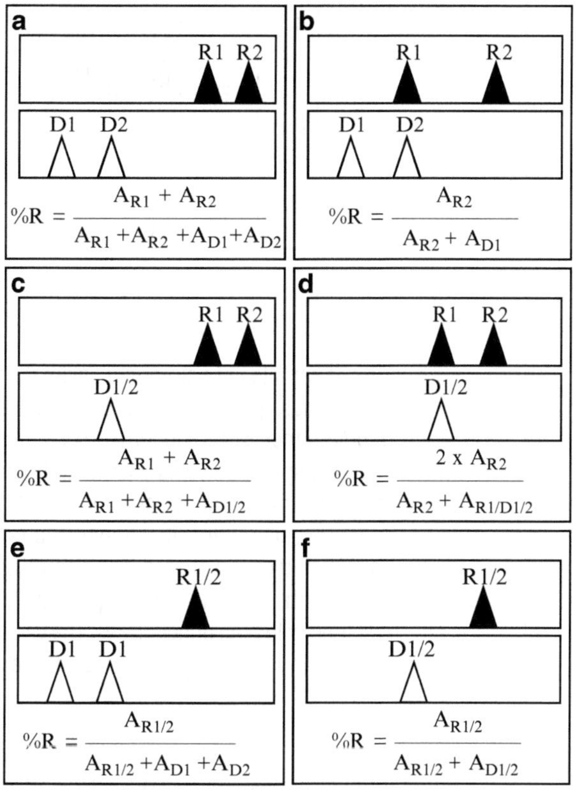

Fig. 1 (**a–f**) Examples of recipient and donor allele patterns that are informative for recipient. The *top panel* represents the capillary electropherogram for the recipient (R, *shaded peaks*), the *bottom panel* for the donor (D, *unshaded peaks*) at a single STR locus. The *x*-axis is size in bases. The *y*-axis is fluorescence intensity. *A* area of the peak. Note that peak height can be used as an alternative to peak area in the calculation. The calculation of %R is multiplied by 100 to give the percentage of recipient in the sample analyzed

6. Two loci and their corresponding calculations are chosen to be used for post-transplant analyses (see Notes 11 and 12). If two informative loci are not identified, additional loci may need to be analyzed (see Note 13).

3.6 Posttransplant Analysis

1. Post-transplant peripheral blood or bone marrow samples are prepared and analyzed as above.
2. Upon reviewing the post-transplant data, the first consideration is whether the sample contains a low amount of donor or low recipient. This will determine what loci and calculations will be used. To do this, review the data from an informative locus and determine if the dominant peaks belong to the donor or recipient.

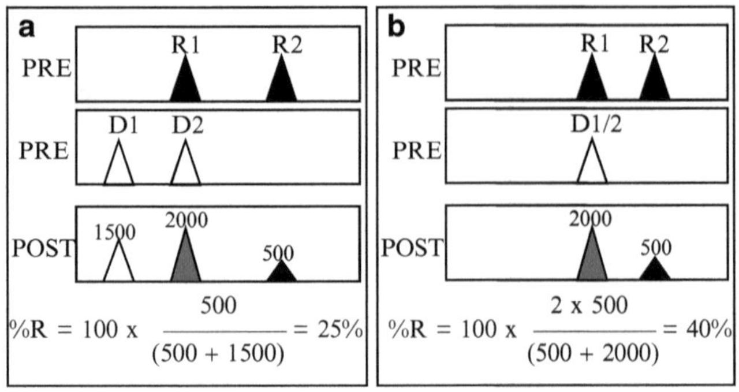

Fig. 2 Examples of chimerism calculations. The *top panel* represents the capillary electropherogram for the pre-transplant recipient (R, *dark shaded peaks*), the *middle panel* for the donor (D, *unshaded peaks*). The *bottom panel* represents a post-transplant analysis with mixed chimerism. Alleles that are shared between the recipient and donor are *light shaded*. The *x*-axis is size in bases. The *y*-axis is fluorescence intensity. In example (**a**), one recipient and one donor allele are unique, and one is shared. The shared allele is disregarded for the calculation. In example (**b**), there is one unique recipient allele, and the second recipient allele is shared with both donor alleles. The value for the unique recipient allele (numerator) must be multiplied by 2 because of the shared alleles

3. The intensity of the peaks to be analyzed must meet two criteria. First, the intensity of the dominant allele used in the calculation must be high enough to ensure the desired limit of detection (see Note 14). Secondly, the peaks to be used in the calculation must be on scale (see Note 15). If the peak heights are too high (off scale) or too low, the sample can be reinjected on the capillary electrophoresis instrument for a decreased or increased amount of time, respectively.
4. The calculations for two loci, which were determined in the comprehensive analysis, are then applied to the post-transplant data. Examples are shown in Fig. 2.
5. The results from the two loci should be concordant (within 10%). If so, average the two values. This is the final result.
6. If the results from the two loci are not concordant, then a third informative locus should be evaluated in order to determine the source of the problem. Discrepancies may be due to genetic alterations in the malignant cells (see Note 11) or may be due to technical problems. There are multiple causes for inferior data. The tips that may help resolve discrepancies due to technical problems related to instrument, software, or sample are presented in Notes 15–18. Please refer to the ABI PRISM 3100 Genetic Analyzer User's Manual and/or the AmpFlSTR Profiler PCR Amplification Kit User's Manual for additional information.

4 Notes

1. In addition to Qiagen, there are several companies that offer reagents for DNA isolation including Roche (Indianapolis, IN), Promega (Madison, WI), Invitrogen (Carlsbad, CA), and Beckman (Fullerton, CA). Automated extraction instruments are also available from these companies.
2. DNA quantification can also be performed using a fluorescent dye such as the Quant-iT PicoGreen dsDNA Reagents (Invitrogen) or qPCR quantification such as the Quantifiler Human DNA Quantification kit (Applied Biosystems). These methods are more expensive and more time consuming, but do yield more accurate quantification, particularly if the sample(s) is highly degraded, or contaminated with RNA.
3. There are multiple manufacturers of thermal cycler instruments. Alternative capillary electrophoresis instruments are also available.
4. Peripheral blood and bone marrow specimens should be anticoagulated in EDTA or heparin. Specimens may be stored at room temperature or 4°C for several days before extraction of DNA. Mix the specimen well prior to DNA extraction. Generally, 0.2 ml of specimen is sufficient for DNA extraction; however, if the patient is severely leukopenic, a larger starting volume may be required. Subsets of leukocytes can be analyzed to determine lineage-specific chimerism. Peripheral blood samples are sorted into fractions using lineage-specific monoclonal antibodies. This can be achieved by flow cytometry or by immunomagnetic bead separation technologies available from Miltenyi Biotec (Auburn, CA), STEMCELL Technologies (Vancouver, British Columbia), and Invitrogen (Carlsbad, CA) (18).
5. Keep AmpFlSTR Profiler reagents at 4°C until ready to use; immediately place them on ice. Primers are light sensitive. Exposure to light should be minimized.
6. Each run should include at least three controls, a pure/not mixed control, a mixed control, and a no template control (NTC). The NTC contains all components of the reaction except DNA, and is used to ensure that the reagents are not contaminated. The mixed control should be a mixture of two genetic patterns that is near the limit of detection of the assay. For example, our laboratory prepared a large quantity of a 5% mixture and analyzed the specimen multiple times in order to determine an acceptable range for the mixture calculations. The pure/not mixed control should be reviewed to ensure that there are no spurious alleles, which may indicate contamination.

7. The number of PCR amplification cycles is critical to the linearity of the assay. Thermal cycling must be terminated while in log phase amplification. It may be necessary to empirically determine thermal cycling conditions if a different thermal cycler is used.
8. Please refer to the ABI PRISM 3100 Genetic Analyzer User's Manual for operation of the ABI3100 instrument.
9. These peaks are called "stutter" peaks or "-4" peaks and occur because Taq polymerase may "slip" on the template and generate a product that is one repeat unit (four bases) smaller than the true allele. The amount of stutter is variable at different loci, and increases with the number of repeat units, but in general, a good rule of thumb is that the stutter peak is usually approximately 5% of the true allele. These stutter peaks further limit the number of informative alleles for follow-up analysis.
10. According to the 2011 College of American Pathologists (CAP) Monitoring Engraftment (ME) B survey, approximately 65% of clinical laboratories use peak area, and the remaining use peak height for engraftment calculations. Subscribing to this survey is an excellent means of monitoring proficiency of chimerism analysis.
11. Two loci are used for analysis (rather than one) because specimens may contain genetic gains or losses, or other abnormalities that may affect an STR locus and cause an erroneous result (19–21). If this occurs, the two loci will give discrepant calculations, which would warrant further follow-up. Thus, analyzing two loci reduces the risk of reporting an erroneous result due to genetic alterations in the sample.
12. It is important to analyze the same two loci using the same calculation for all post-transplant specimens to reduce variability between sequential chimerism analyses.
13. As noted in the introduction, there are multiple commercially available reagents that contain various combinations of STR loci. These include multiple kits from Applied Biosystems (Profiler, Profiler Plus, Cofiler, Identifiler) and from Promega (Powerplex 16 and Powerplex 1.2). If informative loci are not identified using one set of reagents, it may be necessary to run an alternative kit that has additional STR loci.
14. The peak height/area of the dominant allele(s) determines the limit of detection for any given analysis. A minor peak of approximately 100 relative fluorescent units (RFU) can be confidently detected. Thus if the peak height for the dominant allele is 2,000, the limit of detection for the analysis is approximately 5% [100/(2,000 + 100)). If the dominant peak height

is 5,000 RFU, then the limit of detection is approximately 2% [100/(5,000 + 100)). In our laboratory, we require that the peak height of the dominant peak(s) must be over 2,000 RFU to ensure that the limit of detection is at least 5%.

15. The electropherogram must be reviewed to identify off-scale data. Off-scale data are indicated by a red line running through the peaks on the electropherogram. When the fluorescence of a peak is off scale, the RFU value in the tabular data is not accurate. This highlights the importance of reviewing both the electropherogram and the numerical data.
16. Instrument-related problems: Data that do not size properly or have broadened peaks may be due to a bubble or leak in the polymer, or the need to change the capillary(s).
17. Software-related problems: Peaks that have a strong fluorescence intensity can "pull up" or "bleed" into other colors because of the overlapping spectra of emission of the fluorescent dyes. When a peak of one color is superimposed on a peak of another color, one should be suspicious for pull up. This problem can be addressed by simply injecting the sample for a shorter injection time so that the fluorescence intensity is lower and will not pull up other colors. However, if pull up is seen even when the fluorescent intensity of the peaks is relatively low (less than approximately 3,000 RFU), this may indicate that it is necessary to generate new dye matrix files by running the matrix standard samples.
18. Sample-related problems: Samples of poor quality (degraded DNA, or containing contaminating materials) may not PCR amplify and will yield low or no detectable peaks. These samples may need to be re-extracted and/or repurified. Samples that are contaminated with fluorescent material such as eosin may show fluorescent peaks on the electropherogram that are not PCR amplification products (22). This can usually be eliminated by performing additional wash steps during the DNA isolation procedure. Samples of too high a concentration (>2 ng/μl) can cause incomplete non-templated adenosine (A) addition during PCR cycling. This results in the presence of two peaks that differ by just one base, rather than a single peak for each allele. If non-templated A is identified, re-quantify and dilute specimens appropriately.

Acknowledgments

The author would like to thank Dr. Constance Griffin, Michael Hafez, and Penny Spencer for technical assistance and critical reading of this manuscript.

References

1. Antin JH, Childs R, Filipovich AH, Giralt S, Mackinnon S, Spitzer T, Weisdorf D (2001) Establishment of complete and mixed donor chimerism after allogeneic lymphohematopoietic transplantation: recommendations from a workshop at the 2001 tandem meetings of the international bone marrow transplant registry and the American society of blood and marrow transplantation. Biol Blood Marrow Transplant 7:473–485
2. Baron F, Sandmaier BM (2006) Chimerism and outcomes after allogeneic hematopoietic cell transplantation following nonmyeloablative conditioning. Leukemia 20:1690–1700
3. Toor AA, Sabo RT, Chung HM, Roberts C, Manjili RH, Song S et al (2012) Favorable outcomes in patients with high donor-derived T cell count after in vivo T cell-depleted reduced-intensity allogeneic stem cell transplantation. Biol Blood Marrow Transplant 18:794–804
4. Thiede C, Florek M, Bornhauser M, Ritter M, Mohr B, Brendel C, Ehninger G, Neubauer A (1999) Rapid quantification of mixed chimerism using multiplex amplification of short tandem repeat markers and fluorescence detection. Bone Marrow Transplant 23:1055–1060
5. Nuckols JD, Rasheed BK, McGlennen RC, Bigner SH, Stenzel TT (2000) Evaluation of an automated technique for assessment of marrow engraftment after allogeneic bone marrow transplantation using a commercially available kit. Am J Clin Pathol 113:135–140
6. Schichman SA, Suess P, Vertino AM, Gray PS (2002) Comparison of short tandem repeat and variable number tandem repeat genetic markers for quantitative determination of allogeneic bone marrow transplant engraftment. Bone Marrow Transplant 29:243–248
7. Thiede C, Bornhauser M, Ehninger G (2004) Strategies and clinical implications of chimerism diagnostics after allogeneic hematopoietic stem cell transplantation. Acta Haematol 112:16–23
8. Thiede C, Bornhauser M, Ehninger G (2004) Evaluation of STR informativity for chimerism testing–comparative analysis of 27 STR systems in 203 matched related donor recipient pairs. Leukemia 18:248–254
9. Hochberg EP, Miklos DB, Neuberg D, Eichner DA, McLaughlin SF, Mattes-Ritz A, Alyea EP, Antin JH, Soiffer RJ, Ritz J (2003) A novel rapid single nucleotide polymorphism (SNP)-based method for assessment of hematopoietic chimerism after allogeneic stem cell transplantation. Blood 101:363–369
10. Eshel R, Vainas O, Shpringer M, Naparstek E (2006) Highly sensitive patient-specific real-time PCR SNP assay for chimerism monitoring after allogeneic stem cell transplantation. Lab Hematol 12:39–46
11. Maas F, Schaap N, Kolen S, Zoetbrood A, Buno I, Dolstra H, de Witte T, Schattenberg A, van de Wiel-van Kemenade E (2003) Quantification of donor and recipient hemopoietic cells by real-time PCR of single nucleotide polymorphisms. Leukemia 17:621–629
12. Alizadeh M, Bernard M, Danic B, Dauriac C, Birebent B, Lapart C, Lamy T, Le Prise PY, Beauplet A, Bories D, Semana G, Quelvennec E (2002) Quantitative assessment of hematopoietic chimerism after bone marrow transplantation by real-time quantitative polymerase chain reaction. Blood 99:4618–4625
13. Masmas TN, Madsen HO, Petersen SL, Ryder LP, Svejgaard A, Alizadeh M, Vindelov LL (2005) Evaluation and automation of hematopoietic chimerism analysis based on real-time quantitative polymerase chain reaction. Biol Blood Marrow Transplant 11:558–566
14. Jimenez-Velasco A, Barrios M, Roman-Gomez J, Navarro G, Buno I, Castillejo JA, Rodriguez AI, Garcia-Gemar G, Torres A, Heiniger AI (2005) Reliable quantification of hematopoietic chimerism after allogeneic transplantation for acute leukemia using amplification by real-time PCR of null alleles and insertion/deletion polymorphisms. Leukemia 19:336–343
15. Koldehoff M, Steckel NK, Hlinka M, Beelen DW, Elmaagacli AH (2006) Quantitative analysis of chimerism after allogeneic stem cell transplantation by real-time polymerase chain reaction with single nucleotide polymorphisms, standard tandem repeats, and Y-chromosome-specific sequences. Am J Hematol 81:735–746
16. Oliver DH, Thompson RE, Griffin CA, Eshleman JR (2000) Use of single nucleotide polymorphisms (SNP) and real-time polymerase chain reaction for bone marrow engraftment analysis. J Mol Diagn 2:202–208
17. Harries LW, Wickham CL, Evans JC, Rule SA, Joyner MV, Ellard S (2005) Analysis of haematopoietic chimaerism by quantitative real-time polymerase chain reaction. Bone Marrow Transplant 35:283–290
18. Last Willasch A, Eing S, Weber G, Kuçi S, Schneider G, Soerensen J et al (2010) Enrichment of cell subpopulations applying automated MACS technique: purity, recovery and applicability for PCR-based chimerism analysis. Bone Marrow Transplant 45:181–189

19. Zhou M, Sheldon S, Akel N, Killeen AA (1999) Chromosomal aneuploidy in leukemic blast crisis: a potential source of error in interpretation of bone marrow engraftment analysis by VNTR amplification. Mol Diagn 4:153–157
20. Schichman SA, Lin P, Gilbrech LJ, Gray PS, Wilson CS, Sawyer JR (2002) Bone marrow transplant engraftment analysis with loss of an informative allele. J Mol Diagn 4:230–232
21. Swierczynski SL, Hafez MJ, Philips J, Higman MA, Berg KD, Murphy KM (2005) Bone marrow engraftment analysis after granulocyte transfusion. J Mol Diagn 7:422–426
22. Murphy KM, Berg KD, Geiger T, Hafez M, Flickinger KA, Cooper L, Pearson P, Eshleman JR (2005) Capillary electrophoresis artifact due to eosin: implications for the interpretation of molecular diagnostic assays. J Mol Diagn 7:143–148

Chapter 10

Detection of Clonal Immunoglobulin Heavy Chain Gene Rearrangements by the Polymerase Chain Reaction and Capillary Gel Electrophoresis

Hongxin Fan and Ryan S. Robetorye

Abstract

Although well-established diagnostic criteria exist for mature B-cell neoplasms, a definitive diagnosis of a B-cell lymphoproliferative disorder cannot always be obtained using more conventional techniques such as flow cytometric immunophenotyping, conventional cytogenetics, fluorescence in situ hybridization, or immunohistochemistry. However, because B-cell malignancies contain identically rearranged immunoglobulin heavy chain genes, the polymerase chain reaction (PCR) can be a fast, convenient, and dependable option to identify clonal B-cell processes. This chapter describes the use of PCR and capillary electrophoresis to identify clonal immunoglobulin heavy chain (*IGH*) variable and joining region (VH-JH) gene rearrangements (*IGH* VH-JH PCR) using a commercially available method employing multiple multiplex PCR tubes that was originally developed as the result of a large European BIOMED-2 collaborative study (Invivoscribe Technologies). The core protocol involves the use of three separate master mix tubes that target the conserved framework (FR1, FR2, and FR3) and joining (J) regions of the *IGH* gene. Analysis of these three framework regions can detect approximately 88% of clonal *IGH* gene rearrangements.

Key words Immunoglobulin heavy chain gene, Clonality testing, PCR, Capillary gel electrophoresis

1 Introduction

The vast majority of hematolymphoid malignancies are comprised of abnormal B cells. In a significant number of suspected B-cell lymphoproliferative disorders, a definitive diagnosis of malignancy cannot be made without additional evidence of a clonal process. This evidence can often be obtained using flow cytometric immunophenotyping, conventional cytogenetics, fluorescence in situ hybridization, or immunohistochemistry. However, because nearly all B-cell malignancies contain identically rearranged immunoglobulin heavy chain genes, clonality testing using the polymerase chain reaction (PCR) can be a fast, convenient, and dependable option to confirm the presence of clonal B-cell processes.

Magdalena Czader (ed.), *Hematological Malignancies*, Methods in Molecular Biology, vol. 999,
DOI 10.1007/978-1-62703-357-2_10, © Springer Science+Business Media New York 2013

In this chapter, we describe using the PCR and capillary gel electrophoresis to detect clonal immunoglobulin heavy chain (*IGH*) variable and joining region (VH-JH) gene rearrangements (*IGH* VH-JH PCR). The current most commonly used *IGH* VH-JH PCR method involves the use of multiple multiplex PCR tubes and was originally developed as the result of a large European BIOMED-2 collaborative study (BIOMED-2 Concerted Action BMH4-CT98-3936) (1). However, because the production, vialing, and quality control testing of the BIOMED-2 multiplex PCR tubes and controls are time-consuming and not easy to perform by most clinical molecular diagnostic laboratories, the BIOMED-2 primers have been made commercially available in kit form via Invivoscribe Technologies (San Diego, CA, USA; www.invivoscribe.com).

This method requires extraction of DNA from the desired sample to be analyzed, which can originate from a variety of clinical sample types, such as bone marrow aspirate, peripheral blood, fresh (or fresh-frozen) tissue, or formalin-fixed paraffin-embedded (FFPE) tissue. The DNA can be obtained using either manual or automated DNA extraction methods. The isolated DNA then serves as a template for the standardized BIOMED-2 multiplex PCR protocol. The core protocol involves the use of three separate master mixes (Tubes A, B, and C) that target the conserved framework (FR1, FR2, and FR3) and joining (J) regions of the *IGH* gene for the detection of clonal *IGH* gene VH-JH rearrangements. A specimen control size ladder master mix is also included in the kit and serves as a DNA quality and quantity control for each test sample. The PCR products are subsequently analyzed by capillary gel electrophoresis using an Applied Biosystems (ABI) 3130*xl* Genetic Analyzer. Clonality can then be established if a peak(s) is detected in any or all of the three framework regions. Analysis of these three framework regions can detect approximately 88% of clonal *IGH* gene rearrangements (2). Although the BIOMED-2 protocol also includes additional multiplex PCR reactions for the detection of incomplete *IGH* gene diversity and joining region (DH-JH) rearrangements, as well as kappa (*IGK*) and lambda (*IGL*) immunoglobulin light chain gene rearrangements, these reactions will not be further discussed in this chapter (see Note 1).

2 Materials

2.1 Samples

1. Peripheral blood, bone marrow aspirate, fresh or frozen tissue, or FFPE tissue.

2.2 Sample Preparation

2.2.1 DNA Extraction from Fresh Samples

1. Gentra Puregene Blood Kit for 3 or 30 ml blood or bone marrow aspirate (Qiagen, Valencia, CA).
2. Gentra Puregene Tissue Kit for 100 mg tissue (Qiagen, Valencia, CA).
3. 100% isopropanol.
4. 70% ethanol.
5. 1.5 ml microcentrifuge tubes, or 15 ml centrifuge tubes.
6. Pipettes and pipette tips.
7. Liquid nitrogen.
8. Mortar and pestle.
9. General laboratory equipment, including vortex mixer, desktop centrifuge, microcentrifuge, spectrophotometer, and incubators.

2.2.2 DNA Extraction from Formalin-Fixed Paraffin-Embedded Tissue

1. Fisherbrand CitriSolv Clearing Agent (Fisher Scientific Inc., Pittsburgh, PA).
2. Xylene.
3. 100% ethanol.
4. Heating block.
5. Proteinase K (20 mg/ml).
6. Gentra Puregene Cell Lysis Solution 125 ml (Qiagen, cat. no. 158906).
7. Thermomixer or other similar equipment.
8. EZ1 DNA Tissue Kit (Qiagen, Valencia, CA).
9. EZ1 DNA Paraffin Section Card (Qiagen, Valencia, CA).
10. BioRobot® EZ1 workstation (Qiagen, Valencia, CA).

2.3 Multiplex PCR

1. PCR thermal cycler (e.g., GeneAmp® PCR System 9700, Applied Biosystems).
2. PCR tubes or PCR reaction plate (e.g., 0.2 ml MicroAmp® Reaction Tubes with Cap, or MicroAmp Optical 96-well Reaction Plate with MicroAmp™ Optical 8-Cap Strip, Applied Biosystems, Carlsbad, CA).
3. *IGH* Gene Clonality Assay Kit for ABI Fluorescence Detection (Invivoscribe Technologies, San Diego, CA). This kit includes multiplex PCR master mixes and control DNA samples (see Note 2).
4. AmpliTaq Gold DNA Polymerase at 5 units/μl (Applied Biosystems, Carlsbad, CA).
5. Nuclease-free H_2O.

2.4 Capillary Gel Electrophoresis

1. ABI 3130*xl* Genetic Analyzer with 50 cm Capillary Array (Applied Biosystems) (see Note 3).

2. POP-7™ Polymer for ABI 3130/3130*xl* Genetic Analyzer (Applied Biosystems, Carlsbad, CA) (see Note 3).
3. 10× Running Buffer (Applied Biosystems, Carlsbad, CA).
4. GeneScan™ 400HD ROX™ Size Standard (Applied Biosystems, Carlsbad, CA).
5. Hi-Di Formamide (Applied Biosystems, Carlsbad, CA).
6. DS-30 Matrix Standard Kit (Applied Biosystems, Carlsbad, CA).
7. MicroAmp Optical 96-well Reaction Plate (Applied Biosystems, Carlsbad, CA).

3 Methods

3.1 Sample Preparation

DNA can be extracted using either manual or automated methods based on the resources available in individual laboratories. Here, we describe a manual DNA extraction method for fresh samples using Gentra Puregene reagents, and a modified automated DNA extraction method for FFPE samples using the Qiagen EZ1 workstation and EZ1 DNA Tissue Kit (see Note 4).

3.1.1 DNA Extraction from Fresh Samples

1. DNA isolated from a variety of fresh samples may be analyzed using the *IGH* Gene Clonality Assay Kit, including bone marrow aspirate, peripheral blood, and fresh or fresh-frozen tissue.
2. Collect bone marrow (minimum 1 ml) or peripheral blood (minimum 3 ml) samples in EDTA (purple top) tubes and extract DNA using the Gentra Puregene Blood Kit for 3 or 30 ml blood (depending on sample volume) according to the manufacturer's recommendations (3).
3. Fresh tissues should be obtained in a sterile manner, and a minimum of 5 mm^3 representative tumor tissue (see Note 5) is required for molecular testing. Fresh tissue should be transported to the laboratory immediately after excision for processing, or if immediate transport is not possible, then the tissue should either be transported in RPMI 1640 culture medium, or snap frozen in liquid nitrogen or dry ice and transported frozen.
4. Extract DNA from fresh or fresh-frozen tissues using the Gentra Puregene Tissue Kit according to the manufacturer's recommendations (3).
5. After extraction, temporarily store DNA samples at 4°C, or place at −20°C for longer term storage.
6. Measure DNA concentration using a spectrophotometer (see Note 6). Adjust the DNA concentration with nuclease-free H_2O to a concentration of 100–500 ng/μl DNA for subsequent PCR analysis (see Subheading 3.2).

3.1.2 DNA Extraction from Formalin-Fixed Paraffin-Embedded Tissues

1. Many factors can affect the quality of DNA isolated from FFPE tissues (see Note 7). Therefore, fresh or fresh-frozen tissue is recommended for optimal detection of clonal *IGH* gene rearrangements.
2. Cut one to five 10 μm thick sections containing representative tumor (see Note 5) from each FFPE tissue block (e.g., lymph nodes, skin biopsies, gastrointestinal biopsies, or other tissues) using a clean microtome, and place in 1.5 ml microcentrifuge tubes (see Note 8). For fine-needle aspirates or other very small biopsy samples, up to ten sections may be required to obtain sufficient DNA for subsequent clonality testing.
3. Extract the DNA from FFPE tissue samples using the EZ1 DNA Tissue Kit and the EZ1 DNA Paraffin Section Card along with important modifications (see Note 9) involving extra deparaffinization steps using CitriSolv or xylene and the Gentra Puregene Cell Lysis Solution instead of the G2 buffer supplied in the EZ1 DNA Tissue Kit.
4. Add 1 ml of CitriSolv or xylene to each tube containing paraffin sections and mix the tubes by gentle vortexing for 5–10 s.
5. Incubate the tubes at room temperature for 10 min.
6. Pellet the tissue by centrifugation at full speed for 10 min and discard the supernatant.
7. Add 1 ml of 100% ethanol to each tube and mix by inverting the tubes.
8. Pellet tissue by microcentrifugation at full speed for 10 min and discard the supernatant.
9. Repeat the ethanol wash one additional time, and after the last wash, remove as much supernatant as possible.
10. Open the tubes and evaporate the residual ethanol by incubation in a heating block at 56°C for 15–30 min, or until the samples are completely dry.
11. Add 190 μl of Gentra Puregene Cell Lysis Solution and 10 μl of proteinase K (20 mg/ml) solution to the dried sample (see Note 9).
12. Close tubes and incubate at 56°C overnight or up to 72 h (see Note 10) with continuous vigorous mixing (e.g., in a thermomixer) until the samples are completely lysed.
13. After incubation, centrifuge the samples at full speed for 5 min, and then transfer the supernatant to new 2 ml sample tubes.
14. Process supernatant (containing raw DNA) on the BioRobot® EZ1 workstation using the EZ1 DNA Tissue Kit along with the EZ1 DNA Paraffin Section Card according to the manufacturer's instructions (4). Use a starting sample volume of 200 μl; if the sample volume from the above step is less than

200 µl, Gentra Puregene Cell Lysis Solution should be added to 200 µl total volume. The final elution volume from the BioRobot® EZ1 workstation is 50 µl.

15. After extraction, store the DNA sample temporarily at 4°C (see Note 11) or at −20°C for longer term storage until ready to proceed with subsequent multiplex PCR.
16. Measure DNA concentration using a spectrophotometer. DNA recovery from FFPE samples varies widely from sample to sample (see Note 12). Adjust DNA concentration in nuclease-free H_2O, and use 100–500 ng of DNA (see Notes 12 and 17) for each subsequent multiplex PCR.

3.2 Multiplex PCR

In this chapter, we describe the use of multiplex *IGH* VH-JH and specimen control PCR using only the Invivoscribe Technologies core protocol that targets the conserved framework (FR1, FR2, and FR3) and joining (J) regions of the *IGH* gene for the detection of clonal *IGH* gene VH-JH rearrangements (see Note 13).

1. Remove reagents and patient samples from freezer and/or refrigerator. Thaw, if necessary, and keep samples cool on wet ice.
2. Prepare four multiplex PCR master mixes (tubes A, B, C, and specimen control size ladder tube) and adjust master mix volumes based on the total number of samples that will be analyzed—45 µl of master mix and 0.25 µl of AmpliTaq Gold DNA Polymerase are required for each sample.
3. Add 45.25 µl of master mix to each reaction tube (or to each well, if using 96-well plate) and then add 5 µl of patient or control DNA (equivalent DNA amount 100–500 ng) to appropriate tubes or wells. In each run, at least three controls should be included for each master mix (see Subheading 3.4 for additional details). Cap tubes or cover reaction plate with optical 8-cap strip and load tubes or plate on to PCR thermal cycler. An example analysis with four multiplex PCR reactions for two patient samples is illustrated in Table 1.
4. Perform *IGH* VH-JH multiplex PCR using the following conditions: 95°C for 7 min and then, 34 cycles of 95°C for 45 s, 60°C for 45 s, and 72°C for 90 s. The final elongation step should be 72°C for 10 min, and then hold the temperature at 15°C until tubes or plates are removed from the thermal cycler.

3.3 Capillary Gel Electrophoresis

Multiplex PCR products are fractionated and analyzed using an ABI 3130*xl* Genetic Analyzer (see Notes 3 and 14).

1. Set up a denaturing reaction by adding 20 µl of HI-DI Formamide, 0.5 µl of Size Standard GS 400HD ROX, and 1.0 µl of PCR product into each well of a 96-well plate. Heat to 95°C for 2 min, and then quick-chill on wet ice for 5 min.

Table 1
An example of multiplex PCR reactions for two patient samples

Master mix			
Tube A (FRI)	**Tube B (FRII)**	**Tube C (FRIII)**	**Specimen control**
Sample 1	Sample 1	Sample 1	Sample 1
Sample 1	Sample 1	Sample 1	
Sample 2	Sample 2	Sample 2	Sample 2
Sample 2	Sample 2	Sample 2	
5% clonal control	5% clonal control	5% clonal control	5% clonal control
Polyclonal control	Polyclonal control	Polyclonal control	Polyclonal control
No template control	No template control	No template control	No template control

2. Load sample plate on the ABI 3130*xl* and set up the plate in the Data Collection Software according to the manufacturer's instructions (5, 6). Briefly, power on the 3130*xl* instrument and attached computer.
3. Open the Data Collection Software, create and save an *IGH* plate record, select run module Spect50_POP7 and Dye Set D (DS-30 Matrix Standards) (see Note 3), and load sample plate onto the instrument.
4. Operate the instrument according to the manufacturer's instructions (5, 6) by selecting the desired plate record. Link the plate position indicator to the corresponding plate position in the instrument, and run the plate.
5. Data are automatically collected by the Data Collection Software on the ABI 3130*xl* instrument and are analyzed using GeneMapper Analysis Software. After completion of the run, open GeneMapper Analysis Software and analyze the data according to the manufacturer's instructions (see Note 15).
6. View the results of the analysis by selecting Display Plots and choosing the desired wells for each sample. Adjust the viewing scale by setting vertical and horizontal parameters according to PCR product size and print the results.

3.4 Quality Control

1. DNA integrity should be monitored for each test sample by including a separate tube for specimen control size ladder PCR.
2. Multiple controls should also be included in each run for each master mix (see Table 1 for examples), including:
   (a) A clonal and sensitivity control comprised of a 5% mixture of clonal *IGH* gene DNA diluted with polyclonal *IGH*

gene control DNA for each master mix tube. This control monitors assay sensitivity and mimics clinical specimens in which clonal cells are present along with polyclonal background cells (see Note 16).

(b) A polyclonal control: Polyclonal control DNA is supplied in *IGH* Gene Clonality Assay Kit. The polyclonal control helps to establish the PCR product size range for each specific master mix.

(c) Blank or no DNA template control consisting of master mix and nuclease-free H_2O to monitor for possible sample contamination.

3. Replicate samples should be included for *IGH* VH-JH (FR I, II, III) multiplex PCR (see Note 17). Consistent peak patterns should be obtained from replicate samples.

3.5 Result Interpretation

1. The interpretation of *IGH* VH-JH Clonality Assay results should include examination of the technical aspects of each assay as well as all available clinical information. Technical aspects include appropriate positive, negative, and reagent controls in each run; patient sample DNA quantity and quality; and replicate master mix tube results. *IGH* gene clonality results should also be interpreted in the context of available clinical information, tissue morphology, and other laboratory test results such as immunophenotype and cytogenetics.
2. The reagent (no template) controls (Fig. 1a) should not display any peaks in any of the master mix tubes—the presence of any peaks in these tubes indicates a possible contamination problem, and the assay should be repeated. The polyclonal (negative) control should show a bell-shaped peak distribution (Gaussian distribution) pattern (Fig. 1b), and the clonal (positive) control should exhibit a narrow (one to two base pair) dominant peak, with or without a bell-shaped polyclonal peak background (Fig. 1c).
3. PCR amplicons for each of the framework region master mix tubes should have appropriate size ranges (see Note 18). The specimen control size ladder PCR products have a range from 84 to 600 bp in a sample with intact DNA (Fig. 1d) (see Note 19). Samples with amplicons larger than 300 bp in size in the specimen control size ladder PCR tube are considered to have DNA of acceptable quality (Fig. 1e) (see Note 18). Samples with amplicons smaller than 300 bp in size in the specimen control size ladder usually indicate DNA degradation, especially in FFPE tissue samples (Fig. 1f).

a

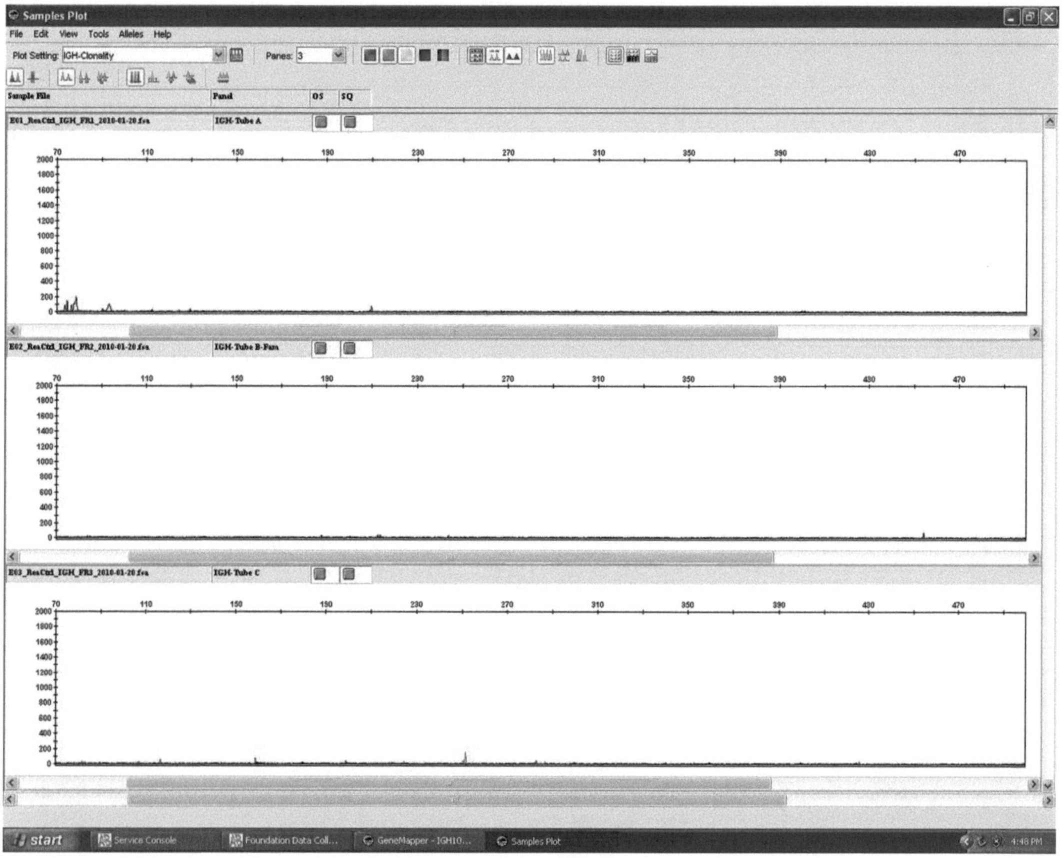

Fig. 1 Examples of results for reagent, negative, positive, and specimen DNA size ladder controls. In all figures FR1 is shown in the *top panel*, FR2 in the *middle panel*, and FR3 in the *lower panel*. (**a**) Reagent control for FR1-3. (**b**) Negative (polyclonal) control for FR1-3. (**c**) Positive (clonal) control for FR1-3. (**d**) Specimen control size ladder with full range of PCR products from 84 to 600 bp. (**e**) Acceptable sample for analysis with DNA size ladder control with peaks at least 300 bp in length. (**f**) Unacceptable (degraded) sample with DNA size ladder control with peaks less than 300 bp in length

4. Clonal peak heights may vary in size (see Note 20). Replicate patient samples should produce similar *IGH* gene rearrangement patterns. If a clonal peak is seen, the peak should be of identical size (in base pairs) and exhibit a similar peak height in replicate samples. In biallelic or biclonal samples, two or more clonal peaks may be present in a single patient sample.
5. The BIOMED-2 *IGH* VH-JH multiplex PCR protocol for framework regions 1–3 is able to detect clonal *IGH* gene rearrangements in about 88% of mature B-cell malignancies (see Note 21) (2).

b

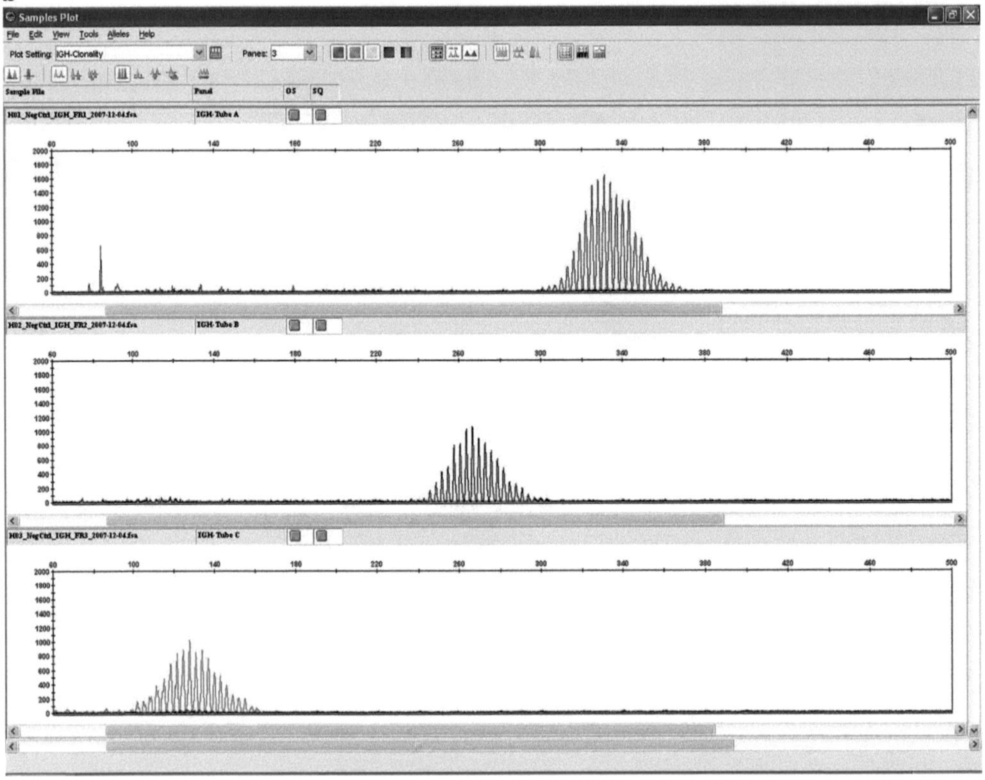

c

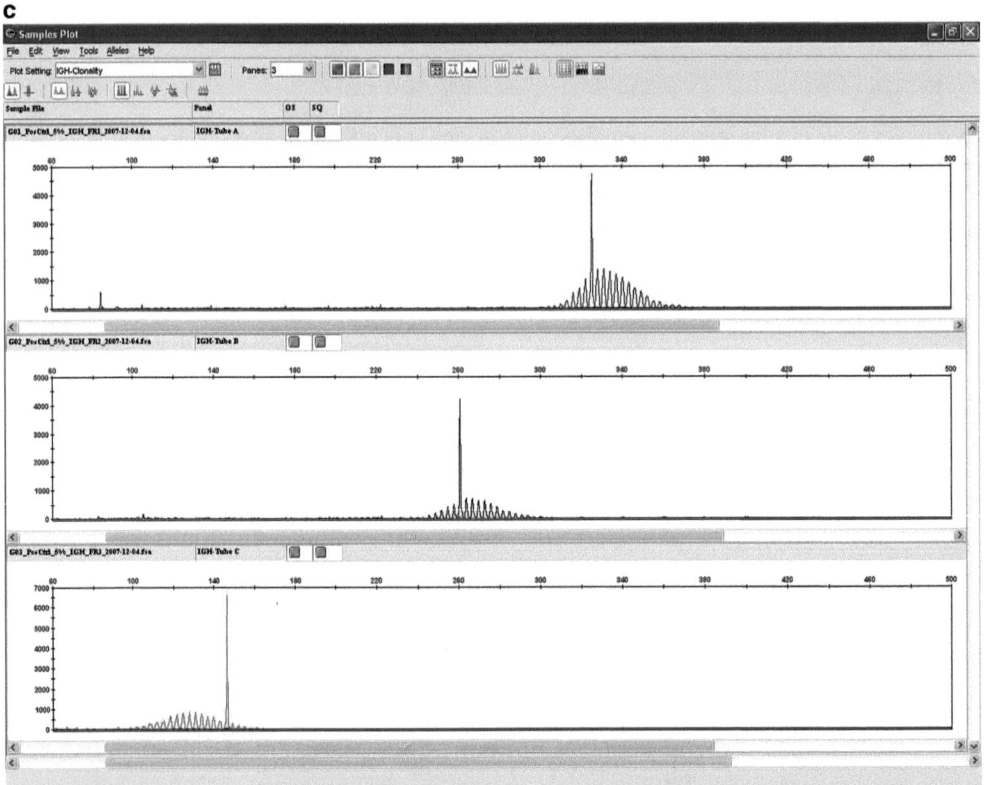

Fig. 1 (continued)

d

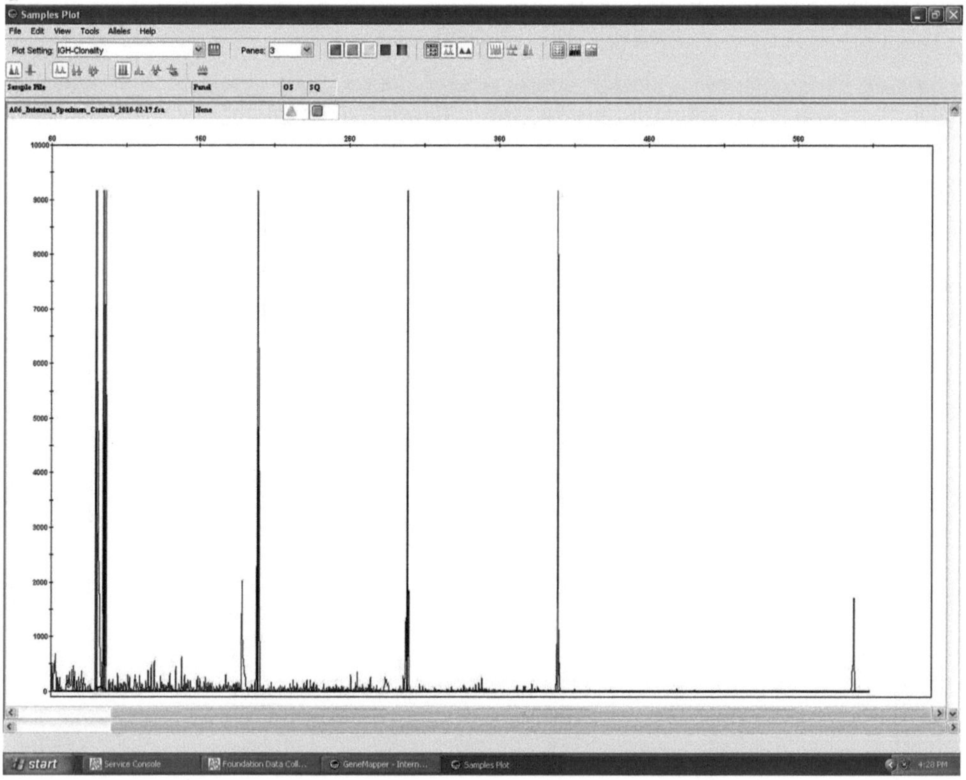

e

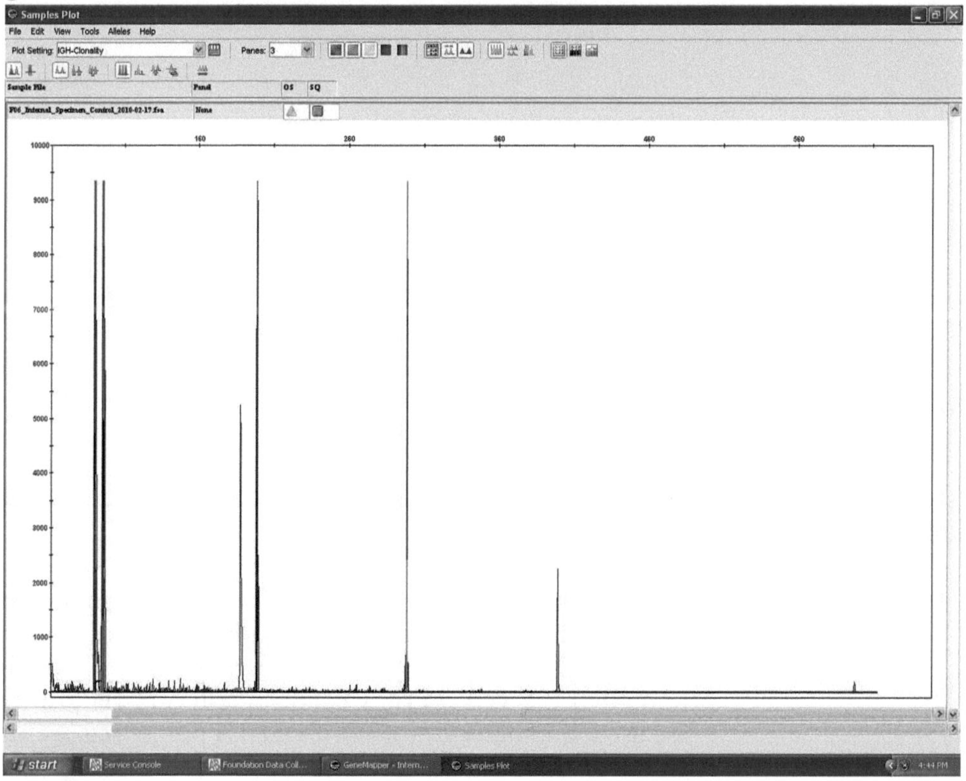

Fig. 1 (continued)

f

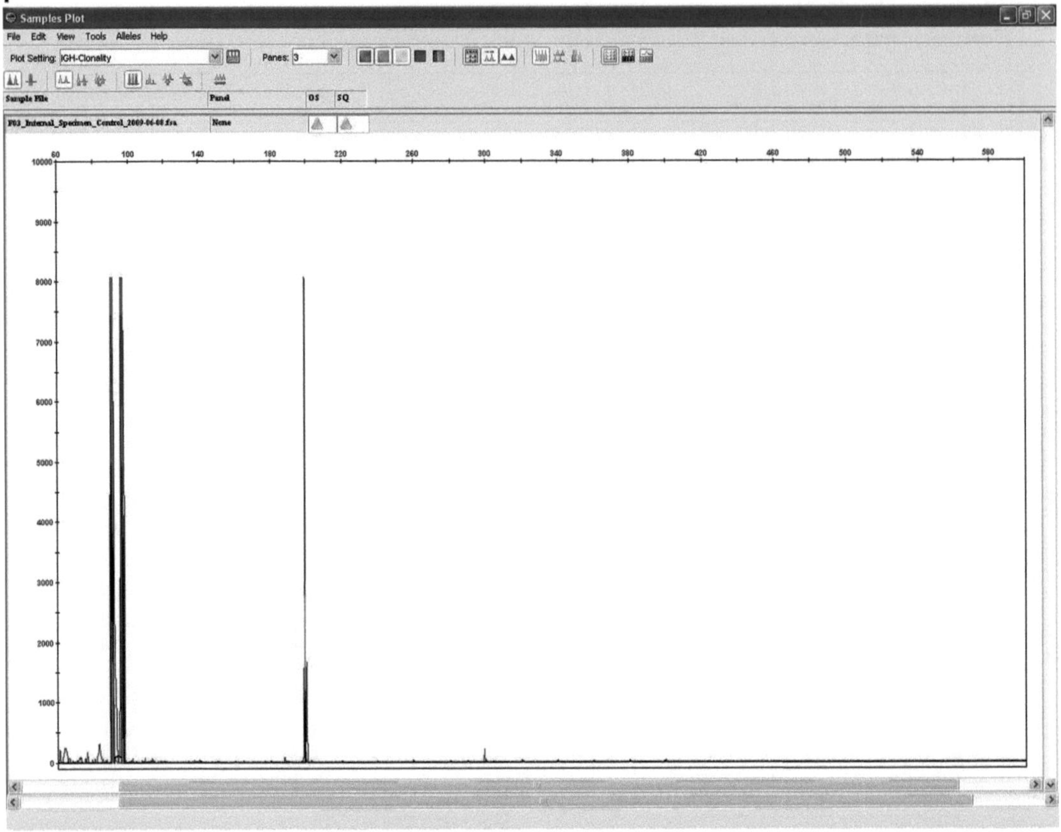

6. The detection of a clonal *IGH* gene rearrangement can be highly suggestive of a B-cell malignancy, but it should not be used as the sole criterion for diagnosis of a lymphoid neoplasm, as clonal *IGH* gene rearrangements are not exclusively detected in malignancies (7). Although *IGH* clonality can help to identify cell lineage, the presence of a B-cell clone does not always indicate B-cell lineage (8, 9).

4 Notes

1. For clonal immunoglobulin gene rearrangement detection, the BIOMED-2 protocol also includes multiplex PCR reactions for DH-JH, *IGK*, and *IGL* rearrangements. The detection rate for B-cell clonality is 88% if only VH-JH primer sets are used, but increases to 91% if DH-JH primer sets are added. If all primer combinations are used (*IGH* VH-JH, *IGH* DH-JH, *IGK*, and *IGL*), the detection rate increases to 99% (2).

See the original 2003 BIOMED-2 Concerted Action review paper and subsequent 2007 publication for detailed protocols and testing strategy for these primer sets (1, 9).

2. Six master mix tubes are provided in the *IGH* Gene Clonality Assay Kit. Tubes A, B, and C contain multiple VH forward primers and one JH consensus reverse primer in each tube that target the FR1, FR2, and FR3 regions. Tubes D and E target the DH and JH region, and a specimen control size ladder tube master mix is used for DNA quality control. In this chapter, we will only discuss methodology for detection of clonal *IGH* gene rearrangement in the FR1, FR2, and FR3 regions and for the use of the specimen control size ladder. Prior to use, the four master mix tubes (tubes A, B, C, and specimen control master mix) should be aliquoted to convenient volumes for one-time use and stored at −80°C. In addition, the master mix tubes should not be subjected to repeated freeze-thaw cycles.

3. In this chapter, we describe the use of the ABI 3130*xl* Genetic Analyzer equipped with a 50 cm capillary array and POP-7 polymer as an example system that works well with the *IGH* Gene Clonality Assay Kit in our molecular diagnostics laboratory. However, different capillary gel electrophoresis systems may also perform just as well for this purpose in other laboratories.

4. Other DNA extraction methods can also be used as long as adequate DNA quality and quantity is maintained. The automated extraction system we use in our laboratory (BioRobot® EZ1 workstation, Qiagen) can process only low-volume (200–350 μl) blood samples. For larger volume fresh samples, we use a manual extraction method (Gentra Puregene reagents) for DNA isolation. For FFPE samples, we use the EZ1 instrument for DNA isolation. We have found that the *IGH* Gene Clonality Assay performs best if DNA isolated from FFPE samples is as pure as possible.

5. Samples that contain representative tumor tissue should be collected for analysis. It is recommended that the tumor cell load should be greater than 15% for the *IGH* Gene Clonality Assay.

6. Our laboratory uses a NanoDrop 1000 Spectrophotometer (Thermo Fisher Scientific, Wilmington, DE) to quantitate DNA samples prior to adjusting the concentration for subsequent PCR analysis because only 1 μl of sample is required for quantitation without prior dilution.

7. Many factors affect DNA quality in FFPE tissues such as fixative type and fixation time. Some FFPE tissues are unacceptable for molecular studies, such as those fixed in Zenker's, B5, or

Bouin's fixatives, as well as formic acid decalcified bone marrow biopsy samples. These fixatives/procedures can produce extensive degradation of DNA, making their use inappropriate for molecular studies.

8. When sectioning FFPE tissue blocks for molecular studies, special precautions should be followed to avoid carry-over DNA contamination from previously cut samples. These precautions may include using new microtome blades for each sample, or cleaning the microtome with xylene and 100% ethanol between samples.

9. For FFPE tissue sections, we do not perform paraffin trimming steps as recommended in the EZ1 DNA Tissue Kit instructions, but rather perform extra deparaffinization steps instead. Paraffin can be completely removed by using either CitriSolv or xylene, and will not interfere with subsequent extraction steps. Also, according to our own validation study, Gentra Puregene Cell Lysis Solution tended to produce better results than the G2 buffer supplied in the EZ1 DNA Tissue Kit.

10. Addition of Gentra Puregene Cell Lysis Solution and/or proteinase K is based on relative sample size and sample type. Samples with relatively large amounts of tissue should be resuspended in more than 200 μl lysis solution with proportional increases in the amount of proteinase K added. For tissue samples that are more difficult to digest, proteinase K concentration can be increased or incubation times can be increased as needed. For example, for skin tissue FFPE samples, we routinely perform a 48–72 h proteinase K incubation step.

11. Compared to genomic DNA isolated from fresh samples or fresh-frozen samples, the DNA isolated from FFPE samples is more prone to degradation. DNA isolated from FFPE samples should be aliquoted in volumes sufficient for one-time use. Remaining DNA aliquots should be stored at −20°C, and repeated freeze-thaw cycles should be avoided.

12. DNA recovery from FFPE samples can vary widely from sample to sample, ranging from as little as a few nanograms up to several hundred nanograms per microliter. We recommend using 100–500 ng of DNA for each multiplex PCR. However, even very small amounts of input DNA can sometimes produce analyzable PCR products as long as the specimen control DNA indicates good DNA quality, and multiplex *IGH* VH-JH PCR amplification produces a clonal peak(s) or an appropriate polyclonal peak distribution. It should also be noted that low-input DNA concentrations may result in false clonal results due to restricted PCR amplification of only a few B cells; however, replicate samples usually show different capillary electrophoresis peak patterns.

13. In this chapter, we will discuss only the use of *IGH* VH-JH for identification of clonal *IGH* gene rearrangements in the conserved FR I, II, and III regions. However, in clinical laboratory practice, DH-JH rearrangement detection assays, as well as immunoglobulin light chain rearrangement (*IGK* and *IGL*) detection assays, may be performed to increase the clonality detection rate if patient samples are negative for a clonal rearrangement in FR I, II and III, but clinical suspicion is high for a B-cell malignancy (see Note 1).
14. Capillary gel electrophoresis (GeneScanning) and heteroduplex analysis can be used for analyzing *IGH* VH-JH PCR products. We will confine discussion to the capillary gel electrophoresis technique in this chapter. Heteroduplex analysis may be considered if analysis of the *IGH* VH-JH PCR product composition and conformation is desired (1). Please note that for heteroduplex analysis there is no need to use fluorochrome-labeled PCR primers.
15. Please refer to the GeneMapper® Software Version 4.0 Quick Reference Guide (10) for additional information on how to use the GeneMapper Software. We use the Microsatellite setting for multiplex *IGH* VH-JH PCR analysis (11).
16. Assay sensitivity may differ for each master mix and for different analysis systems. In our molecular diagnostics laboratory, assay sensitivities among three *IGH* VH-JH (FR I, II, and III) PCRs range from 1 to 5%, so we use a 5% mixture of clonal *IGH* gene DNA diluted with polyclonal *IGH* gene control DNA as a clonality and sensitivity control. You will need to validate the assay sensitivity in your laboratory, and include that determined sensitivity control in each clinical run.
17. For DNA extracted from fresh or fresh-frozen samples, identical DNA concentrations may be used for replicate testing. For DNA extracted from FFPE samples, it may be useful to perform replicate testing with one tube of the original DNA solution and additional tubes with diluted DNA (e.g., 1:5 or 1:10 diluted DNA) in order to overcome the effects of possible PCR inhibitors. However, our assay validation study has shown that EZ1 extraction of FFPE samples usually produces DNA of sufficient purity for subsequent *IGH* VH-JH PCR analysis so that no DNA dilution step is required.
18. In the *IGH* VH-JH Clonality Assay, the amplicons from the three framework regions should range in size from 100 to 170 bp in the FR3 region, 250 to 295 bp in the FR2 region, and 310 to 360 bp in the FR1 region. Therefore, adequate interrogation of all three of the framework regions requires the DNA sample template to be greater than 300 bp in length. Amplicons outside of the expected size ranges may represent

actual rearranged clones, but such clones should be confirmed by DNA sequencing (12).

19. The specimen control size ladder PCR products should be 84, 96, 200, 300, 400, 500, and 600 bp in length in a sample with intact DNA.
20. Peak heights may be of variable size in different samples. Peak height is relatively proportional to the percentage of tumor cells in a specific sample, but it cannot be used reliably for estimation of tumor burden.
21. Although a recent BIOMED-2 study (2) showed that *IGH* VH-JH PCR assays that included primers for FR1-FR3 could detect clonal *IGH* gene rearrangements in 88% of mature B-cell malignancies, it should be noted that only fresh or fresh-frozen tissue samples were analyzed in this study. The detection rate for clonal B-cell proliferations is likely to be lower if FFPE tissues are analyzed. However, the detection rate in FFPE specimens may be enhanced with additional application of the BIOMED-2 *IGK* primer sets (*IGK* Tubes A and B) along with all of the primer sets that target the FR1, FR2, and FR3 regions of the *IGH* gene (*IGH* Tubes A, B, and C), as demonstrated in a recent study of follicular lymphomas (13). Demonstration of clonality in follicular lymphomas has traditionally been challenging due to the presence of somatic hypermutations in the *IGH* gene framework regions.

Acknowledgment

The authors would like to thank Kumari Vadlamudi for her excellent technical assistance.

References

1. van Dongen JJ, Langerak AW, Brüggemann M, Evans PA, Hummel M, Lavender FL et al (2003) Design and standardization of PCR primers and protocols for detection of clonal immunoglobulin and T-cell receptor gene recombinations in suspect lymphoproliferations: report of the BIOMED-2 Concerted Action BMH4-CT98-3936. Leukemia 17: 2257–2317
2. Evans PA, Pott C, Groenen PJ, Salles G, Davi F, Berger F et al (2007) Significantly improved PCR-based clonality testing in B-cell malignancies by use of multiple immunoglobulin gene targets. Report of the BIOMED-2 Concerted Action BHM4-CT98-3936. Leukemia 21:207–214
3. Gentra® Puregene® Handbook. For purification of archive-quality DNA from human whole blood, bone marrow, buffy coat, buccal cells, body fluids, cultured cells, tissue, mouse tail, yeast, bacteria (June 2011) Qiagen. Third Edition. http://www.qiagen.com/literature
4. EZ1® DNA Handbook. For EZ1 DNA Blood 200 μl Kit and EZ1 DNA Blood 350 μl Kit (April 2010) Qiagen. http://www.qiagen.com/literature
5. Applied Biosystems 3130/3130*xl* Genetic Analyzers Getting Started Guide (2004) Applied Biosystems. Part number 4352715 Rev. B. http://www3.appliedbiosystems.com
6. Applied Biosystems 3130/3130*xl* Genetic Analyzers Maintenance, Troubleshooting and

Reference Guide (2004) Applied Biosystems. Part number 4352716 Rev. B. http://www3.appliedbiosystems.com

7. Langerak AW, Molina TJ, Lavender FL, Pearson D, Flohr T, Sambade C et al (2007) Polymerase chain reaction-based clonality testing in tissue samples with reactive lymphoproliferations: usefulness and pitfalls. A report of the BIOMED-2 Concerted Action BMH4-CT98-3936. Leukemia 21:222–229
8. Brüggemann M, White H, Gaulard P, Garcia-Sanz R, Gameiro P, Oeschger S et al (2007) Powerful strategy for polymerase chain reaction-based clonality assessment in T-cell malignancies Report of the BIOMED-2 Concerted Action BHM4 CT98-3936. Leukemia 21: 215–221
9. van Krieken JH, Langerak AW, Macintyre EA, Kneba M, Hodges E, Sanz RG et al (2007) Improved reliability of lymphoma diagnostics via PCR-based clonality testing: report of the BIOMED-2 Concerted Action BHM4-CT98-3936. Leukemia 21:201–206
10. GeneMapper® Software Version 4.0 Quick Reference Guide (2005) Applied Biosystems. Part Number 4362816. http://www3.appliedbiosystems.com
11. GeneMapper® Software Version 4.0 Microsatellite Analysis Getting Started Guide (2005) Applied Biosystems. Part Number 4363095 Rev. B. http://www3.appliedbiosystems.com
12. Langerak AW (2008) Undersized, oversized? It is not one-size-fits-all in lymphoid clonality detection. Leuk Res 32:203–204
13. Berget E, Helgeland L, Molven A, Vintermyr OK (2011) Detection of clonality in follicular lymphoma using formalin-fixed, paraffin-embedded tissue samples and BIOMED-2 immunoglobulin primers. J Clin Pathol 64: 37–41

Chapter 11

Detection of Clonal T-Cell Receptor Beta and Gamma Chain Gene Rearrangement by Polymerase Chain Reaction and Capillary Gel Electrophoresis

Hongxin Fan and Ryan S. Robetorye

Abstract

Although established diagnostic criteria exist for mature T-cell neoplasms, a definitive diagnosis of a T-cell lymphoproliferative disorder cannot always be obtained using more conventional techniques such as flow cytometric immunophenotyping, conventional cytogenetics, fluorescence in situ hybridization, or immunohistochemistry. However, because T-cell malignancies contain identically rearranged T-cell receptor gamma (*TCRG*) and/or beta (*TCRB*) genes, the polymerase chain reaction (PCR) can be a fast, convenient, and dependable option to identify clonal T-cell processes. This chapter describes the use of PCR and capillary electrophoresis to identify clonal *TCRB* and *TCRG* gene rearrangements (*TCRB* and *TCRG* PCR) using a commercially available method employing multiple multiplex PCR tubes that was originally developed as the result of a large European BIOMED-2 collaborative study (Invivoscribe Technologies). The core protocol for the TCRB assay involves the use of three separate multiplex master mix tubes. Tubes A and B target the framework regions within the variable and joining regions of the *TCRB* gene, and Tube C targets the diversity and joining regions of the *TCRB* gene. The core protocol for the TCRG assay utilizes two multiplex master mix tubes (Tubes A and B) that target the variable and joining regions of the *TCRG* gene. Use of the five BIOMED-2 *TCRB* and *TCRG* PCR multiplex tubes in parallel can detect approximately 94% of clonal *TCR* gene rearrangements.

Key words T-cell receptor beta and gamma genes, Clonality testing, PCR, Capillary gel electrophoresis

1 Introduction

In a significant number of suspected T-cell lymphoproliferative disorders, a definitive diagnosis of malignancy cannot be made without additional evidence of a clonal process. This evidence can sometimes be obtained using flow cytometric immunophenotyping, conventional cytogenetics, or fluorescence in situ hybridization. However, because nearly all T-cell malignancies contain identically rearranged T-cell receptor genes, clonality testing using the polymerase chain reaction (PCR) can be a fast, convenient, and dependable option to confirm the presence of clonal T-cell processes.

Magdalena Czader (ed.), *Hematological Malignancies*, Methods in Molecular Biology, vol. 999,
DOI 10.1007/978-1-62703-357-2_11, © Springer Science+Business Media New York 2013

Here, we describe utilization of the PCR and capillary gel electrophoresis to detect clonal T-cell receptor beta (*TCRB*) and T-cell receptor gamma (*TCRG*) chain gene rearrangements (*TCRB* and *TCRG* PCR). The *TCRB* and *TCRG* PCR protocols were originally developed by the Europe Against Cancer Program (BIOMED-2 protocol) (1), and now are manufactured by a commercial vendor (Invivoscribe Technologies, San Diego, CA, USA; www.Invivoscribe.com). These methods require extraction of DNA from the desired sample to be analyzed, which can originate from a variety of clinical sample types, such as bone marrow aspirate, peripheral blood, fresh (or fresh-frozen) tissue, or formalin-fixed paraffin-embedded (FFPE) tissue. The DNA can be obtained using either manual or automated DNA extraction methods. The isolated DNA then serves as a template for the standardized BIOMED-2 multiplex PCR protocols. The Invivoscribe multiplex PCR protocol for *TCRB* gene rearrangement detection (*TCRB* PCR) includes three master mix tubes that target the conserved variable (Vβ), diversity (Dβ), joining (Jβ) regions, and detects Vβ–Jβ and Dβ–Jβ rearrangements. The Invivoscribe multiplex PCR protocol for *TCRG* gene rearrangement detection (*TCRB* PCR) includes two master mix tubes that target the conserved variable (Vγ) and joining (Jγ) regions and detects Vγ–Jγ rearrangements. PCR products are analyzed by capillary gel electrophoresis using an ABI 3130*xl* Genetic Analyzer. Clonality can be established if an appropriate peak(s) is detected in any of these master mixes tubes. Use of the five BIOMED-2 *TCRB* and *TCRG* PCR multiplex tubes in parallel can detect approximately 94% of clonal *TCR* gene rearrangements (2, 3). A Specimen Control Size Ladder master mix that targets multiple genes is also included to serve as a DNA quality and quantity control for each test sample. Although the BIOMED-2 protocol also includes an additional available multiplex PCR tube for the detection of clonal T-cell receptor Delta (*TCRD*) gene rearrangements, this assay is not recommended for routine T-cell clonality studies (2, 3) and is not further discussed in this chapter (see Note 1).

2 Materials

2.1 Samples

1. Peripheral blood, bone marrow aspirate, fresh or frozen tissue, or FFPE tissue.

2.2 Sample Preparation

2.2.1 DNA Extraction from Fresh Samples

1. Gentra Puregene Blood Kit for 3 or 30 ml blood (Qiagen, Valencia, CA).
2. Gentra Puregene Tissue Kit for 100 mg tissue (Qiagen, Valencia, CA).
3. 100% isopropanol.

4. 70% ethanol.
5. 1.5 ml microcentrifuge tubes, or 15 ml centrifuge tubes.
6. Pipettes and pipette tips.
7. Liquid nitrogen.
8. Mortar and pestle.
9. General laboratory equipment, including vortex mixer, desktop centrifuge, microcentrifuge, spectrophotometer, and incubators.

2.2.2 DNA Extraction from Paraffin-Embedded Tissues

1. Fisherbrand CitriSolv Clearing Agent (Fisher Scientific Inc., Pittsburgh, PA).
2. Xylene.
3. 100% ethanol.
4. Heating block.
5. Proteinase K (20 mg/ml).
6. Gentra Puregene Cell Lysis Solution 125 ml (Qiagen, Valencia, CA).
7. Thermomixer or other similar equipment.
8. EZ1 DNA Tissue Kit (Qiagen, Valencia, CA).
9. EZ1 DNA Paraffin Section Card (Qiagen, Valencia, CA).
10. BioRobot® EZ1 workstation (Qiagen, Valencia, CA).

2.3 Multiplex PCR

1. PCR thermocycler (e.g., GeneAmp® PCR System 9700, Applied Biosystems).
2. PCR tube or PCR reaction plate (e.g., 0.2 ml MicroAmp® Reaction Tube with Cap, or MicroAmp Optical 96-well Reaction Plate with MicroAmp™ Optical 8-Cap Strip, Applied Biosystems).
3. *TCRB* Gene Clonality Assay for ABI Fluorescence Detection (Invivoscribe Technologies, San Diego, CA). The kit includes multiplex PCR master mixes and control DNA samples (see Notes 2 and 3).
4. *TCRG* Gene Clonality Assay for ABI Fluorescence Detection (Invivoscribe Technologies, San Diego, CA). The kit includes multiplex PCR master mixes and control DNA samples (see Notes 3 and 4).
5. AmpliTaq Gold DNA Polymerase at 5 units/μl (Applied Biosystems, Carlsbad, CA).
6. Nuclease-free H_2O.

2.4 Capillary Gel Electrophoresis

1. ABI 3130*xl* Genetic Analyzer with 50 cm Capillary Array (Applied Biosystems, Carlsbad, CA) (see Note 5).
2. POP-7™ Polymer for ABI 3130/3130*xl* Genetic Analyzers (Applied Biosystems, Carlsbad, CA) (see Note 5).

3. 10× Running Buffer (Applied Biosystems, Carlsbad, CA).
4. GeneScan™ 400HD ROX™ Size Standard (Applied Biosystems, Carlsbad, CA).
5. Hi-Di Formamide (Applied Biosystems, Carlsbad, CA).
6. DS-30 Matrix Standard Kit (Applied Biosystems, Carlsbad, CA).
7. MicroAmp Optical 96-well Reaction Plate (Applied Biosystems, Carlsbad, CA).

3 Methods

3.1 Sample Preparation

DNA can be extracted using either manual or automated methods based on the resources available in individual laboratories. Here, we describe a manual DNA extraction method for fresh samples using Gentra Puregene reagents, and a modified automated DNA extraction method for FFPE samples using the Qiagen EZ1 workstation and EZ1 DNA Tissue Kit (see Note 6).

3.1.1 DNA Extraction from Fresh Samples

1. DNA isolated from a variety of fresh samples may be analyzed using the *TCRB* and *TCRG* Gene Clonality Assay Kits, including bone marrow aspirate, peripheral blood, and fresh or fresh-frozen tissue.
2. Collect bone marrow (minimum 1 ml) or peripheral blood (minimum 3 ml) samples in EDTA (purple top) tubes and extract DNA using the Gentra Puregene Blood Kit for 3 or 30 ml blood (depending on sample volume) according to the manufacturer's recommendations (4).
3. Fresh tissues should be obtained in a sterile manner, and a minimum of 5 mm^3 representative tumor tissue (see Note 7) is required for molecular testing. Fresh tissue should be transported to the laboratory immediately after excision for processing, or if immediate transport is not possible, then the tissue should either be transported in RPMI 1640 culture medium, or snap-frozen in liquid nitrogen or dry ice and transported frozen.
4. Extract DNA from fresh or fresh-frozen tissues using the Gentra Puregene Tissue Kit according to the manufacturer's recommendations (4).
5. After extraction, temporarily store DNA samples at 4°C, or place at −20°C for longer term storage.
6. Measure DNA concentration using a spectrophotometer (see Note 8). Adjust the DNA concentration with nuclease-free H_2O to a concentration of 100–500 ng/μl DNA for subsequent PCR analysis (see Subheading 3.2).

3.1.2 DNA Extraction from Formalin-Fixed Paraffin-Embedded Tissues

1. Many factors can affect the quality of DNA isolated from FFPE tissues (see Note 9). Therefore, fresh or fresh-frozen tissue is recommended for optimal detection of clonal *TCRB* and *TCRG* gene rearrangements.
2. Cut one to five 10-μm-thick sections containing representative tumor (see Note 7) from each FFPE tissue block (e.g., lymph nodes, skin biopsies, gastrointestinal biopsies, or other tissues) using a clean microtome, and place in 1.5 ml microcentrifuge tubes (see Note 10). For fine-needle aspirates or other very small biopsy samples, up to ten sections may be required to obtain sufficient DNA for subsequent clonality testing.
3. Extract the DNA from FFPE tissue samples using the EZ1 DNA Tissue Kit and the EZ1 DNA Paraffin Section Card along with important modifications (see Note 11) involving extra deparaffinization steps using CitriSolv or xylene and the Gentra Puregene Cell Lysis Solution instead of the G2 buffer supplied in the EZ1 DNA Tissue Kit.
4. Add 1 ml of CitriSolv or xylene to each tube containing paraffin sections and mix the tubes by gentle vortexing for 5–10 s.
5. Incubate the tubes at room temperature for 10 min.
6. Pellet the tissue by centrifugation at full speed for 10 min and discard the supernatant.
7. Add 1 ml of 100% ethanol to each tube and mix by inverting the tubes.
8. Pellet tissue by microcentrifugation at full speed for 10 min and discard the supernatant.
9. Repeat the ethanol wash one additional time, and after the last wash, remove as much supernatant as possible.
10. Open the tubes and evaporate the residual ethanol by incubation in a heating block at 56°C for 15–30 min, or until the samples are completely dry.
11. Add 190 μl of Gentra Puregene Cell Lysis Solution and 10 μl of proteinase K (20 mg/ml) solution to the dried sample.
12. Close tubes and incubate at 56°C overnight or up to 72 h (see Note 12) with continuous vigorous mixing (e.g., in a thermomixer) until the samples are completely lysed.
13. After incubation, centrifuge the samples at full speed for 5 min, and then transfer the supernatant to new 2 ml sample tubes.
14. Process supernatant (containing raw DNA) on the BioRobot® EZ1 workstation using the EZ1 DNA Tissue Kit along with the EZ1 DNA Paraffin Section Card according to the manufacturer's instructions (5). Use a starting sample volume of 200 μl; if the sample volume from above step is less than 200 μl, Gentra Puregene Cell Lysis Solution should be added to 200 μl

total volume. The final elution volume from the BioRobot® EZ1 workstation is 50 μl.

15. After extraction, store the DNA sample temporarily at 4°C (see Note 13) or at −20°C for longer term storage until ready to proceed with subsequent multiplex PCR.
16. Measure DNA concentration using a spectrophotometer. DNA recovery from FFPE samples varies widely from sample to sample (see Note 14). Adjust DNA concentration in nuclease-free H_2O, and use 100–500 ng of DNA (see Notes 14 and 18) for each subsequent multiplex PCR.

3.2 Multiplex PCR

In this chapter, we describe multiplex *TCRB*, *TCRG*, and Specimen Control Size Ladder PCR using the Invivoscribe Technologies core protocols that target the variable and joining regions and diversity and joining regions of the *TCRB* gene and the variable and joining regions of the *TCRG* gene for the identification of clonal *TCRB* and *TCRG* gene rearrangements (see Note 1).

1. Remove reagents and patient samples from freezer and/or refrigerator. Thaw, if necessary, and keep samples cool on wet ice.
2. For *TCRB* PCR, prepare four multiplex PCR master mixes (Tubes A, B, C, and specimen control size ladder tube) and adjust master mix volumes based on the total number of samples that will be analyzed—45 μl of master mix and 0.45 μl of AmpliTaq Gold DNA Polymerase for Tubes A and B, and 45 μl of master mix and 0.25 μl of AmpliTaq Gold DNA Polymerase to Tube C and the Specimen Control Size Ladder tube.
3. For *TCRG* PCR, prepare three multiplex PCR master mixes (Tubes A, B, and Specimen Control Size Ladder) and adjust master mix volumes based on the total number of samples that will be analyzed—to each PCR reaction, add 45 μl of master mix and 0.25 μl of AmpliTaq Gold DNA Polymerase.
4. For both *TCRB* and *TCRG* PCR reactions, pipette 45 μl of master mix to each reaction tube (or to each well, if using 96-well plate) and then add 5 μl of patient or control DNA (equivalent DNA amount 100–500 ng) to appropriate tubes or wells. In each run, at least three controls should be included for each master mix (see Subheading 3.4 for additional details).
5. Cap tubes or cover reaction plate with optical 8-cap strip and load tubes or plate on to PCR thermal cycler. An example analysis with four multiplex *TCRB* PCR reactions for two patient samples is illustrated in Table 1.
6. Perform *TCRB* and *TCRG* multiplex PCR reactions using the following thermal cycling conditions: 95°C for 7 min; then, 34 cycles of 95°C for 45 s, 60°C for 45 s, and 72°C for 90 s. The final elongation step should be 72°C for 10 min; and then

Table 1
***TCRB* multiplex PCR setup**

Master mix			
Tube A	**Tube B**	**Tube C**	**Specimen control**
Sample 1	Sample 1	Sample 1	Sample 1
Sample 1	Sample 1	Sample 1	
Sample 2	Sample 2	Sample 2	Sample 2
Sample 2	Sample 2	Sample 2	
10% Clonal control	10% Clonal control	10% Clonal control	10% Clonal control
Polyclonal control	Polyclonal control	Polyclonal control	Polyclonal control
No template control	No template control	No template control	No template control

hold the temperature at 15°C until tubes or plates are removed from the thermal cycler.

3.3 Capillary Gel Electrophoresis

Multiplex PCR products are fractionated and analyzed using an ABI 3130*xl* Genetic Analyzer (see Notes 5 and 15).

1. Set up denature reaction: add 20 μl of HI-DI Formamide, 0.5 μl of Size Standard GS 400HD ROX, and 1.0 μl of PCR product into each well of a 96-well plate. Heat to 95°C for 2 min and then quick-chill on ice for 5 min.
2. Load sample plate on the ABI 3130*xl* and set up the plate in the Data Collection Software according to the manufacturer's instructions (6, 7). Briefly, power on the 3130*xl* instrument and attached computer. Open the Data Collection Software; create and save a *TCRB* or *TCRG* plate record, select run module Spect50_POP7 and Dye Set D (DS-30 Matrix Standards) (see Note 5), and load the sample plate onto the instrument.
3. Operate the instrument according to the manufacturer's instructions (6, 7) by selecting the desired plate record. Link the plate position indicator to the corresponding plate position in the instrument, and run the plate.
4. Data are automatically collected by the Data Collection Software on the ABI 3130*xl* instrument and are analyzed using GeneMapper Analysis Software. After completion of the run, open the GeneMapper Analysis Software and analyze the data according to manufacturer's instructions (see Note 16).

5. View the results of the analysis by selecting Display Plots and choosing the desired wells for each sample. Adjust the viewing scale by setting vertical and horizontal parameters according to PCR product size and print the results.

3.4 Quality Control

1. DNA integrity should be monitored for each test sample by including a separate tube for Specimen Control Size Ladder PCR.
2. Multiple controls should be included in each run for each master mix (see Table 1 for examples), including: (1) Clonal and sensitivity controls comprised of a 10% or a 5% mixture of clonal *TCRB* or *TCRG* gene DNA, respectively, diluted with polyclonal control DNA for each master mix tube (see Note 17). These controls monitor assay sensitivity and mimic clinical specimens in which clonal cells are present along with normal background cells. (2) Polyclonal control DNA samples as supplied in the *TCRB* and *TCRG* Gene Clonality Assay Kits. Polyclonal controls help to establish the PCR product size range for each specific master mix. (3) Blank or no DNA template control consisting of master mix and nuclease-free H_2O to monitor for possible sample contamination.
3. Replicate samples should be included for *TCRB* or *TCRG* multiplex PCR. You can use identical or different DNA concentration for replicates (see Note 18). Consistent peak patterns should be obtained from replicate samples.

3.5 Result Interpretation

1. The interpretation of *TCRB* and *TCRG* PCR assay results should include examination of the technical aspects of each assay as well as all available clinical information. Technical aspects include appropriate positive, negative, and reagent controls in each run, patient sample DNA quantity and quality, and replicate master mix tube results. *TCRB and TCRG* PCR results should also be interpreted in the context of available clinical information, tissue morphology, and other laboratory test results such as immunophenotype and cytogenetics. In select instances such as cutaneous T-cell lymphomas, a comparison of the results of *TCRB* and *TCRG* PCR assays from different sites (two different skin biopsies) may be helpful.
2. The reagent (no template) controls (Fig. 1a) should not display any peaks in any of the master mix tubes—the presence of any peaks in these tubes indicates a possible contamination problem, and the assay should be repeated. The polyclonal (negative) controls should show a bell-shaped peak distribution (Gaussian distribution) pattern (Fig. 1b, c), and the clonal (positive) controls should exhibit a narrow (one to two base pair) dominant peak, with or without a bell-shaped polyclonal peak background (Fig. 1d, e).

a

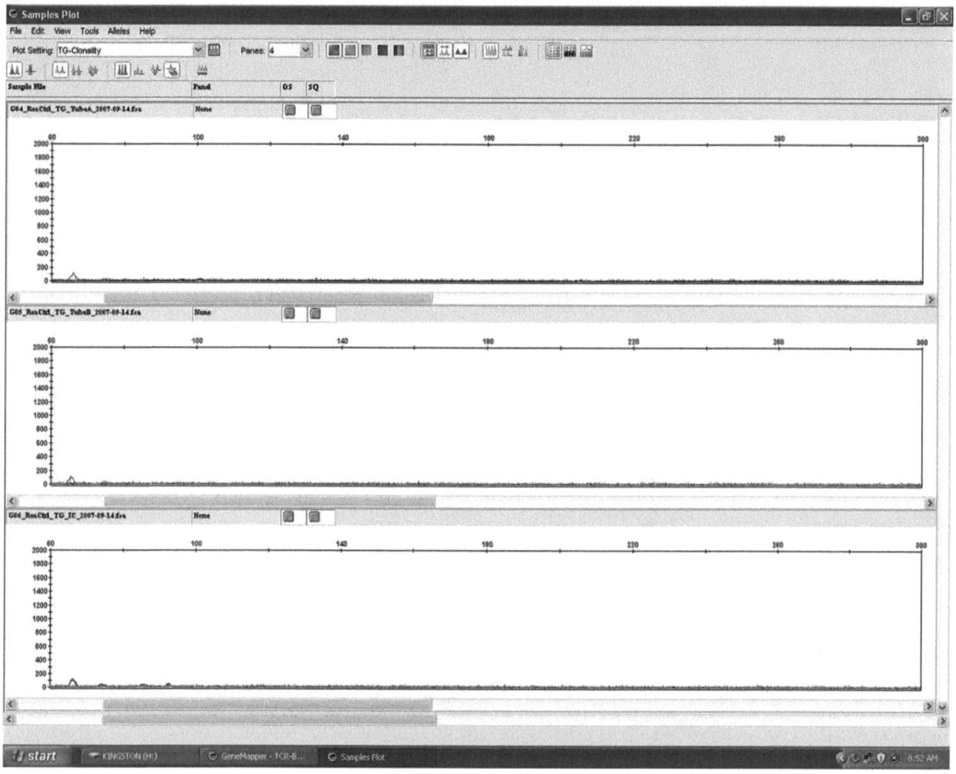

Fig. 1 Examples of results for reagent, negative, positive, and specimen DNA size ladder controls. (**a**) Reagent (no template) control for *TCRG* PCR. (**b**) Negative (polyclonal) control for *TCRB* PCR. (**c**) Negative (polyclonal) control for *TCRG* PCR. (**d**) Positive (clonal) control for *TCRB* PCR. (**e**) Positive (clonal) control for *TCRG* PCR. (**f**) Fully intact specimen DNA size ladder control. (**g**) Acceptable sample for analysis with DNA size ladder control with peaks at least 300 bp in length. (**h**) Unacceptable (degraded) sample with DNA size ladder control with peaks less than 300 bp in length

3. The specimen control size ladder PCR products have a range from approximately 100–600 bp in a sample with intact DNA (Fig. 1f) (see Note 19). Samples with amplicons larger than 300 bp in size in the specimen control size ladder PCR tube are considered to have good quality DNA (Fig. 1g). Samples with amplicons smaller than 300 bp in size in the specimen control size ladder usually indicate DNA degradation, especially in FFPE tissue samples (Fig. 1h).
4. Verify that polyclonal and positive control sample amplified products are consistent with expected amplicon sizes. Expected amplicon size information is found in the *TCRB* and *TCRG* Gene Clonality Assay Kit inserts (8, 9) (see Note 20).
5. Evaluate patient sample results using the same expected amplicon size criteria as for the controls (see Note 21).
6. One or two prominent peaks in the valid size range should be considered evidence of the presence of a clonal T-cell receptor

b

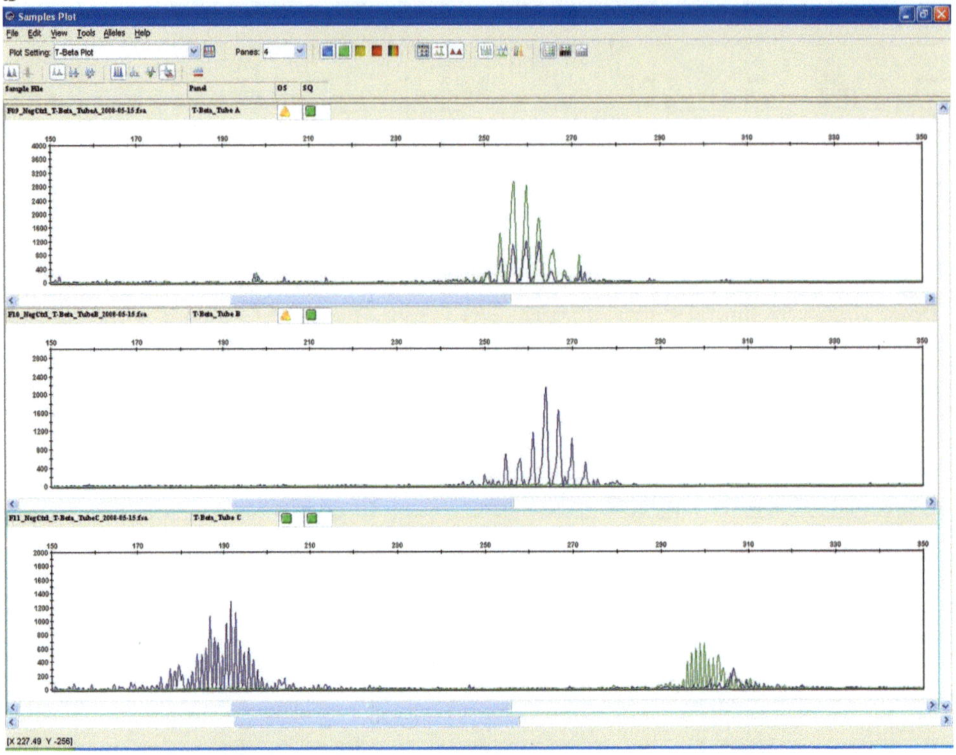

c

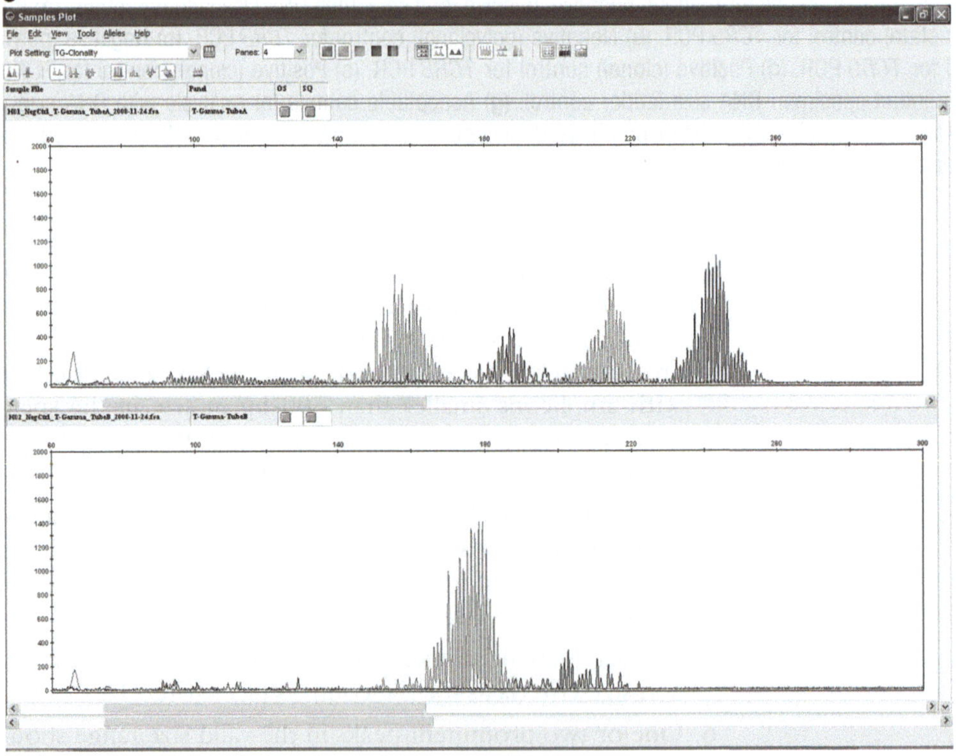

Fig. 1 (continued)

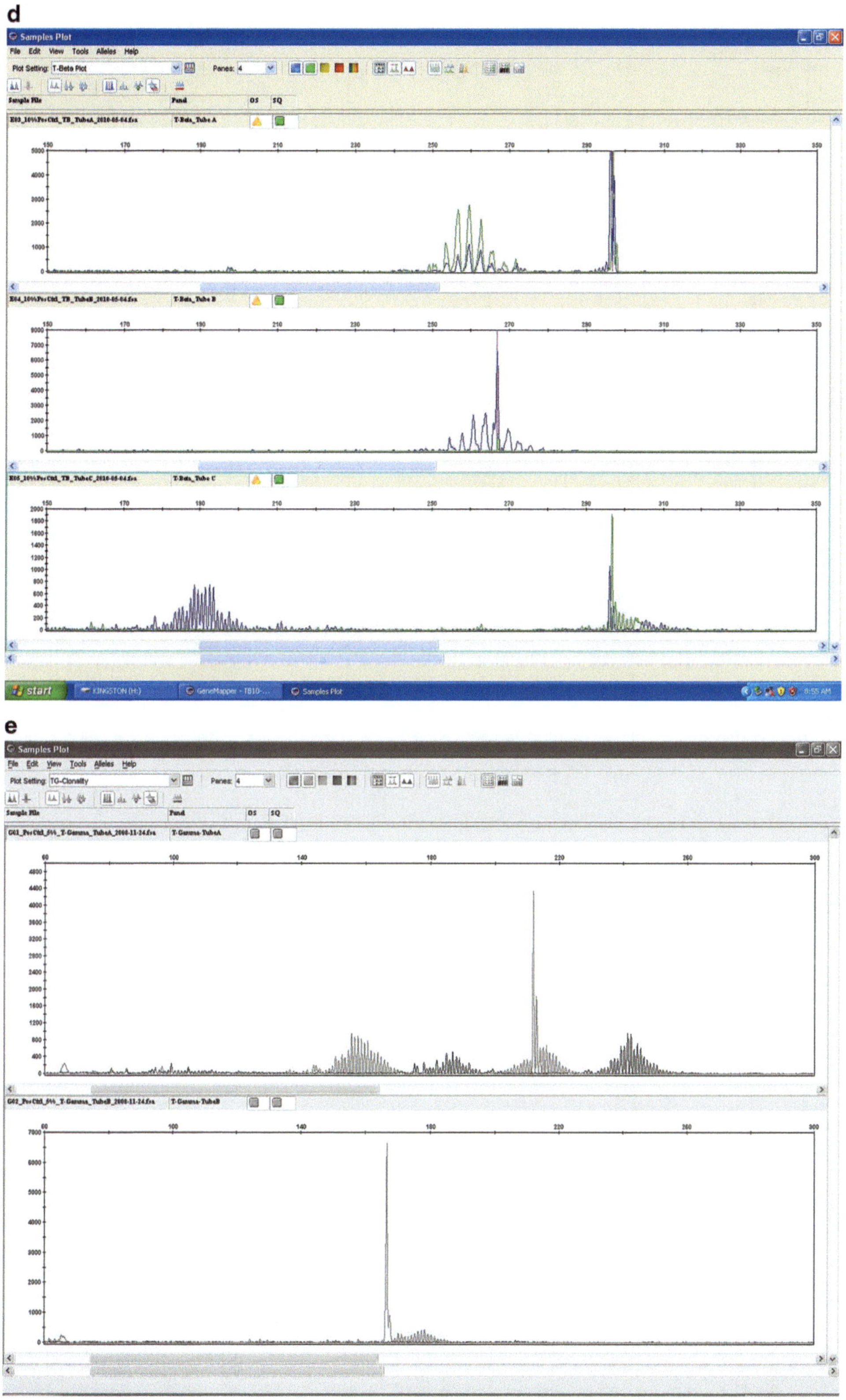

Fig. 1 (continued)

f

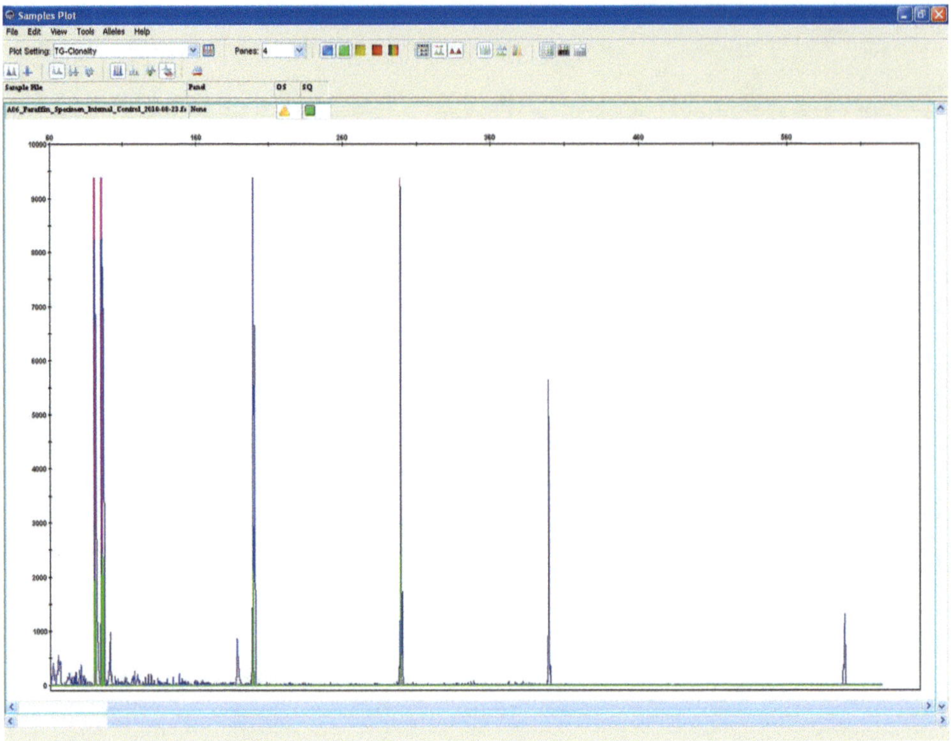

g

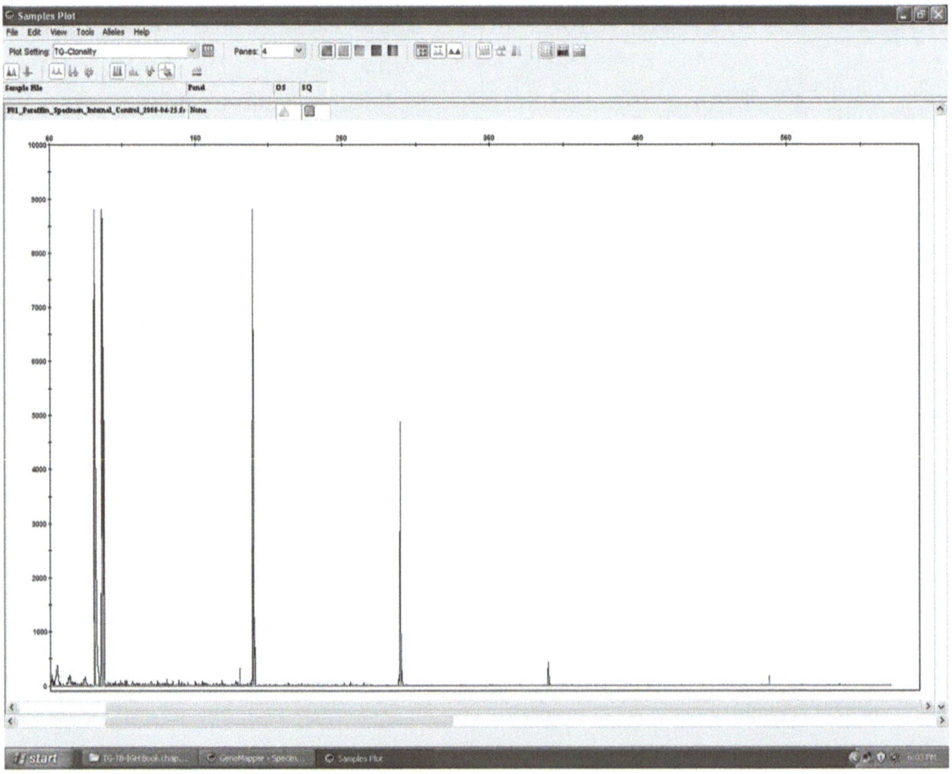

Fig. 1 (continued)

h

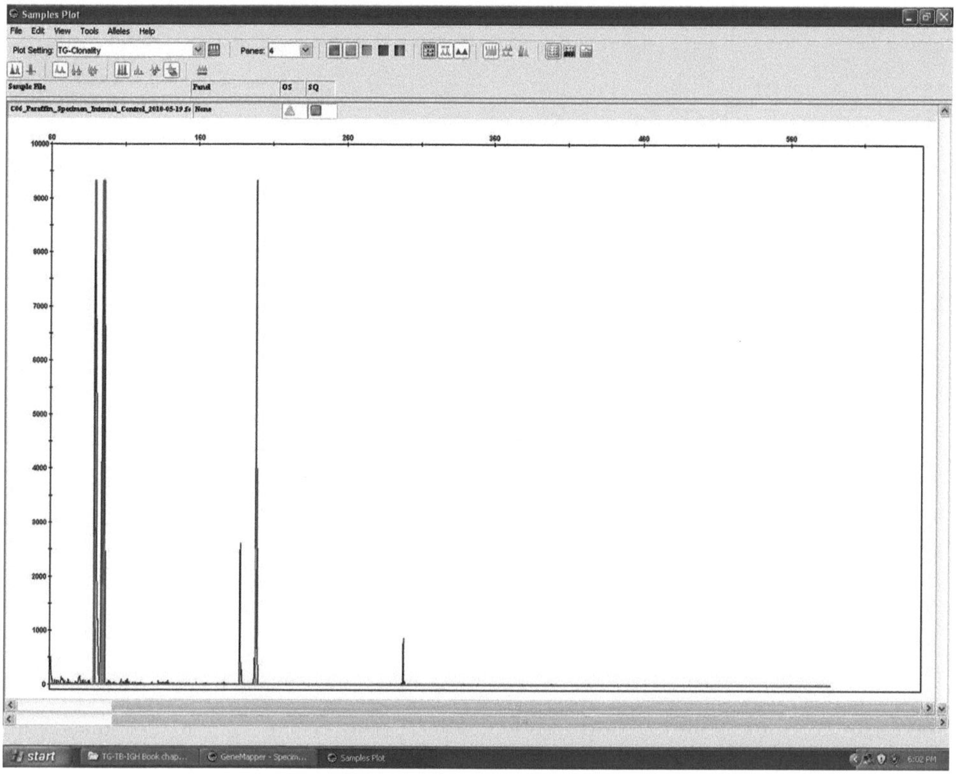

beta or gamma chain gene rearrangement (see Note 22). Replicate patient samples should produce similar *TCRB* or *TCRG* gene amplification peak patterns. If a clonal peak is seen, the peak should be of identical size (in base pairs) and exhibit a similar peak height in replicate samples. In biallelic or biclonal samples, two or more clonal peaks may be present in a single patient sample (3).

7. Clonal peak heights may vary in size (see Note 23). Pseudoclonal peaks are relative common in *TCRB* and *TCRG* assays, and appropriate caution should be exercised when interpreting these results (see Note 24). Examples of clonal *TCRB* and *TCRG* results are shown in Fig. 2a, b.
8. The BIOMED-2 *TCRB* or *TCRG* multiplex PCR protocols are able to detect about 91% or 89% of T-cell malignancies, respectively, according to a BIOMED-2 study. If both assays are used in combination, the clonality detection rate can be increased to 94% (see Note 1) (2, 3). However, lower detection rates have been reported for FFPE skin biopsy samples of cutaneous T-cell lymphomas (10).

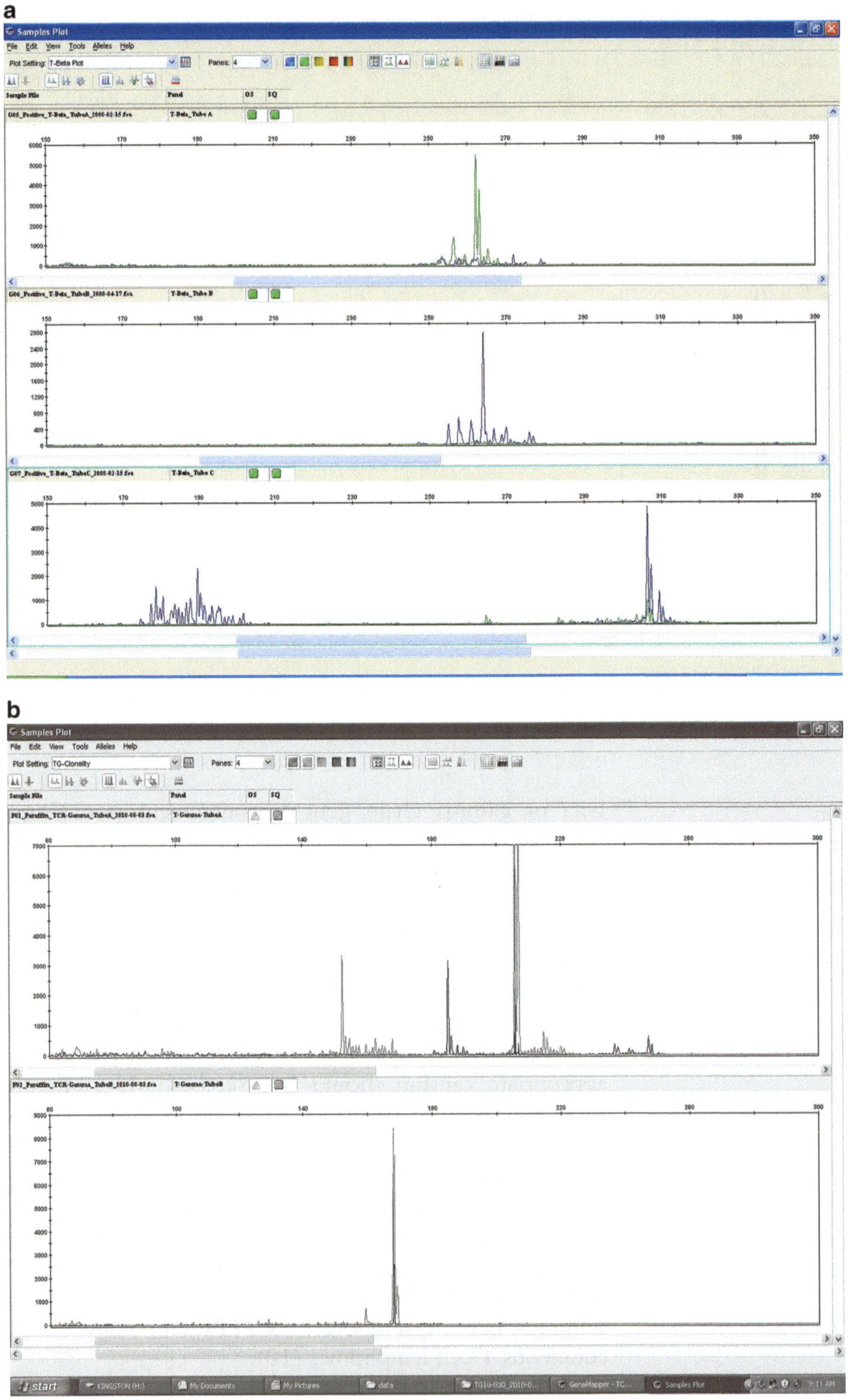

Fig. 2 Examples of positive (clonal) results for *TCRB* and *TCRG* PCR. (**a**) Positive *TCRB* PCR result. (**b**) Positive *TCRG* PCR result

9. The detection of clonal rearrangement of the *TCRB* and/or *TCRG* genes is highly suggestive of malignancy, but should not be used as the sole criterion for diagnosis of a lymphoid neoplasm, as clonal *TCRB* or *TCRG* rearrangements are not exclusively detected in malignancies (11, 12). In addition, *TCRB* or *TCRG* clonality can help to identify cell lineage and to exclude morphologically and immunophenotypically overlapping NK-cell malignancies, but the presence of a T-cell clone does not always indicate T-cell lineage (11–13).

4 Notes

1. The BIOMED-2 protocol also includes a multiplex PCR reaction tube for the detection of TCR Delta (*TCRD*) gene rearrangements. In the BIOMED-2 study, utilization of *TCRB* or *TCRG* clonality detection assays allowed detection of 91% and 89% of T-cell malignancies, respectively. If the *TCRB* and *TCRG* PCR assays are used in combination, the detection rate can be increased to 94% (2, 3). Use of a *TCRD* rearrangement assay adds value for the detection of clonal immature T-cell and TCRγδ+T-cell proliferations but is not recommended for routine T-cell clonality studies (2, 3). Please refer to original BIOMED-2 publications for a detailed protocol and test strategy (1–3). Note that the BIOMED-2 study used only fresh or fresh frozen tissue samples for analysis. TCR clonality detection rates are likely to be lower if fixed FFPE tissues are analyzed.
2. Four master mix tubes are provided in the *TCRB* Gene Clonality Assay Kit. Tubes A and B target the Vβ, Jβ1 and Jβ2 regions of the *TCRB* gene, and Tube C targets the Dβ and Jβ regions. A fourth master mix tube consists of a Specimen Control Size Ladder that targets multiple genes to generate a series of amplicons from approximately 100–600 bp in length to serve as a DNA quality and quantity control.
3. Prior to use, all the master mixes tubes contained in the *TCRB* and *TCRG* Gene Clonality Assay Kits should be aliquoted to convenient volumes for one-time use and stored at −80°C. In addition, the master mix tubes should not be subjected to repeated freeze-thaw cycles. The *TCRB* and *TCRG* Gene Clonality Assay Kits also include clonal and polyclonal control DNAs for use in the assays; these controls should be used as recommended by the manufacturer.
4. Three master mix tubes are provided in the *TCRG* Gene Clonality Assay Kit. Tubes A and B target four Vγ genes and all Jγ regions of the *TCRG* gene. A third master mix tube consists of a Specimen Control Size Ladder that targets multiple genes to generate a

series of amplicons from approximately 100–600 bp in length to serve as a DNA quality and quantity control.

5. In this chapter, we describe the use of the ABI 3130*xl* Genetic Analyzer equipped with a 50 cm capillary array and POP-7 polymer as an example system that works well with the *TCRB* and *TCRG* Gene Clonality Assay Kits in our molecular diagnostics laboratory. However, different capillary gel electrophoresis systems may also perform just as well for this purpose in other laboratories.

6. Other DNA extraction methods can also be used as long as adequate DNA quality and quantity is maintained. The automated extraction system we use in our laboratory (BioRobot® EZ1 workstation, Qiagen) can process only low volume (200–350 μl) blood samples. For larger volume fresh samples, we use a manual extraction method (Gentra Puregene reagents) for DNA isolation. For FFPE samples, we use the EZ1 instrument for DNA isolation. We have found that the *TCRB* and *TCRG* Gene Clonality Assay Kits perform best if DNA isolated from FFPE samples is as pure as possible.

7. Samples that contain representative tumor tissue should be collected for analysis. It is recommended that the tumor cell load should be greater than 15% for the *TCRB* and *TCRG* Gene Clonality Assay Kits.

8. Our laboratory uses a NanoDrop 1000 Spectrophotometer (Thermo Fisher Scientific, Wilmington, DE) to quantitate DNA samples prior to adjusting the concentration for subsequent PCR analysis because only one microliter of sample is required for quantitation without prior dilution.

9. Many factors affect DNA quality in FFPE tissues such as fixative type and fixation time. Some FFPE tissues are unacceptable for molecular studies, such as those fixed in Zenker's, B5, or Bouin's fixatives, as well as formic acid decalcified bone marrow biopsy samples. These fixatives/procedures can produce extensive degradation of DNA, making their use inappropriate for molecular studies.

10. When sectioning FFPE tissue blocks for molecular studies, special precautions should be followed to avoid carry-over DNA contamination from previously cut samples. These precautions may include using new microtome blades for each sample, or cleaning the microtome with xylene and 100% ethanol between samples.

11. For FFPE tissue sections, we do not perform paraffin trimming steps as recommended in the EZ1 DNA Tissue Kit instructions, but rather perform extra deparaffinization steps instead. Paraffin can be completely removed by using either CitriSolv or xylene, and will not interfere with subsequent extraction steps.

Also, according to our own validation study, Gentra Puregene Cell Lysis Solution tended to produce better results than the G2 buffer supplied in the EZ1 DNA Tissue Kit.

12. Addition of Gentra Puregene Cell Lysis Solution and/or proteinase K is based on relative sample size and sample type. Samples with relatively large amounts of tissue should be resuspended in more than 200 μl lysis solution with proportional increases in the amount of proteinase K added. For tissue samples that are more difficult to digest, proteinase K concentration can be increased or incubation times can be increased as needed. For example, for skin tissue FFPE samples, we routinely perform a 48–72 h proteinase K incubation step.
13. Compared to genomic DNA isolated from fresh samples or fresh-frozen samples, the DNA isolated from FFPE samples is more prone to degradation. DNA isolated from FFPE samples should be aliquoted in volumes sufficient for one-time use. Remaining DNA aliquots should be stored at -20°C, and repeated freeze-thaw cycles should be avoided.
14. DNA recovery from FFPE samples can vary widely from sample to sample, ranging from as little as a few nanograms up to several hundred nanograms per microliter. We recommend using 100–500 ng of DNA for each multiplex PCR. However, even very small amounts of input DNA can sometimes produce analyzable PCR products as long as the specimen control DNA indicates good DNA quality, and multiplex *TCRB* and *TCRG* PCR assays produce a clonal peak(s) or an appropriate polyclonal peak distribution. It should also be noted that low input DNA concentrations may result in false clonal results due to restricted PCR amplification of only a few T-cells (see Note 24); however, replicate samples usually show different capillary electrophoresis peak patterns.
15. Capillary gel electrophoresis (GeneScanning) and heteroduplex analysis can also be used for analyzing *TCRB* and *TCRG* PCR products. We confine our discussion to the capillary gel electrophoresis technique in this chapter. Heteroduplex analysis may be considered if analysis *TCRB* or *TCRG* PCR product composition and conformation is desired (1). Please note that for heteroduplex analysis there is no need to use fluorochrome-labeled PCR primers.
16. Please refer to GeneMapper® Software Version 4.0 Quick Reference Guide (14) for additional information on how to use the GeneMapper Software. We use the Microsatellite setting for multiplex *TCRB* and *TCRG* PCR analysis (15).
17. Assay sensitivity may differ for each master mix and for different analysis systems. In our molecular diagnostics laboratory, assay sensitivities range from 1–10% to 1–5% for *TCRB* and

TCRG assays, respectively, when testing different master mixes and clonal DNA control samples. Therefore, we use mixtures of 10% clonal *TCRB* gene DNA diluted with polyclonal DNA, and 5% clonal *TCRG* gene DNA diluted with polyclonal DNA, as clonal and sensitivity controls for *TCRB* and *TCRG* assays, respectively. However, assay sensitivities must be determined in each individual laboratory, and appropriate sensitivity controls should be included in each analysis.

18. For DNA extracted from fresh or fresh-frozen samples, identical DNA concentrations may be used for replicate testing. For DNA extracted from FFPE samples, it may be useful to perform replicate testing with one tube of the original DNA solution and additional tubes with diluted DNA (e.g., 1:5 or 1:10 diluted DNA) in order to overcome the effects of possible PCR inhibitors. However, our assay validation study has shown that EZ1 extraction of FFPE samples usually produces DNA of sufficient purity for subsequent *TCRB* and *TCRB* PCR analysis, so that no DNA dilution step is required.
19. The specimen control size ladder PCR products should be 84, 96, 200, 300, 400, and 600 bp in length in a sample with intact DNA (see Fig. 1f).
20. The expected amplicon sizes listed in the *TCRB* and *TCRG* PCR Clonality Kit inserts were determined using an ABI 3100 Genetic Analyzer. Amplicon sizes observed on different capillary electrophoresis instruments may differ from 1 to 4 nucleotides from those listed in the inserts. However, once the expected sizes have been determined, the amplicon sizes should be consistent from run to run.
21. Amplicons outside of expected size ranges may represent actual rearranged clones, but such clones should be confirmed by DNA sequencing (11).
22. The BIOMED-2 multiplex PCR approach has become a standard protocol for identification of TCR clonality detection. The TCRB and TCRG Gene Clonality Assay Kit inserts recommend that amplicons generated from diagnostic samples that fall within the valid size range and that are at least three times the size of the third largest peak in the polyclonal background be considered clonal peaks (8, 9). Guidelines for interpretation and reporting of Ig/TCR clonality testing have also been recently published (16). However, criteria for determining clonality should be established in each individual laboratory. For example, in our molecular diagnostics laboratory, we found that amplicons generated from diagnostic samples that fell within the valid size range and that were at least three times the size of the second largest peak in the polyclonal background were the most reliable criteria for indentifying clonal peaks in our specific patient population.

23. Peak heights may be of variable size in different samples. Peak height is relatively proportional to percentage of tumor cells in a specific sample, but it cannot be reliably used for estimation of tumor burden. Peak height ratio calculations may be helpful for identification of clonality in some difficult cases (17–19), but these results should be correlated with available clinical information.

24. Pseudoclonal peaks may result from restricted amplification of small numbers of T-cells in the test sample. Small T-cell populations (or small amounts of T-cell DNA) may be present due to the following: (1) limited specimen volume (e.g., fine needle aspiration and small core biopsy samples), (2) small amounts of DNA or degraded DNA (e.g., DNA from FFPE samples), (3) limited normal T-cell rearrangements (see Note 14), or (4) the presence of only a few reactive T-cells in the sample, or the presence of subclonal reactive T-cells from a site of active infection. In addition, we have reported clonal *TCRB* and *TCRG* rearrangements in peripheral blood samples obtained from normal blood donors (20–21). These findings stress the importance of interpreting clonal results in the appropriate clinical context.

Acknowledgments

The authors would like to thank Kumari Vadlamudi for her excellent technical assistance.

References

1. van Dongen JJ, Langerak AW, Brüggemann M, Evans PA, Hummel M, Lavender FL et al (2003) Design and standardization of PCR primers and protocols for detection of clonal immunoglobulin and T-cell receptor gene recombinations in suspect lymphoproliferations: report of the BIOMED-2 Concerted Action BMH4-CT98-3936. Leukemia 17: 2257–2317
2. van Krieken JH, Langerak AW, Macintyre EA, Kneba M, Hodges E, Sanz RG et al (2007) Improved reliability of lymphoma diagnostics via PCR-based clonality testing: report of the BIOMED-2 Concerted Action BHM4-CT98-3936. Leukemia 21:201–206
3. Brüggemann M, White H, Gaulard P, Garcia-Sanz R, Gameiro P, Oeschger S et al (2007) Powerful strategy for polymerase chain reaction-based clonality assessment in T-cell malignancies Report of the BIOMED-2 Concerted Action BHM4 CT98-3936. Leukemia 21:215–221
4. Gentra® Puregene® Handbook. For purification of archive-quality DNA from human whole blood, bone marrow, buffy coat, buccal cells, body fluids, cultured cells, tissue, mouse tail, yeast, bacteria (June 2011) Qiagen. Third Edition. http://www.qiagen.com/literature
5. EZ1® DNA Handbook. For EZ1 DNA Blood 200 μl Kit and EZ1 DNA Blood 350 μl Kit (April 2010) Qiagen. http://www.qiagen.com/literature
6. Applied Biosystems 3130/3130*xl* Genetic Analyzers Getting Started Guide (2004) Applied Biosystems. Part number 4352715 Rev. B. http://www3.appliedbiosystems.com
7. Applied Biosystems 3130/3130*xl* Genetic Analyzers Maintenance, Troubleshooting and Reference Guide (2004) Applied Biosystems. Part number 4352716 Rev. B. http://www3.appliedbiosystems.com
8. *TCRB* Gene Clonality Assay Kit insert. Invivoscribe Technologies. http://catalog.invivoscribe.com
9. *TCRG* Gene Clonality Assay Kit insert. Invivoscribe Technologies. http://catalog.invivoscribe.com

10. Lukowsky A, Muche JM, Mobs M, Assaf C, Humme D, Hummel M et al (2010) Evaluation of T-cell clonality in archival skin biopsy samples of cutaneous T-cell lymphomas using the Biomed-2 PCR Protocol. Diagn Mol Pathol 19:70–77
11. Langerak AW (2008) Undersized, oversized? It is not one-size-fits-all in lymphoid clonality detection. Leuk Res 32:203–204
12. Langerak AW, Molina TJ, Lavender FL, Pearson D, Flohr T, Sambade C et al (2007) Polymerase chain reaction-based clonality testing in tissue samples with reactive lymphoproliferations: usefulness and pitfalls. A report of the BIOMED-2 Concerted Action BMH4-CT98-3936. Leukemia 21:222–229
13. Evans PA, Pott C, Groenen PJ, Salles G, Davi F, Berger F et al (2007) Significantly improved PCR-based clonality testing in B-cell malignancies by use of multiple immunoglobulin gene targets. Report of the BIOMED-2 Concerted Action BHM4-CT98-3936. Leukemia 21:207–214
14. GeneMapper® Software Version 4.0 Quick Reference Guide (2005) Applied Biosystems. Part Number 4362816. http://www3.appliedbiosystems.com
15. GeneMapper® Software Version 4.0 Microsatellite Analysis Getting Started Guide (2005) Applied Biosystems. Part Number 4363095 Rev. B. http://www3.appliedbiosystems.com
16. Langerak AW, Groenen PJ, Brüggemann M, Beldjord K, Bellan C, Bonello L et al (2012) EuroClonality/BIOMED-2 guidelines for interpretation and reporting of Ig/TCR clonality testing in suspected lymphoproliferations. Leukemia 26(10):2159–2171
17. Lee SC, Berg KD, Racke FK, Griffin CA, Eshleman JR (2000) Pseudo-spikes are common in histologically benign lymphoid tissues. J Mol Diagn 2:145–152
18. Greiner TC, Rubocki RJ (2002) Effectiveness of capillary electrophoresis using fluorescent-labeled primers in detecting T-cell receptor gamma gene rearrangements. J Mol Diagn 4:137–143, Erratum in: J Mol Diagn. 2003 Aug;5(3):195
19. Kuo FC, Hall D, Longtine JA (2007) A novel method for interpretation of T-cell receptor gamma gene rearrangement assay by capillary gel electrophoresis based on normal distribution. J Mol Diagn 9:12–19
20. Beyer GM, Vadlamudi K, Robetorye RS, Ehsan A, Wang Y, Cho C et al (2007) Detection of clonal T-cell receptor gamma gene rearrangements in peripheral blood sample from normal blood donors using *TCRG* gene clonality (BIOMED-2) and T cell receptor gamma gene rearrangement kits. J Mol Diagn 9:664, Abstract
21. Fulton RL, Vadlamudi K, Robetorye RS, Wang Y, Cho C, Fan H (2008) Detection of clonal T-cell receptor beta gene rearrangements in peripheral blood samples from normal blood donors using the Invivoscribe *TCRB* gene clonality (BIOMED-2) assay. J Mol Diagn 10:576, Abstract

Chapter 12

Detection of Genetic Translocations in Lymphoma Using Fluorescence In Situ Hybridization

Kaaren K. Reichard and Sheldon Robinett

Abstract

Certain lymphoma types are characterized by recurring genetic translocations. Detection of these translocations enables confirmation of a suspected diagnosis and provides a genetic marker which can be subsequently monitored and followed. Rapid and reliable identification of these molecular rearrangements is a key component in the workup of lymphoma. While conventional cytogenetics may be a useful tool in this regard, fluorescence in situ hybridization (FISH) offers additional advantages including the ability to use formalin-fixed tissues, no requirement for dividing cells, ability to score many cells, improved sensitivity, and faster turnaround time for results.

Key words Lymphoma, Translocation, FISH

1 Introduction

Recurring genetic translocations are hallmark features of a variety of lymphomas (Table 1) (1, 2). These translocations can be detected via conventional cytogenetic methods, although in routine clinical practice FISH is more practical, more sensitive and specific, and does not require fresh tumor cells (3–5). Identification of these molecular events provides valuable insight into lymphoma pathogenesis but also allows for the confirmation of a suspected diagnosis in an otherwise diagnostically challenging case. Compared with PCR-based molecular techniques, FISH is generally more sensitive in identifying the presence of these genetic alterations (3, 6).

The identification of certain recurring genetic translocations aids in the confirmation of a suspected lymphoma diagnosis and also allows for more sensitive minimal residual testing if required. The *IGH@-BCL2* fusion, associated with the cytogenetic finding of t(14;18)(q32;q21), is detected in 85–90% of follicular lymphomas. Particularly with small or suboptimal biopsies, detection of this fusion may be the final piece of data required to confidently establish the morphologic diagnosis. Importantly however, it must

Magdalena Czader (ed.), *Hematological Malignancies*, Methods in Molecular Biology, vol. 999,
DOI 10.1007/978-1-62703-357-2_12, © Springer Science+Business Media New York 2013

Table 1
Selected recurring translocations in lymphomas

Translocation	Genes involved	Lymphoma type	FISH probe detection strategy	Comments/caveats
t(14;18)(q32;q21)	*IGH@*, *BCL2*	Follicular lymphoma	Dual color, dual fusion	Subset of DLBCL "double-hit" lymphomas
t(11;14)(q13;q32)	*CCND1*, *IGH@*	Mantle cell lymphoma	Dual color, dual fusion	Subset of myeloma
t(11;18)(q22;q21)	*BIRC3*, *MALT1*	Subset of gastric MALT	Dual color, dual fusion	Subset of pulmonary MALT
t(v;2p23)	*ALK*	Anaplastic large cell lymphoma, ALK positive	Break-apart probe	Subset of DLBCL, inflammatory myofibroblastic tumor, lung carcinoma
t(8;14)(q24;q32)	*MYC*, *IGH@*	Burkitt lymphoma	Tricolor, dual fusion	Subset of transformed lymphomas, myeloma, "double-hit" lymphoma
t(2;8)(p11.2;q24)	*IGK@*, *MYC*		Break-apart (*MYC*)	
t(8;22)(q24;q11.2)	*MYC*, *IGL@*			

DLBCL diffuse large B-cell lymphoma, *FISH* fluorescence in situ hybridization, *MALT* extranodal marginal zone lymphoma of mucosa-associated lymphoid tissue

be recalled that the *IGH@-BCL2* fusion is also seen in a subset of de novo diffuse large B-cell lymphomas (approximately 25%) and double-hit lymphomas. Thus, the identification of this fusion in isolation cannot be used to establish a diagnosis without appropriate morphologic and clinical data.

The *CCND1-IGH@* fusion, associated with the cytogenetic finding of t(11;14)(q13;q32), is the molecular hallmark of mantle cell lymphoma. Only very rare cases are reported to be *CCND1-IGH@* negative. As mentioned before with the *IGH@-BCL2* fusion, the detection of this molecular abnormality does not automatically confer a diagnosis of mantle cell lymphoma in the absence of appropriate morphologic, laboratory, and/or immunophenotypic data. The *CCND1-IGH@* fusion is also present in approximately 25% of plasma cell myeloma cases.

A fusion product of the *MYC* gene (8q24) with an immunoglobulin gene [*IGH@* (14q32), *IGK@* (2p11.2), *IGL@* (22q11.2)] is the hallmark of Burkitt lymphoma. The *MYC-IGH@* fusion, associated with the cytogenetic finding of t(8;14)(q24;q32), is the most common finding, seen in more than 80% of cases. As stated before with other lymphoma fusion genes, this molecular finding is not specific for Burkitt lymphoma and requires morphologic, immunophenotypic, and often, additional genetic, correlation. The *MYC-IGH@* fusion may be seen in transformed lymphoma (e.g., follicular lymphoma, large B-cell lymphoma) as well as progressive plasma cell myeloma and the highly aggressive "double-hit" lymphomas. The latter most often demonstrate concurrent *MYC-IGH@* and *IGH@-BCL2* fusions.

The *BIRC3-MALT1* fusion, associated with the cytogenetic finding t(11;18)(q21;q21), is specifically associated with extranodal marginal zone lymphomas (MALT) with variable detection frequencies depending on the anatomic location (~25% gastric, ~40% lung, others). Detection of this abnormality is unique in the stomach in that it predicts for advanced stage of disease and resistance to *Helicobacter pylori* eradication.

Rearrangements of the anaplastic lymphoma kinase gene (*ALK*) on 2p23 occur in ALK+anaplastic large cell lymphomas (ALCL). A variety of partner genes are known (e.g., *NPM1*, clathrin), and, as a consequence, the FISH probe of choice is a break-apart (see below). ALK+ALCL has an overall reported better prognosis than ALK(-); thus demonstration of its rearrangement is of clinical importance.

Translocations in lymphoma are best detected with FISH using either a dual color dual fusion probe (DCDF) strategy or a break-apart (BA) probe strategy (Table 1). DCDF probes target the two genes/genetic loci of interest and assess for the abnormal production of two fusion signals (Fig. 1a, b). BA probes are used to detect a rearrangement of a particular gene (e.g., anaplastic lymphoma kinase, *ALK*) that typically has a variety of different translocation partners (usually more than five) (Fig. 2a, b). Assessment for

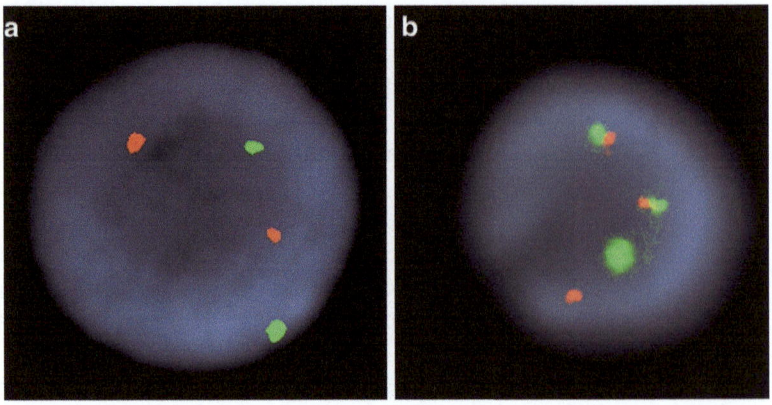

Fig. 1 Dual color dual fusion FISH probes in interphase preparations. (**a**) Normal pattern of two *orange* and two *green* signals in a single interphase nucleus. (**b**) Typical abnormal pattern of two fused (*yellow*) signals and one *orange* and one *green* signal in a single interphase nucleus

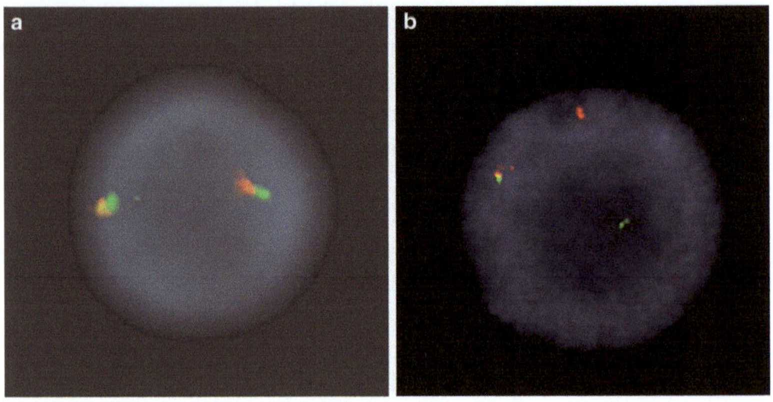

Fig. 2 Break-apart FISH probes in interphase preparations. (**a**) Normal pattern of two fused (*yellow*) signals in a single interphase nucleus. (**b**) Typical abnormal pattern of one fused, one *orange,* and one *green* signal in a single interphase nucleus

each possible translocation partner is not readily available, time-consuming, impractical, and expensive.

The establishment of reference ranges is vital for accurately reporting the results of a FISH test. Per suggested guidelines, the reference range for each probe type used in each different tissue type/site should be independently established (7). An adequate number of normal and abnormal samples should be evaluated in this process. In addition, a subsequent and ongoing reassessment of continued analytic accuracy should be performed. Determining references ranges on formalin-fixed paraffin-embedded tissue whole sections is more challenging. One must work closely with the instrumentation parameters and utilize sufficient numbers of normal and abnormal tissues to determine the reference ranges. In this regard, it is the authors' opinion that detection of minimal residual disease is more challenging in such cases.

2 Materials

Detection of recurrent genetic rearrangement by fluorescence in situ hybridization can be performed in peripheral blood, bone marrow aspirate, fresh or frozen tissue, or formalin-fixed paraffin-embedded (FFPE) tissue (see Notes 1–3).

2.1 Sample Preparation in Fresh Specimens

1. Microscope slides.
2. Coverslips: 22 × 22, 24 × 40, 24 × 50, or circles.
3. 0.075 M KCl, expiration: 2 weeks from preparation date.
4. Carnoy's fixative: 9 ml analytical reagent grade methanol, 3 ml analytical reagent grade glacial acetic acid. Store at −20°C, make up fresh daily.
5. 20× SSC (Saline Sodium Citrate): 132 g Saline Sodium Citrate, make 500 ml solution with distilled H_2O, pH to 7.0. Expiration 1 year from preparation date.
6. 2× SSC (Saline Sodium Citrate) pH to 7.0. Expiration 1 year from preparation date.
7. Pepsin working solution: 20 μl 10% pepsin solution, 40 ml 0.01 N HCl. Expiration 6 months from preparation date.
8. 0.01 N HCl.
9. 70% ETOH. Expiration 6 months from preparation date.
10. 80% ETOH. Expiration 6 months from preparation date.
11. 95% ETOH. Expiration 6 months from preparation date.

2.2 Sample Preparation for FFPE Non-decalcified Tissues

1. 4–5 μm thick tissue sections, mounted on the positive side of an organosaline-coated slide.
2. 1 H&E-stained section for review for presence of tumor.
3. VP-2000 Processor (Abbott Molecular, Des Plaines, IL).
4. Citri-Solv (similar to xylene).
5. 100% ETOH.
6. 0.2 N HCl.
7. 2× SSC.
8. Protease solution: 0.25 g Protease (Abbott Laboratories, Des Plaines, IL), 500 ml 2 M (100×) $MgCl_2$, 370 ml 1× phosphate-buffered saline. Store at 2–8°C. Expiration 6 months from preparation.
9. 10% buffered formalin.
10. 70% EtOH.
11. 85% EtOH.

2.3 Probe Hybridization in Fresh Specimens

1. Probes: store at −20°C, protect from light (see Note 4).
2. Hybridization buffer (comes with purchased probes): store at −20°C, protect from light.
3. DAPI II counterstain reagent: store at −20°C, protect from light.
4. HYBrite™ hybridization system.
5. Coverslips.
6. Rubber cement.
7. 0.4× SSC/0.3% Igepal CA-630 (Sigma, St. Louis, MO): 20 ml of 2× SSC (Saline Sodium Citrate), 3 ml of Igepal. Prepare 1 l of solution with distilled H_2O and adjust pH to 7.0. Expiration 1 year from preparation date.
8. 2× SSC/0.1% Igepal CA-630 (Sigma, St. Louis, MO): 100 ml 20× SSC, 1 ml Igepal. Prepare 1 l of solution with distilled H_2O and adjust pH to 7.0. Expiration 1 year from preparation date.

2.4 Probe Hybridization in FFPE Non-decalcified Tissues

1. Probes: store at −20°C, protect from light (see Note 4).
2. Hybridization buffer (comes with purchased probes): store at −20°C, protect from light.
3. DAPI I counterstain reagent: store at −20°C, protect from light.
4. HYBrite™ hybridization system.
5. Coverslips.
6. Rubber cement.
7. 2× SSC/0.3% Igepal CA-630.

2.5 Probe Visualization and Enumeration

1. Fluorescence microscope with imaging system for fresh specimens (see Note 5).
2. Automated image analysis system (e.g., MetaSystems™) for FFPE non-decalcified tissues (see Note 6).

3 Methods

3.1 Sample Preparation for Fresh Specimens

1. Label 15 ml centrifuge tube with accession number and patient name.
2. Pipette 0.5–1 ml of sample into the centrifuge tube.
3. Add 10 ml of 0.075 M KCl.
4. Place in 37°C incubator for 15 min.
5. Remove sample from incubator and prefix with 1 ml of Carnoy's fixative.
6. Mix sample and centrifuge at 244,9 ×g for 8 min.

7. Remove supernatant.
8. Slowly add 10 ml of cold Carnoy's fixative.
9. Mix and centrifuge at 244,9×g for 8 min.
10. Remove supernatant.
11. Add 10 ml of cold Carnoy's fixative.
12. Mix and centrifuge at 244,9×g for 8 min.
13. Remove supernatant.
14. Label slide with patient accession number, name, probe, and date. Mark the areas to be hybridized by scratching the edge of the slide with a diamond scribe, approximately in the middle of the hybridization area.
15. Drop cell suspension on slide and let dry.
16. Warm slides on 60°C slide warmer for 5 min. Allow to cool.
17. Age slides in 2× SSC at 37°C for 30 min.
18. Place slides in pepsin working solution at 37°C for 13 min.
19. Dehydrate slides through ethanol series (70, 80, 95%, 2 min each).
20. Air-dry.
21. FISH may be performed on a previously Wright-stained smear (see Notes 7 and 8).

3.2 Sample Preparation for FFPE Non-decalcified Specimen

1. Bake slides at 56°C (±2°C) on a HYBrite for at least 2 h and up to overnight, before deparaffinizing. Be sure to include control slides as well as patient samples (see Note 4).
2. FISH may be performed on a previously H&E-stained slide (see Note 7).
3. Place slides in VP-2000 Processor.
4. Fill VP-2000 basins appropriately.
5. Run VP-2000.
   (a) 20 min Citri-Solv.
   (b) 10 min Citri-Solv. Agitate.
   (c) 10 min 100% EtOH.
   (d) Air-dry, 5 min, 47°C.
   (e) 0.2 N HCl 20 min.
   (f) Water rinse, 3 min.
   (g) 2× SSC, 3 min.
   (h) 1 M sodium thiocyanate, 30 min, 80°C.
   (i) Water rinse, 1 min.
   (j) 2× SSC, 10 min.

(k) Protease solution, 60 min, 37°C.
(l) 2× SSC, 10 min.
(m) Air-dry, 5 min, 47°C.
(n) 10% buffered formalin,10 min.
(o) 2× SSC, 10 min.
(p) Water rinse, 2 s.
(q) 70% ETOH, 1 min.
(r) 85% ETOH, 1 min.
(s) 100% ETOH, 1 min.
(t) Air-dry, 5 min, 47°C.

3.3 Probe Hybridization for Fresh Specimen

1. Thaw the probe components at room temperature in the dark.
2. Prepare probe mix per manufacturer's instruction in a clean microcentrifuge tube.

   Typical mixture: 7 μl hybridization buffer, 1 μl probe, and 2 μl sterile DI H_2O (to bring the total volume up to 10 μl). If preparing a mixture of more than one probe, add 1 μl of each probe and decrease the amount of water by the same volume. The total volume should be 10 μl of probe mix.
3. Apply 10 μl of probe solution to target area.
4. Coverslip immediately with 22 × 22 coverslip.
5. Apply rubber cement to outer edge of coverslip with a syringe.
6. Place on HYBrite™. Run 74°C for 1 min followed by 37°C for 6 h to overnight (see Note 9).
7. Remove slides from HYBrite™.
8. Remove rubber cement from slides using forceps.
9. Carefully remove coverslip from slides.
10. Place slides in 0.4× SSC/0.3% Igepal at 73°C for 2 min. Do not wash more than three slides at a time (see Note 9).
11. Rinse slides in 2× SSC/0.1% Igepal at room temperature for 1 min.
12. Stand slides on end in a dark drawer and allow to air-dry.
13. Apply 10 μl of DAPI II to each hybridization area.
14. Apply 22 × 40 mm coverslip (or a 24 × 50 mm coverslip if two hybridization areas are to be covered).
15. Store in slide holder at 4°C until analysis.

3.4 Probe Hybridization for FFPE Non-decalcified Specimen

1. Prepare probe mix per manufacturer's instruction.
2. Add 10 μl of probe mix to the sample area of the slide corresponding to the area(s) on the H&E-stained slide marked by a pathologist.

3. Place a 22 × 22 mm coverslip (or a 24 × 40 mm coverslip if the tissue section is very large) over the section and seal the edges with rubber cement.
4. Place slide on HYBrite™: denature at 73°C for 6 min; hybridize at 37°C for 16–20 h (see Note 9).
5. Add 2× SSC/0.3% Igepal to each of two Coplin jars. Prewarm one jar (plastic) in a 72°C water bath for at least 30 min; second one, room temperature (see Note 9).
6. Mark the boundaries of the hybridization area on the back of the slide with a diamond scribe or HistoPrep pen if the whole tissue section is not covered by the coverslip.
7. Remove the rubber cement seal from the slides by gently pulling up on the sealant with forceps.
8. Immerse slides in post-hybridization wash buffer at room temperature and float off coverslips. Place slides in the dark while the coverslips are soaking off.
9. Remove excess liquid by blotting off the edges of the slides and immerse slides in 2× SSC/0.3% Igepal at 72°C for 2 min (up to three slides per jar).
10. Remove slides from wash buffer and air-dry the slides in the dark in an upright position.
11. Apply 10–15 μl of DAPI I counterstain to the target area of the slides and place a 24 × 40 mm or 24 × 50 mm coverslip.
12. After removing from 4°C storage, allow slides to reach room temperature prior to viewing using fluorescence microscopy.
13. Archive slides at −20°C.

3.5 Probe Enumeration and Result Interpretation in Fresh Specimen

1. Score two hundred interphase cells per probe, one hundred nuclei each by two qualified technologists (see Notes 10–13, Table 2).
2. On the imaging system, capture one image for assays with normal results and two images for assays with abnormal results and label with patient name, accession number, and FISH probes used.
3. Combine the two sets of scores (200 cells total) and determine positive or negative results based on prior determination of reference ranges (see Notes 14 and 15).
4. If a result is close to a cutoff value, consideration for a third reader is suggested (300 cells to reach a total of 500).

3.6 Probe Visualization and Enumeration in FFPE Non-decalcified Specimen

1. Load slide into slide frame on automated image analysis system.
2. Place a drop of immersion oil on area to be scanned.
3. Select tumor areas to be scanned and enter into computer.
4. Select and run appropriate program for analysis depending on probe set utilized. Analyze at least 1,000 nuclei if possible.

Table 2
Troubleshooting tips

Problem	Possible cause	Solution
High background fluorescence	Glass slides not sufficiently cleaned Cellular debris in pellet Slide inadequately washed following hybridization	Rinse slides in EtOH prior to using Wash pellet in fresh fixative three times and re-drop. Ensure wash solutions were made correctly and pH is 7.0 Remove coverslip and rewash. Increase wash time in 0.4× SSC/0.3% Igepal up to 4 min
Weak or no signal	Slide not adequately denatured Slide not adequately aged Probe not added Probe mix dried too much on slide Air bubbles were trapped under coverslip during hybridization Hybridization conditions were inappropriate Wash conditions or solutions incorrect Probes or specimen slides stored improperly Wrong counterstain used, counterstain is too bright (DAPI I for paraffin used) Slides viewed using inappropriate filter sets	Ensure melt temperature of HYBrite is 73 ± 1 °C. Increase melt temperature to 74 °C. Increase melt time to 2 min Age slide at least 24 h at ambient temperature Prepare new probe mixture, allow probe to thaw completely, vortex and centrifuge to mix, pipette probe slowly. Ensure pipettes are calibrated correctly Immediately place coverslip on probe area, ensure rubber cement seal completely surrounds coverslip Press out visible bubbles with pencil eraser Ensure temperature of HYBrite is 37 °C and that hybridization program was started Ensure wash solutions were made correctly and pH is 7.0. Ensure wash temperature of 0.4× SSC/0.3% Igepal is 73 ± 1 °C before washing slides. Ensure thermometers and pH meters are calibrated correctly Store probes at −20 °C protected from light. Store hybridized slides at 4 °C short term, −20 °C long term protected from light Remove coverslip, immerse slides in 2× SSC/0.1% Igepal at ambient temperature for 5 min with occasional agitation, dehydrate through alcohol series, air-dry and apply DAPI II Multi-bandpass filter sets provide less light than single bandpass filter sets, probe signals may appear fainter when viewed through multi-bandpass filter sets Use correct filter for viewing specified fluorophore

(continued)

Table 2 (continued)

Problem	Possible cause	Solution
Diffuse signal, signal speckling	Probes diluted inappropriately, too much probe in the assay Inappropriate hybridization conditions Wash temp. too low Wash stringency too low Cross-hybridization	Ensure probe mixture was made according to protocol Ensure hybridization temperature of HYBrite is 37°C. Ensure hybridization buffer was added to the probe mixture in proper amount Maintain the wash temperature of 0.4× SSC/0.3% Igepal at 73 ± 1°C Ensure wash solutions were made according to protocol Increase temperature of 0.4× SSC/0.3% Igepal by 2°C. Increase more if necessary. Decrease melt temperature by 2°C
Bright or weak counterstain	Weak counterstain due to oil droplets under coverslip Wrong counterstain applied (Note: DAPI I counterstain is eight times more concentrated than DAPI II counterstain) Counterstain too old or exposed to light for extended periods	Remove coverslip, immerse slides in 2× SSC/0.1% Igepal at ambient temperature for 5 min with occasional agitation, dehydrate through alcohol series, air-dry and reapply DAPI II. Store counterstain at −20°C protected from light and when using. Ensure counterstain is not expired

5. Archive image(s) (Figs. 3 and 4).
6. Review histograms upon completion of analysis to determine positive or negative results based on prior establishment of normal reference ranges (see Note 14).
7. Visually review the screen shots of the analyzed areas to ensure adequate probe hybridization, nuclear morphology, probe signal intensity, and crispness (see Notes 15 and 16, Table 2).

3.7 Quality Control (QC)

1. All new lot numbers for each kit are tested for probe specificity using a PHA-stimulated peripheral blood sample from a known karyotypically normal male (see Note 17).
2. Analyze five metaphase spreads. Use reverse DAPI image analysis to confirm that the signals reside on the appropriate chromosome location.
3. Capture one demonstrative metaphase image and label with the QC lot number and probe used.

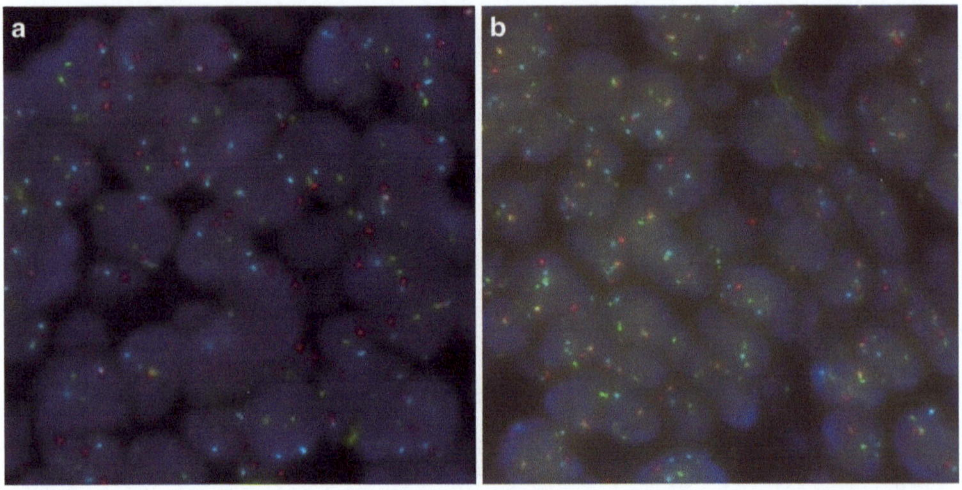

Fig. 3 Tricolor dual fusion FISH probe (*MYC* (*orange*), *IGH@* (*green*), CEP8 (*aqua*)) in formalin-fixed, paraffin-embedded tissue sections. (**a**) Normal pattern of two *orange*, two *green*, and two *aqua* signals is seen in a subset of nuclei. Other nuclei may appear abnormal; however, this is due to sectioning/truncation artifact. (**b**) Typical abnormal pattern of two fused (*yellow*) and two *aqua* signals and one *orange* and one *green* signal seen in a subset of nuclei. Other nuclei may appear different; however, this is due to sectioning/truncation artifact

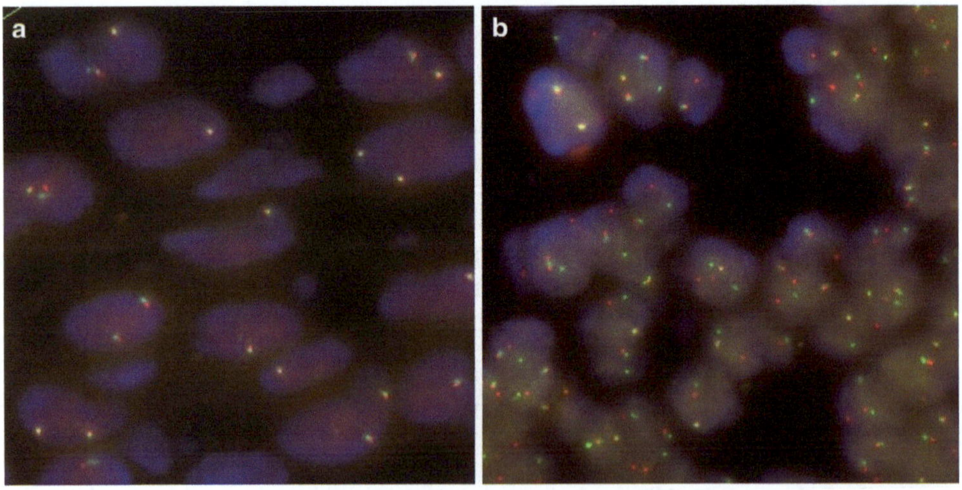

Fig. 4 Break-apart FISH probe (*ALK*) in formalin-fixed, paraffin-embedded tissue sections. (**a**) Normal pattern of two fused (*yellow*) signals seen in a subset of nuclei. Other nuclei may appear abnormal; however this is due to sectioning/truncation artifact. (**b**) Typical abnormal pattern of one fused (*yellow*), one *orange,* and one *green* signal seen in a subset of nuclei. Other nuclei may appear different; however this is due to sectioning/truncation artifact

4. If a known abnormal case is available for the probe being tested, process this sample with the metaphase QC slide and count 50 interphase cells.
5. Establish your laboratory normal reference ranges for each probe set in each assayed tissue site as per published recommendations (7).

4 Notes

1. Cellular enrichment techniques for the cells of interest increase diagnostic yield; however, separate validation studies and determination of reference ranges are required (if previously performed) with a change in technique. Combined FISH with fluorescent cellular markers (e.g., CD138) is feasible and serves as an alternative in situ cell enrichment technique.
2. Intact, single nuclei can be extracted from FFPE tissues to perform FISH assays (8).
3. Confirmation by a pathologist or other valid designee that the cells of interest are present on a slide for FISH is recommended.
4. The use of controls for non-FDA-approved probes is at the discretion of the laboratory director.
5. Verify that all fluorescent microscopes have identical filter sets to ensure similar results.
6. Manual scoring of FISH hybridization signals on FFPE tissues can be performed but is more troublesome than automation due to interpreter bias, truncation of nuclei, signal variability, and time requirement (5).
7. FISH may also be performed on previously H&E- or Wright-stained smears. Stained slides should be soaked in acetone or xylene until the coverslip is easily removed or falls off the slide. This can take up to 48 h. Subsequently, slide is washed in fresh xylene for 5 min to remove residual glue, and placed in acetic acid for 30 s to 1 min to destain. After air-drying follow steps in Subheading 3.3.
8. To perform FISH on a previously air-dried smear follow these steps: place slides in 3:1 Carnoy's fixative for 15 min, exchange with fresh fixative after the first 5 min; air-dry and age slides in 2× SSC at 37°C for 30 min; place slides in pepsin working solution at 37°C for 13 min; dehydrate slides through ethanol series (70, 80, 95%, 2 min each); and air-dry.
9. Confirm temperature accuracy of hybridization chambers and warmed solutions for consistent results.

10. Knowledge of atypical abnormal signal patterns is of crucial importance when assessing for the presence of a translocation/ rearrangement.
11. Diagnostic accuracy and inter-reader comparisons are facilitated by having two separate readers scan, score, and record data independently of one another.
12. If two readers have significant disparate results (i.e., one is positive and one is negative), have a third reader confirm both results by reviewing both slide areas initially scanned.
13. Consider designating and training certain members of your laboratory to focus specifically on all process related to FISH to ensure consistency in processing and scanning.
14. Knowledge of your laboratory's analytical detection sensitivities for different probes is crucial to ensuring an accurate result.
15. Utilize ISCN 2009 FISH nomenclature for reporting as appropriate. Implement use of standardized comments/interpretations as appropriate for typical normal and abnormal cases for improved efficiency, synoptic reporting, and error reduction.
16. If results are suboptimal (e.g., nuclear morphology, signal morphology, signal intensity, background, cell density) or readers are concerned with the validity of results, do not hesitate to repeat the procedure.
17. Appropriate probe validation and ongoing quality studies are necessary for quality assurance.

References

1. Nussenzweig A, Nussenzweig MC (2010) Origin of chromosomal translocations in lymphoid cancer. Cell 141:27–38
2. Kurtin PJ (2009) Indolent lymphomas of mature B lymphocytes. Hematol Oncol Clin North Am 23:769–790
3. Belaud-Rotureau MA, Parrens M, Carrere N, Turmo M, Ferrer J, de Mascarel A et al (2007) Interphase fluorescence in situ hybridization is more sensitive than BIOMED-2 polymerase chain reaction protocol in detecting *IGH-BCL2* rearrangement in both fixed and frozen lymph node with follicular lymphoma. Hum Pathol 38:365–372
4. Ventura RA, Martin-Subero JI, Jones M, McParland J, Gesk S, Mason DY et al (2006) FISH analysis for the detection of lymphoma-associated chromosomal abnormalities in routine paraffin-embedded tissue. J Mol Diagn 8:141–151
5. Reichard KK, Hall BK, Corn A, Foucar MK, Hozier J (2006) Automated analysis of fluorescence in situ hybridization on fixed, paraffin-embedded whole tissue sections in B-cell lymphoma. Mod Pathol 19: 1027–1033
6. Belaud-Rotureau MA, Parrens M, Dubus P, Garroste JC, de Mascarel A, Merlio JP (2002) A comparative analysis of FISH, RT-PCR, PCR, and immunohistochemistry for the diagnosis of mantle cell lymphomas. Mod Pathol 15:517–525
7. Wiktor AE, Van Dyke DL, Stupca PJ, Ketterling RP, Thorland EC, Shearer BM et al (2006) Preclinical validation of fluorescence in situ hybridization assays for clinical practice. Genet Med 8:16–23
8. Paternoster SF, Brockman SR, McClure RF, Remstein ED, Kurtin PJ, Dewald GW (2002) A new method to extract nuclei from paraffin-embedded tissue to study lymphomas using interphase fluorescence in situ hybridization. Am J Pathol 160:1967–1972

Chapter 13

Molecular Detection of t(14;18)(q32;q21) in Follicular Lymphoma

C. Cameron Yin and Rajyalakshmi Luthra

Abstract

The t(14;18)(q32;q21) can be detected in approximately 80% of cases of follicular lymphoma (FL). This translocation juxtaposes the *BCL2* oncogene at 18q21 with the *IGH@* at 14q32, and leads to overexpression of BCL2 protein which protects the cells from apoptosis. The high degree of sequence homology among the 3′ portion of the J_H segments and the clustering of breakpoints on chromosome 18 make the *IGH@/BCL2* very amenable to polymerase chain reaction (PCR) detection. We describe two multiplex TaqMan-based real-time PCR assays which can be used to detect and quantify the major and minor breat-point cluster regions of *IGH@/BCL2* fusion products in newly diagnosed FL, and to monitor minimal residual disease during treatment or early relapse.

Key words Follicular lymphoma, t(14;18)(q32;q21), PCR

1 Introduction

Chromosomal translocations occur in many types of B-cell and T-cell lymphomas and play an important role in lymphomagenesis. These translocations can be subdivided into two types. In the first type, an oncogene is activated or overexpressed through juxtaposition with another gene, usually antigen receptor genes. Examples of this type include the t(8;14)(q24;q32) in Burkitt lymphoma/leukemia, the t(11;14)(q13;q32) in mantle cell lymphoma, and the t(14;18)(q32;q21) in follicular lymphoma. In the second type, two genes are disrupted, and portions of each gene are juxtaposed, resulting in the formation of a fusion gene and a chimeric protein. This type of translocation occurs in some types of non-Hodgkin lymphoma, such as the t(2;5) in anaplastic large cell lymphoma, but is more commonly seen in acute and chronic myeloid leukemias (1). The detection of these translocations is helpful for the diagnosis and classification of malignant lymphomas and leukemias, as well as monitoring residual disease following therapy.

Magdalena Czader (ed.), *Hematological Malignancies*, Methods in Molecular Biology, vol. 999,
DOI 10.1007/978-1-62703-357-2_13, © Springer Science+Business Media New York 2013

In this and the following chapters, we describe the molecular methodology using polymerase chain reaction (PCR) for the detection of selected chromosomal translocations that are commonly seen in several types of malignant lymphomas.

Follicular lymphoma (FL) is a neoplasm of follicle center B-cells and is characterized by the t(14;18)(q32;q21), detected in approximately 80% of FL cases at the time of initial diagnosis (2, 3). This translocation juxtaposes the *BCL2* oncogene at 18q21 with the *IGH@* gene at 14q32, and results in overexpression of BCL2 protein which protects the cells from apoptosis and confers the cells survival advantage. In the remaining 10–20% of FL cases, the t(14;18) is not detectable using any available method, suggesting the existence of other mechanisms for the pathogenesis of FL. The t(14;18) is also present in 20–30% of diffuse large B-cell lymphomas (DLBCL) with presumably follicular center cell origin (4). The t(14;18)(q32;q21) has been identified in a small subset of healthy individuals (5). The significance of this finding is uncertain in the absence of appropriate clinical history.

The t(14;18)(q32;q21) involving *IGH@* and *BCL2* genes should not be confused with the cytogenetically identical, but molecularly distinct t(14;18)(q32;q21) that involves *IGH@* at 14q32 and *MALT1* at 18q21 seen in extranodal marginal zone lymphoma of mucosa-associated lymphoid tissue (MALT lymphoma). Both translocations can be detected by conventional karyotyping, fluorescence in situ hybridization (FISH), Southern blot hybridization, or PCR.

The breakpoints on chromosome 14 are tightly clustered, occurring immediately 5′ to the J_H regions. The majority of *BCL2* breakpoints on chromosome 18 are also clustered; most (60–70%) occur in the 3′ noncoding region, in a 150 base pair (bp) span termed the major breakpoint cluster region (M-bcr), and approximately 10–20% occur more than 20 kb downstream within the minor breakpoint cluster region (m-bcr) (6). The remainder are scattered between the M-bcr and m-bcr regions, with a third breakpoint cluster region, intermediate cluster region (icr), identified in 5–15% of FL cases (7, 8). The high degree of sequence homology among the 3′ portion of the J_H segments and the clustering of breakpoints on chromosome 18 make the *IGH@/BCL2* very amenable to PCR detection.

The purpose of this PCR assay is to (1) determine the presence or absence of *IGH@/BCL2* gene rearrangement in newly diagnosed cases of FL and other lymphomas (e.g., DLBCL), (2) in positive cases, test whether the M-bcr or m-bcr breakpoint region is involved, and (3) monitor minimal residual disease (MRD) during treatment or early relapse.

We developed two multiplex TaqMan-based real-time PCR assays for the detection and quantification of the M-bcr and m-bcr *IGH@/BCL2* fusion products, separately (9, 10). Target Taqman probes for M-bcr/m-bcr labeled with 6-FAM and reference cyclophilin probes labeled with VIC reporter dye are compared. Standard curves of known amounts of both target and cyclophilin allow the calculation of the quantity of the specific target and the endogenous control. The results are reported as a percentage ratio of target to internal control. The PCR product is also sized by capillary electrophoresis to assess the particular size of the patient *IGH@/BCL2* rearrangement.

2 Materials

2.1 Specimen Requirements

1. Bone marrow (1–2 ml) or peripheral blood (5–10 ml) collected in EDTA tubes and delivered to the lab on cold pack within 48 h of collection (see Note 1).
2. Tissues in sterile containers on dry ice.
3. Formalin-fixed, paraffin-embedded tissue sections.

2.2 Reagents

1. DNA isolation using Qiagen kit and protocols appropriate for specimen type (Qiagen, Valencia, CA).
2. Primers and probes sequences are presented in Table 1 (see Note 2). The non-labeled primers are purchased from Invitrogen Corporation (Carlsbad, CA). The fluorescently labeled primers and TaqMan probes are purchased from Applied Biosystems (Foster City, CA). All primers and probes are stored at −20°C and are stable for 1 year.
3. TaqMan Universal PCR Master Mix with uracil N-glycosylase (UNG, Applied Biosystems, Foster City, CA).

Table 1
Primer and probe sequences for *IGH@/BCL2* PCR analysis

Primer/probe	Sequence
M-bcr forward primer (M-bcr-F)	5′-GCTTTACGTGGCCTGTTTCA-3′
m-bcr forward primer (m-bcr-F)	5′-CCTGGCTTCCTTCCCTCTGT-3′
J_H reverse primer (J_H-NED-R)	5′-NED-ACCTGAGGAGACGGTGACC-3′
Cyclophilin forward primer (cyclo-F)	5′-TGAGACAGCAGATAGAGCCAAGC-3′
Cyclophilin reverse primer (cyclo-R)	5′-TCCCTGCCAATTTGACATCTTC3′
M-bcr probe (M-bcr-P)	5′-FAM-AGGGCTCTGGGTGGGTCTGTGTTG-TAMRA-3′
m-bcr probe (m-bcr-P)	5′-FAM-TCTCTGGGGAGGAGTGGAAAGGAAGG-TAMRA-3′
Cyclophilin probe (cyclo-P)	5′-VIC-AGCACCAATATTCAGTACACAGCTTAAAGCTAT-TAMRA-3′

4. Performance optimized polymer.
5. Deionized formamide.
6. GeneScan Rox 500 size standard (Perkin Elmer, Waltham, MA).

2.3 Equipment

1. ABI 7500 Real-Time PCR System.
2. ABI 3100 Genetic Analyzer.
3. 96-well optical plate (VWR LabShop, Batavia, IL).

3 Methods

3.1 DNA Extraction and Quantification

1. Extract and quantify DNA using standard method. The amount of DNA required for PCR testing is 1 μg.

3.2 PCR Amplification

1. Prepare the following reaction mix for M-bcr (final concentration): TaqMan Universal PCR Master Mix with UNG (1×) (see Note 3), M-bcr-F (0.2 μM), J_H-NED-R (0.2 μM), cyclo-F (40 nM), cyclo-R (40 nM), M-bcr-P (0.1 μM), cyclo-P (0.04 μM).
2. Prepare the following reaction mix for m-bcr (final concentration): TaqMan Universal PCR Master Mix with UNG (1×), m-bcr-F (0.2 μM), J_H-NED-R (0.2 μM), cyclo-F (40 nM), cyclo-R (40 nM), m-bcr-P (0.1 μM), cyclo-P (0.04 μM).
3. Add 15 μl of the reaction mix to each well of a 96-well optical plate.
4. Pipette 10 μl of patient DNA (1 μg), standards, or controls into the appropriate wells (see Notes 4–6).
5. Cover the wells with optical caps, vortex plate, and quick-spin the plate to ensure that no bubbles are present at the bottom of the wells.
6. Perform PCR amplification on a thermocycler (e.g., ABI 7500) as follows:
   (a) 50°C for 2 min.
   (b) 95°C for 10 min.
   (c) Repeat 42 cycles of: 95°C for 15 s, 57°C for 45 s, 72°C for 45 s.
7. After PCR, remove the plate from the thermocycler and place it in −20°C freezer until ready for the next step.

3.3 Capillary Electrophoresis

1. Make a 1:20 dilution of the PCR product with water.
2. Prepare a 96-well reaction plate by adding a 20 μl of a mixture of deionized formamide and 0.08 μl GS Rox 500 size standard per well.

3. Add 1 μl of the diluted PCR product to each well.
4. Cover the plate, quick-spin, and denature by heating at 95°C for 5 min followed by rapid cooling to 4°C.
5. Spin the plate to collect the product in the bottom of the wells. Be sure there are no bubbles on the bottom of the wells.
6. Load samples on the Genetic Analyzer (e.g., ABI 3100) for electrophoresis.

3.4 Result Interpretation and Reporting

1. The normalized reporter (Rn) on the *Y*-axis represents the level of detected fluorescence. The threshold cycle (Ct) on the *X*-axis represents the PCR cycle number at which the fluorescence is greater than the baseline signal.
2. The threshold will be set automatically, though it can be adjusted manually.
3. Adjust the threshold in such a way that the line is above the noise level. Amplification above the threshold is indicative of accumulated target, whereas that below the threshold is indicative of no amplification.
4. If unknown DNA samples are run with known DNA standards, the amount of DNA in the unknown samples can be quantified.
5. The accuracy of the standards can be determined from the correlation co-efficient by selecting "Standard Curve" from the "Analysis" menu. A slope value of 3.33 and an *R* value close to 1.0 is optimal.
6. For positive cases, the size of the products can be achieved by the GeneScan Analysis software (see Note 7).

4 Notes

1. Heparin is an inhibitory agent for PCR; specimens should not be collected in heparinized tubes.
2. Breakpoints other than M-bcr and m-bcr are not detected by this assay, but would be best detected by FISH. PCR including primers for icr, or long-range PCR also gives a higher detection rate for the t(14;18). However, this technique requires high-quality DNA and has not yet been implemented as a routine detection method in most laboratories. Southern blot hybridization represents another method, but the sensitivity is only 5% and would not detect the small numbers of FL cells typically found in blood or bone marrow aspirates.
3. To prevent contamination of the specimen by amplicon carry over, we utilize UNG to degrade specifically PCR products from previous PCR amplifications. This is achieved when dTTP is replaced by dUTP in the PCR. Other procedures, such as

separation of pre- and post-PCR area, adherence to sterile technique, as well as never return aliquots to original container, should also be practiced.

4. The following controls are included:
   - (a) Positive controls from M-bcr- and m-bcr-positive patient samples.
   - (b) Negative control (HL-60 cell line) is used to assure the specificity of the assay. Only the internal control should be observed in the negative control.
   - (c) Internal control (cyclophilin) is used to assess the quality of each PCR reaction. An internal control target must be amplified in all negative samples in order to rule out false negatives due to poor specimen quality (e.g., due to inappropriate tissue fixatives) or PCR failure. Specimens with fewer than 10,000 copies of cyclophilin amplified will be signed out with a comment indicating that the low control amplification observed will limit the accuracy and/or sensitivity of M-bcr or m-bcr detection. Specimens with very low cyclophilin control amplification levels will be regarded as inadequate for quantitation for a positive test or inadequate for reporting for a negative result.
   - (d) No template reagent control is used to assure that there is no template contamination of the PCR reagents. Nothing should be observed in the reagent control.
   - (e) Sensitivity controls are used to assure that the stated sensitivity of the assay is reached when conditions are ideal. If the sensitivity control using the positive control does not reveal the adequate reported sensitivity, the assay may be repeated, or the results may be reported with a caveat about reduced sensitivity.
5. Reactions in duplicate are used to rule out false positive results due to contamination, or false negative results due to sampling error or PCR failure.
6. To minimize nonspecific products, once pre-PCR is set up, it is necessary to run the samples as soon as possible. In addition, probe breakdown or nonspecific probe binding may occasionally give low signal at high cycles.
7. There is considerable variation in the length of PCR products due to random insertion of variable numbers of extra nucleotides at the breakpoint junction during crossover and the variability of the breakpoints in the *BCL2* fusion gene and the six J_H segments. The size of the PCR products usually ranges from 100 to 270 bp for the M-bcr and the m-bcr. Therefore, not only the presence but also the particular size of the *IGH@/BCL2* PCR product is important in the monitoring of MRD.

References

1. Vega F, Medeiros LJ (2003) Chromosomal translocation involved in non-Hodgkin lymphomas. Arch Pathol Lab Med 127: 1148–1160
2. Yunis JJ, Frizzera G, Oken MM, McKenna J, Theologides A, Armesen M (1987) Multiple recurrent genomic defects in follicular lymphoma. A possible model for cancer. N Engl J Med 316:79–84
3. Leich E, Ott G, Rosenwald A (2011) Pathology, pathogenesis and molecular genetics of follicular NHL. Best Pract Res Clin Haematol 24:95–109
4. Jacobson JO, Wilkes BM, Kwaiatkowski DJ, Medeiros LJ, Aisenberg AC, Harris NL (1993) Bcl-2 rearrangements in de novo diffuse large cell lymphoma. Association with distinctive clinical features. Cancer 72:231–236
5. Aster JC, Kobayashi Y, Shiota M, Mori S, Sklar J (1992) Detection of the t(14;18) at similar frequencies in hyperplastic lymphoid tissues from American and Japanese patients. Am J Pathol 141:291–299
6. Tsujimoto Y, Cossman J, Jaffe ES, Croce CM (1985) Involvement of the bcl-2 gene in human follicular lymphoma. Science 228:1440–1443
7. Albinger-Hegyi A, Hochreutener B, Abdou MT, Hegyi I, Durs-Zimmermann MT, Kurrer MO, Heitz PU, Zimmermann DR (2002) High frequency of t(14;18)-translocation breakpoints outside of major breakpoint and minor cluster regions in follicular lymphomas: improved polymerase chain reaction protocols for their detection. Am J Pathol 160: 823–832
8. Batstone PJ, Goodlad JR (2005) Efficacy of screening the intermediate cluster region of the bcl2 gene in follicular lymphomas by PCR. J Clin Pathol 58:81–82
9. Cleary ML, Smith SD, Sklar J (1986) Cloning and structural analysis of cDNAs for bcl2 and a hybrid bcl2/immunoglobulin transcript resulting from the t(14;18) translocation. Cell 47: 19–28
10. Sanchez-Vega B, Vega F, Hai S, Medeiros LJ, Luthra R (2002) Real-time t(14;18)(q32;q21) PCR assay combined with high-resolution capillary electrophoresis: a novel and rapid approach that allows accurate quantitation and size determination of bcl-2/JH fusion sequences. Mod Pathol 15:448–453

Chapter 14

Molecular Detection of t(11;14)(q13;q32) in Mantle Cell Lymphoma

C. Cameron Yin and Rajyalakshmi Luthra

Abstract

Mantle cell lymphoma (MCL) is characterized by the presence of t(11;14)(q13;q32) which juxtaposes *CCND-1* gene (also known as *BCL-1*, *PRAD-1*) at 11q13 with an enhancer of the *IGH@* gene at 14q32. The resultant overexpression of cyclin D1 plays an essential role in the pathogenesis of MCL. The breakpoints on chromosome 14 occur 5′ to one of six J_H segments, whereas only 30–50% of the breakpoints on chromosome 11 are localized within a 1 kb region called the major translocation cluster (MTC) which can be easily assessed by polymerase chain reaction (PCR). The remainder of the breakpoints are widely scattered over approximately 120 kb, making PCR analysis infeasible. We describe a TaqMan-based real-time PCR assay to detect and quantify *IGH@/BCL1* fusion products in newly diagnosed MCL, and to monitor minimal residual disease during treatment or early relapse in MTC-positive cases.

Key words Mantle cell lymphoma, t(11;14)(q13;q32), PCR

1 Introduction

Mantle cell lymphoma (MCL) is a clinically aggressive B-cell lymphoma associated with the t(11;14)(q13;q32). This translocation juxtaposes *CCND-1* gene (also known as *BCL-1*, *PRAD-1*) at 11q13 with an enhancer of the *IGH@* gene at 14q32 and results in cyclin D1 overexpression. The latter plays an important role in the pathogenesis of MCL by forming complexes with either cyclin-dependent kinase (CDK)-4 or CDK-6, phosphorylating (inactivating) *RB* gene, and promotes cell cycle progression from G1 to S phase (1). The *IGH@/BCL1* rearrangement is not specific for MCL. It also occurs in a subset of multiple myeloma. However, there are usually no diagnostic problems caused by this overlap (2).

The reported frequency of the t(11;14) in MCL depends greatly on the method used for detection. Fluorescence in situ hybridization (FISH) detects *IGH@/BCL1* fusion in more than 95% of MCLs. Lower ranges are reported for conventional

Magdalena Czader (ed.), *Hematological Malignancies*, Methods in Molecular Biology, vol. 999,
DOI 10.1007/978-1-62703-357-2_14, © Springer Science+Business Media New York 2013

karyotyping (80–90%), Southern blot using multiple probes (70–80%), and PCR (major translocation cluster, 30–50%) (3). These differences are largely explained by the relatively long distance between *CCND-1* gene and the *JH* gene, approximately 130 kb, with the breakpoints on chromosome 11 scattered throughout this distance (3). The breakpoints on chromosome 14 occur 5′ to one of six J_H segments. On chromosome 11, approximately 30–50% of the t(11;14) breakpoints are localized within a 1 kb region called the major translocation cluster (MTC), which can be easily assessed by routine PCR methods (4, 5). However, the remainder of the breakpoints are widely scattered over approximately 120 kb, making PCR analysis not feasible in at least half of MCL cases.

We developed a TaqMan-based real-time PCR assay to detect and quantify *IGH@/BCL1* fusion products using two separate PCR reactions for *IGH/BCL1* and for cyclophilin, respectively (6). Target Taqman probe for MTC labeled with 6-FAM and reference cyclophilin probe labeled with VIC reporter dye are compared. Standard curves of known amounts of both target and cyclophilin allow the calculation of the quantity of the specific target and the endogenous control. The results are reported as a percentage ratio of target to internal control. The PCR product is also sized by capillary electrophoresis to assess the particular size of the patient *IGH@/BCL1* rearrangement.

The purpose of this assay is to (1) determine the presence or absence of *IGH@/BCL1* gene rearrangement in newly diagnosed cases of MCL, and (2) monitor minimal residual disease (MRD) during treatment or early relapse in MTC-positive cases.

2 Materials

2.1 Specimen Requirements

1. Bone marrow (1–2 ml) or peripheral blood (5–10 ml) collected in EDTA tubes and delivered to the lab on cold pack within 48 h of collection (see Note 1).
2. Fresh unfixed tissues in sterile containers on dry ice.
3. Formalin-fixed, paraffin-embedded tissue sections.

2.2 Primers and Probes

1. The sequences of primers and probes are presented in Table 1 (see Note 2). The non-labeled primers are purchased from Invitrogen Corporation (Carlsbad, CA). The fluorescently labeled primers and TaqMan probes are purchased from Applied Biosystems (Foster City, CA). All primers and probes are stored at −20°C and are stable for 1 year.
2. 10× PCR reaction buffer (Applied Biosystems, Foster City, CA).
3. 50 mM $MgCl_2$.
4. 10 mM dNTP mix.
5. AmpliTaq Gold 5 U/ml (Applied Biosystems, Foster City, CA).

Table 1
Primer and probe sequences for *IGH@/BCL1* PCR analysis

Primer/probe	Sequence
BCL1 MTC forward primer (MTC-F)	5′-TTGGATAAAGGCGAGGAGCA-3′
J_H reverse primer (J_H-NED-R)	5′-NED-ACTCACCTGAGGAGACGGTGAC-3′
Cyclophilin forward primer (cyclo-F)	5′-TGAGACAGCAGATAGAGCCAAGC-3′
Cyclophilin reverse primer (cyclo-R)	5′-TCCCTGCCAATTTGACATCTTC-3′
BCL1 MTC probe (MTC-P)	5′-FAM-AATTGCTGCACTGCATATTCGGTTAGACTGTG-TAMRA-3′
Cyclophilin probe (cyclo-P)	5′-VIC-AGCACCAATATTCAGTACACAGCTTAAAGCTAT-TAMRA-3′

6. Tween 20 (enzyme grade, Fisher Scientific, Pittsburgh, PA).
7. Gelatin, type A (from porcine skin, Sigma Aldrich, St. Louis, MO).
8. Performance optimized polymer.
9. Deionized formamide.
10. GeneScan Rox 500 size standard (Perkin Elmer, Waltham, MA).

2.3 Equipment

1. ABI 7500 Real-Time PCR System.
2. ABI 3100 Genetic Analyzer.

3 Methods

3.1 DNA Extraction and Quantification

1. Extract and quantify DNA using standard method. We use the Qiagen kits for DNA extraction from a variety of specimen types (Qiagen, Valencia, CA). The amount of DNA required for PCR testing is 1 μg.

3.2 PCR Amplification (See Note 3)

1. Prepare 10× Tween 20/Gelatin mix: 0.0164 g of Tween 20 and 0.0513 g of Gelatin in 10 ml distilled water.
2. Prepare the following reaction mix (final concentration):
   (a) For MTC: PCR reaction buffer (1×), $MgCl_2$ (4 mM), dNTP mix (0.8 mM), Tween 20/Gelatin (1×), MTC-F (0.12 μM), J_H-NED-R (0.12 μM), MTC-P (0.15 μM), AmpliTaq Gold (1.5 U).

(b) For cyclophilin: PCR reaction buffer (1×), $MgCl_2$ (4 mM), dNTP mix (0.8 mM), Tween 20/Gelatin (1×), cyclo-F (0.1 μM), cyclo-R (0.1 μM), cyclo-P (0.1 μM), AmpliTaq Gold (1.5 U).

3. Add 40 μl of the reaction mix to each well of a 96-well optical plate.
4. Pipette 10 μl of patient DNA (1 μg), standards, or controls into the appropriate wells (see Notes 4 and 5).
5. Cover the wells with optical caps, vortex plate, and quick-spin the plate to ensure that no bubbles are present at the bottom of the wells (see Note 6).
6. Perform PCR amplification on a thermocycler (e.g., ABI 7500) as follows:
   (a) 50°C for 2 min.
   (b) 95°C for 10 min.
   (c) Repeat 45 cycles of: 95°C for 15 s, 60°C for 1 min.
7. After PCR, remove the plate from the thermocycler and place it in −20°C freezer until ready for the next step.

3.3 Capillary Electrophoresis

1. Make a 1:20 dilution of the MTC PCR product with autoclaved water.
2. Prepare a 96-well reaction plate by adding a 20 μl of a mixture of deionized formamide and 0.08 μl GS Rox 500 size standard per well.
3. Add 1 μl of the diluted PCR product to each well.
4. Cover the plate, quick-spin, and denature by heating at 95°C for 5 min followed by rapid cooling to 4°C.
5. Spin the plate to collect the product in the bottom of the wells. Be sure there are no bubbles on the bottom of the wells.
6. Load samples on the Genetic Analyzer (e.g., ABI 3100) for electrophoresis.

3.4 Result Interpretation and Reporting

1. The normalized reporter (Rn) on the *Y*-axis represents the level of detected fluorescence. The threshold cycle (Ct) on the *X*-axis represents the PCR cycle number at which the fluorescence is greater than the baseline signal.
2. The threshold will be set automatically, though it can be adjusted manually.
3. Adjust the threshold in such a way that the line is above the noise. Amplification above the threshold is indicative of accumulated target, whereas that below the threshold is indicative of no amplification.
4. If unknown DNA samples are run with known DNA standards, the amount of DNA in the unknown samples can be quantified.

5. The accuracy of the standards can be determined from the correlation co-efficient by selecting "Standard Curve" from the "Analysis" menu. A slope value of 3.33 and an *R* value close to 1.0 are optimal.
6. For positive cases, the size of the products can be achieved by the GeneScan Analysis software (see Note 7).

4 Notes

1. Heparin is an inhibitory agent for PCR; specimens should not be collected in heparinized tubes.
2. In approximately 50–70% of MCL cases, the 11q13 breakpoints are widely distributed over an approximately 120 kb region, making PCR analysis infeasible. However, the t(11;14) in these cases can be detected by FISH or Southern blot hybridization. Detection of cyclin D1 mRNA by quantitative reverse transcription (RT)-PCR assay on fresh or frozen tissue distinguishes low levels of cyclin D1 derived from non-overexpressing lymphomas or normal cells from high levels of cyclin D1 mRNA characteristic of MCL and thus detects increased cyclin D1 mRNA in a high percentage of MCL (7, 8). However, there is little application for this cumbersome RT-PCR assay when FISH is faster, is more specific, and can be performed on paraffin-embedded tissue.
3. Stringent procedures to prevent contamination, such as separation of pre- and post-PCR area, adherence to sterile technique, as well as never return aliquots to original container, should be practiced.
4. Reactions in duplicate are used to rule out false positive results due to contamination, or false negative results due to sampling error or PCR failure.
5. The following controls are included:
   (a) Positive controls from MTC-positive patient specimens.
   (b) Negative control (HL-60 cell line) is used to assure the specificity of the assay. Only the internal control should be observed in the negative control.
   (c) Internal control (cyclophilin) is used to assess the quality of each PCR reaction. An internal control target must be amplified in all negative samples in order to rule out false negatives due to poor specimen quality (e.g., due to inappropriate tissue fixatives) or PCR failure. Specimens with fewer than 10,000 copies of cyclophilin amplified will be signed out with a comment indicating that the low control amplification observed will limit the accuracy and/or sensitivity of MTC detection. Specimens with very low

cyclophilin control amplification levels will be regarded as inadequate for quantitation for a positive test or inadequate for reporting for a negative result.

(d) No template reagent control is used to assure that there is no template contamination of the PCR reagents. Nothing should be observed in the reagent control.

(e) Sensitivity controls are used to assure that the stated sensitivity of the assay is reached when conditions are ideal. Sensitivity controls are made by serial dilution of the positive control with the negative control. If the sensitivity control using the positive control does not reveal the adequate reported sensitivity, the assay may be repeated, or the results may be reported with a caveat about reduced sensitivity.

6. To minimize nonspecific products, once pre-PCR is set up, it is necessary to run the samples as soon as possible. In addition, probe breakdown or nonspecific probe binding may occasionally give low signal at high cycles.

7. There is considerable variation in the length of PCR products due to random insertion of variable numbers of extra nucleotides at the breakpoint junction during crossover and the variability of the breakpoints in the *BCL1* fusion gene and the six *JH* segments. The size of the PCR products usually ranges from 80 bp to 300 bp for the MTC amplicons. Not only the presence but also the particular size of the *IGH/BCL1* PCR product is important in MRD monitoring.

References

1. Swerdlow SH, Campo E, Seto M, Muller-Hermelink HK (2008) Mantle cell lymphoma. In: Swerdlow SH, Campo E, Harris NL, Jaffe ES, Pileri SA, Stein H et al (eds) WHO classification of tumours of haematopoietic and lymphoid tissues. IARC, Lyon, pp 229–232
2. Lorsbach RB, His ED, Dogan A, Fend F (2011) Plasma cell myeloma and related neoplasms. Am J Clin Pathol 136:168–182
3. Yin CC (2011) Mantle cell lymphoma. In: Medeiros LJ (ed) Diagnostic pathology. Lymph nodes and spleen with extranodal lymphomas, Amirsys Publishing, Inc. pp 6:42–45
4. Williams ME, Swerdlow SH, Rosenberg CL, Arnold A (1993) Chromosome 11 translocation breakpoints at the PRAD1/cyclin D1 gene locus in centrocytic lymphoma. Leukemia 7:241–245
5. Luthra R, Hai S, Pugh WC (1995) Polymerase chain reaction detection of the t(11;14) translocation involving the bcl-1 major translocation cluster in mantle cell lymphoma. Diagn Mol Pathol 4:4–7
6. Luthra R, Sarris AH, Hai S, Paladugu AV, Romaguera JE, Cabanilla FF et al (1999) Real-time 5′–3′ exonuclease-based PCR assay for detection of the t(11;14)(q13;q32). Am J Clin Pathol 112:524–530
7. Medeiros LJ, Hai S, Thomazy VA, Estalilla OC, Romaguera J, Luthra R (2002) Real-time RT-PCR assay for quantifying cyclin D1 mRNA in B-cell non-Hodgkin's lymphomas. Mod Pathol 15:556–564
8. Hui P, Howe JG, Crouch J, Nimmakayalu M, Qumsiyeh MB, Tallini G et al (2003) Real-time quantitative RT-PCR of cyclin D1 mRNA in mantle cell lymphoma: comparison with FISH and immunohistochemistry. Leuk Lymphoma 44:1385–1394

Chapter 15

Detection of t(2;5)(p23;q35) in Anaplastic Large-Cell Lymphoma by Long-Range Nested Polymerase Chain Reaction Assay

C. Cameron Yin and Rajyalakshmi Luthra

Abstract

Anaplastic large-cell lymphoma (ALCL) is characterized by molecular abnormalities involving *ALK* gene located at 2p23 which results in an overexpression of ALK. Nine different rearrangements of *ALK* gene have been reported; the t(2;5)(p23;q35) is the most common. The t(2;5) fuses the *NPM* gene at 5q35 with the *ALK* gene. *NPM/ALK*, as well as *ALK* activation via other molecular abnormalities, plays an important role in the pathogenesis of ALCL. The lack of tight clustering within the involved *NPM* and *ALK* genes precludes analysis using standard PCR methods. We describe a long-range nested PCR assay to detect *NPM/ALK* gene rearrangements.

Key words Anaplastic large-cell lymphoma, t(2;5)(p23;q35), PCR

1 Introduction

Anaplastic large-cell lymphoma (ALCL) is a neoplasm of T- or null-cell lineage. It includes a subset of tumors characterized by molecular abnormalities involving *ALK* located at 2p23, leading to overexpression of ALK (1). Nine different abnormalities involving *ALK* have been reported to date (2, 3). Of these, the t(2;5)(p23;q35) is the most common, identified in 60–85% of ALCL, more commonly in tumors that occur in younger patients (4). The t(2;5) fuses the nucleophosmin gene (*NPM*), at 5q35 with the anaplastic lymphoma kinase gene (*ALK*) at 2p23 (3, 5). The *NPM/ALK* fusion gene is composed of the 5′ end of *NPM* and the 3′ end of *ALK*. The N-terminus of *NPM* has a strong promoter that drives *NPM/ALK* overexpression (6). In other rare translocations, *ALK* fuses with other genes including *TPM3* at 1q25, *TFG* at 3q21, *ATIC* at 2q35, *MSN* at xq11-12, and *CTLC* at 17q23, which also results in *ALK* overexpression (7). *NPM/ALK*, as well as *ALK* activation via other molecular abnormalities, is oncogenic in vitro and in vivo (8, 9).

Magdalena Czader (ed.), *Hematological Malignancies*, Methods in Molecular Biology, vol. 999,
DOI 10.1007/978-1-62703-357-2_15, © Springer Science+Business Media New York 2013

Detection of ALK expression by immunohistochemistry is the most commonly used method due to its ease, rapidity, specificity, and low cost (10). The pattern of immunostaining (nuclear versus cytoplasmic) may also be suggestive of the presence of specific translocations. Large lymphoma cells with both nuclear and cytoplasmic staining are seen in cases with t(2;5)/*NPM-ALK*, whereas in cases with variant tranlocations, the ALK staining may be membranous or cytoplasmic. Conventional cytogenetic analysis also allows detection of not only the t(2;5) but also other variant translocations involving *ALK*. However, it requires viable dividing cells. FISH method can be used to detect the t(2;5) or other *ALK* rearrangements and can be applied to nondividing cells. Southern blot analysis using genomic probes derived from either *ALK* or *NPM* can also be applied. However, this approach is labor intensive. The lack of tight clustering within the involved *NPM* and *ALK* genes precludes analysis using standard PCR methods, but RT or long-range PCR methods can be used (11). Real-time quantitative RT-PCR has been employed to monitor minimal residual disease in ALCL (12). However, RT-PCR requires RNA and generates amplicons of identical size, making it difficult to exclude contamination if it occurs. Long-range PCR has the advantages that RNA is not required and amplicons of distinct size for each case are generated. However, high-quality DNA is necessary for this approach (10). To detect *NPM/ALK* gene rearrangements, we developed a long-range nested PCR assay using a 5′ forward primer derived from the *NPM* gene and a 3′ reverse primer derived from the *ALK* gene (13). This methodology is presented in this chapter.

2 Materials

2.1 Specimen Requirements

1. Bone marrow (1–2 ml) or peripheral blood (5–10 ml) collected in EDTA tubes and delivered to the lab on cold pack within 48 h of collection (see Note 1).
2. Fresh unfixed tissues in sterile containers on dry ice.
3. Formalin-fixed, paraffin-embedded tissue sections.

2.2 Primers

The primers are purchased from Invitrogen (Carlsbad, CA), stored at –20°C and are stable for 1 year.

1. *NPM/ALK* forward primer (*NPM/ALK*-F).
   5′-TCCCTTGGGGGCTTTGAAATAACACC-3′.
2. *NPM/ALK* reverse primer (*NPM/ALK*-R).
   5′-CGAGGTGCGTGAGCTTGCTCAGC-3′.

3. Nested *NPM/ALK* forward primer (nested *NPM/ALK*-F).
   5′-ACCAGTGGTCTTAAGGTTGA-3′.
4. Nested *NPM/ALK* reverse primer (nested *NPM/ALK*-R).
   5′-TTGTACTCAGGGCTCTGCA-3′.
5. β-globin internal control forward primer (β-globin-F).
   5′-GAAGAGCCAAGGACAGGTAC-3′.
6. β-globin internal control reverse primer (β-globin-R).
   5′-GTTTGATGTAGCCTCACTTC-3′.

2.3 Other Reagents

GeneAmp XL PCR kit (Applied Biosystems, Foster City, CA) including:

1. PCR 3.3× XL buffer II.
2. 10 mM dNTP mix.
3. 25 mg $Mg(OAc)_2$ solution.
4. rTth DNA polymerase, XL 2.0 U/μl.

2.4 Equipment

1. ABI 7500 real-time PCR system.
2. Bio-Rad gel electrophoresis apparatus (Hercules, CA).
3. Bio-Rad Gel Doc System.

3 Methods

3.1 DNA Extraction and Quantification

Extract and quantify DNA using standard method (e.g., Qiagen kits, Qiagen, Valencia, CA). Adjust the concentration of DNA to 1 μg/μl (see Note 2).

3.2 XL (Extra Long) PCR Amplification (See Notes 3–6)

1. Prepare the following reaction mix (final concentration): PCR XL buffer II (1×), $Mg(OAc)_2$ (1.5 mM), dNTP mix (0.4 mM), *NPM/ALK*-F (0.1 μM), *NPM/ALK*-R (0.1 μM), β-globin-F (0.06 μM), β-globin-R (0.06 μM), rTth DNA polymerase (1 U).
2. Add 45 μl of the reaction mix to each well of a 96-well optical plate.
3. Pipette 5 μl of patient DNA or controls into the appropriate wells.
4. Cover the wells with optical caps, vortex plate, and quick-spin the plate to ensure that no bubbles are present at the bottom of the wells.
5. Perform PCR amplification on a thermocycler (e.g., ABI 7500) as follows:
   (a) 80°C for 5 min.

(b) 92°C for 1 min.

(c) Repeat 35 cycles of 92°C for 30 s, 56°C for 15 s, 68°C for 2 min 30 s.

(d) 72°C for 5 min.

6. After PCR, remove the plate from the thermocycler and place it in 4°C until ready for the nested PCR.

3.3 Nested PCR Amplification

1. Prepare the following reaction mix (final concentration): PCR XL buffer II (1×), $Mg(OAc)_2$ (1.5 mM), dNTP mix (0.4 mM), nested *NPM/ALK*-F (0.1 μM), nested *NPM/ALK*-R (0.1 μM), rTth DNA polymerase (1 U).
2. Add 49 μl of the reaction mix to each well of a 96-well optical plate.
3. Pipette 1 μl of XL PCR product or controls into the appropriate wells.
4. Cover the wells with optical caps, vortex plate, and quick-spin the plate to ensure that no bubbles are present at the bottom of the wells.
5. Perform PCR amplification on a thermocycler (e.g., ABI 7500) as follows:

   (a) 80°C for 5 min.

   (b) 92°C for 1 min.

   (c) Repeat 20 cycles of 92°C for 30 s, 56°C for 15 s, 68°C for 2 min 30 s.

   (d) 72°C for 5 min.
6. After PCR, remove the plate from the thermocycler and place it in 4°C until ready to load on the gel.

3.4 Gel Electrophoresis and Imaging

1. Load 18 μl of XL PCR products, nested PCR products or appropriate controls, and 2 μl of 10× gel loading buffer to each well on a 0.8% agarose gel.
2. Run the gel at 70 V for 1 h.
3. Prepare a gel image using the Bio-Rad Gel Doc System.

3.5 Result Interpretation and Reporting

1. A positive result is obtained when a band is visible both in the XL PCR lane and in the corresponding nested PCR lane.
2. Size of the positive amplicon can range from 0.8 to 10 kb. The amplicons obtained from the XL PCR primers should be larger than that obtained from the nested PCR primers for the same specimen.
3. A 3 kb β-globin band should be visible in all XL PCR product lanes indicating amplifiable DNA.

4 Notes

1. Heparin is an inhibitory agent for PCR; specimens should not be collected in heparinized tubes.
2. Since this test employs a long-range PCR assay, good quality DNA is required for successful amplification of the high molecular weight amplicons. After DNA extraction, each sample is quantified using a spectrophotometer to determine the DNA concentration. Samples with high protein contamination should be re-extracted.
3. Stringent procedures to prevent contamination, such as separation of pre- and post-PCR area, adherence to sterile technique, as well as never return aliquots to original container, should be practiced.
4. Reactions in duplicate are used to rule out false-positive results due to contamination, or false-negative results due to sampling error or PCR failure.
5. The following controls are included:
   (a) Positive controls from *ALK*-positive patient specimens.
   (b) Negative control (HL-60 cell line) is used to assure the specificity of the assay. Only the internal control should be observed in the negative control.
   (c) Internal control (β-globin) is used to assess the quality of each PCR reaction. An internal control target must be amplified in all negative samples in order to rule out false negatives due to poor DNA quality or PCR failure.
   (d) No-template reagent control is used to assure that there is no template contamination of the PCR reagents. Nothing should be observed in the reagent control.
6. To minimize nonspecific products, once pre-PCR is set up, it is necessary to run the samples as soon as possible.

References

1. Delsol G, Falini B, Muller-Hermelink HK et al (2008) Anaplastic large cell lymphoma (ALCL), ALK-positive. In: Swerdlow SH, Campo E, Harris NL et al (eds) WHO classification of tumours of haematopoietic and lymphoid tissues. IARC, Lyon, pp 312–316
2. Medeiros LJ, Elenitoba-Johnson KS (2007) Anaplastic large cell lymphoma. Am J Clin Pathol 127:707–722
3. Pulford K, Morris SW, Turturro F (2004) Anaplastic lymphoma kinase proteins in growth control and cancer. J Cell Physiol 199:330–358
4. Medeiros LJ (2008) Anaplastic large-cell lymphoma. In: Ioachim HL, Medeiros LJ (eds) Ioachim's lymph node pathology. Lippincott Williams & Wilkins, Philadelphia, pp 504–516
5. Falini B (2001) Anaplastic large cell lymphoma: pathological, molecular, and clinical features. Br J Haematol 114:741–760
6. Drexler HG, Gignac SM, von Wasielewski R, Werner M, Dirks WG (2000) Pathobiology of NPM-ALK and variant fusion genes in anaplastic large cell lymphoma and other lymphomas. Leukemia 14:1533–1559

7. Duyster J, Bai RY, Morris SW (2001) Translocations involving anaplastic lymphoma kinase (ALK). Oncogene 20:5623–5637
8. Kuefer MU, Look AT, Pulford K, Behm FG, Pattengale PK, Mason DY et al (1997) Retrovirus-mediated gene transfer of NPM-ALK causes lymphoid malignancy in mice. Blood 90:2901–2910
9. Chiarle R, Gong JZ, Guasparri I, Pesci A, Cai J, Liu J et al (2003) NPM-ALK transgenic mice spontaneously develop T-cell lymphomas and plasma cell tumors. Blood 101:1919–1927
10. Vega F, Medeiros LJ (2003) Chromosomal translocation involved in non-Hodgkin lymphomas. Arch Pathol Lab Med 127:1148–1160
11. Sarris AH, Luthra R, Cabanillas F, Morris SW, Pugh WC (1998) Genomic DNA amplification and the detection of t(2;5)(p23;q35) in lymphoid neoplasms. Leuk Lymphoma 29:507–514
12. Kalinova M, Krskova L, Brizova H, Kabickova E, Kepak T, Kodet R (2008) Quantitative PCR detection of NPM/ALK fusion gene and CD30 gene expression in patients with anaplastic large cell lymphoma-residual disease monitoring and a correlation with the disease status. Leuk Res 32:25–32
13. Luthra R, Sarris AH, Papadimitracopoulou V, Waasdorp M, Dimopoulos MA, McBride JA et al (1997) Long-range amplification of genomic DNA detects the t(2;5)(p23;q35) in anaplastic large-cell lymphoma, but not in other non-Hodgkin's lymphomas, Hodgkin's disease, or lymphomatoid papulosis. Ann Oncol 8(Suppl 2):59–63

Chapter 16

EBER In Situ Hybridization for Epstein–Barr Virus

Lawrence M. Weiss and Yuan-Yuan Chen

Abstract

Epstein–Barr encoding region (EBER) in situ hybridization is the methodology of choice for the detection of the Epstein–Barr virus (EBV) in tissue sections. Because of the large numbers of copies of EBERs present in latently infected cells, non-isotopic methods can be used. Positive studies show staining in the nuclei of the EBV-infected cells, accentuating the chromatin and often excluding the nucleolus. False-negative results are most often the result of RNA degradation in the tissues, a finding that may be detected through the use of a polyT probe as a control for RNA preservation.

Key words EBER, EBV, In situ hybridization, Malignant lymphoma, Hodgkin lymphoma

1 Introduction

The Epstein–Barr virus (EBV) is a ubiquitous human virus that is present in nearly all adults. Although it starts as a lytic infection, EBV rapidly enters a latent phase within 48 h. Latent infection involves the expression of a limited number of viral proteins, the two small noncoding RNAs Epstein–Barr encoding region (EBER)-1 and EBER-2, as well as several *Bam*H1-A rightward transcripts (1). The utility of EBER as a molecular target for detecting EBV in specimens resides in its ubiquity in expression in all known EBV latency states and its "in vivo" amplification at greater than 10^6 copies per infected cell. EBERs are not essential for the EBV-induced transformation of B-lymphocytes, although they may provide an advantage in transforming ability, play a role in apoptosis, and are known to be associated with the induction of several cytokines (2). There have been publications reporting negativity of EBERs in EBV-infected tissues (3), but these are exceptional, and EBER in situ hybridization is still considered to be the gold standard in detection of a latent infection. However, it has been clearly established that EBER may be negative in exclusively lytic infections, such as may be seen in hairy leukoplakia in human immunodeficiency virus (HIV)-infected patients.

Magdalena Czader (ed.), *Hematological Malignancies*, Methods in Molecular Biology, vol. 999,
DOI 10.1007/978-1-62703-357-2_16, © Springer Science+Business Media New York 2013

In normal lymphoid tissues from EBV serology-positive individuals, EBERs can be detected in between about 1:10^3 to 1:10^4 B-cells, and a higher number can be detected in tissues from immunosuppressed patients (4, 5). Although controversial, EBERs may occasionally be detected in extremely rare T-cells as well. Numerous EBER-positive cells are seen in tissues from patients with EBV-associated acute infectious mononucleosis. EBV has been associated with a number of human neoplasms, and EBERs may be identified in these tissues as well. These neoplasms include nasopharyngeal carcinoma and other lymphoepithelioma-like carcinomas of foregut origin; a subset of gastric carcinoma; a wide variety of B-cell lymphoproliferative disorders, including immunodeficiency-associated lymphomas (such as post-transplantation lymphomas, primary central nervous system lymphoma, primary effusion lymphoma, and plasmablastic lymphoma), endemic and a subset of non-endemic Burkitt lymphoma, EBV-positive diffuse large B-cell lymphoma of the elderly, lymphomatoid granulomatosis, pyothorax-associated lymphoma, and a subset of Hodgkin lymphoma; peripheral T-cell lymphomas, including extranodal NK/T-cell lymphoma of nasal type, systemic EBV-positive T-cell lymphoproliferative disease of childhood, hydroa vacciniforme-like lymphoma, and other mature T-cell lymphomas in which the EBV is primarily in non-neoplastic B-cells; and some mesenchymal neoplasms, such as HIV-associated smooth muscle neoplasms and a subset of inflammatory pseudotumors (6).

A variety of other methodologies are also available for the detection of EBV, and each has its own advantages and disadvantages (7). Polymerase chain reaction (PCR) has the sensitivity to detect EBV in any tissues from seropositive individuals containing B-cells. Therefore, quantitative PCR is much more informative, and is commonly used clinically to evaluate EBV burden in patients. Southern blot analysis of the EBV terminal repeat probe can be used to determine the clonality of the cells harboring EBV. Immunohistochemical detection of specific EBV latent proteins is helpful in determining the latency pattern of the infected cells.

2 Materials

2.1 Preparation of Slides

1. Pronase E stock: Weigh 60 mg of pronase E (Sigma) and add 10 ml of 50 mM Tris–HCl, pH 7.4, 5 mM EDTA. Aliquots of 0.5 ml may be stored in 1.5 ml microcentrifuge tubes at −80°C for up to 1 year.
2. Washing buffer: 0.1 M Tris–HCl, pH 7.5, 0.1 M NaCl with 2 mg/ml of glycine.

2.2 Preparation of Probes

1. EBER1 probe: 5′ AGA CAC CGT CCT CAC CAC CCG GGA CTT GTA 3′.

2. Non-EBV probe: 5′ AGA GTG CGT GGA CAC GTG CCG CCT GAA GTA 3′.
3. PolyT probe: 5′ TTT TTT TTT TTT TTT TTT TTT TTT TTT TTT 3′.
4. Terminal deoxyribonucleotide transferase (TdT) and 5× tailing buffer (Invitrogen, Carlsbad, CA).
5. Biotin-dUTP (16-biotin-dUTP, 1 mM (Roche Applied Science, Indianapolis, IN).
6. 25 mg/ml yeast tRNA: 50 mg tRNA (Invitrogen) added to 2 ml TE buffer to make a 25 mg/ml tRNA solution. TE buffer is made by adding 1 ml 1 M Tris–HCl, pH 7.5, and 0.4 ml 150 mM EDTA, pH 8.0–98.4 ml double-distilled water.
7. 3 M sodium acetate: Dissolve 24.62 g sodium acetate (Sigma, Inc., St. Louis, MD) in double-distilled water to a final volume of 100 ml.

2.3 Hybridization

1. 50× Denhardt's solution: Dissolve 0.1 g of polyvinylprolidone (PVP-40), 0.1 g of bovine serum albumin, and 0.1 g of Ficoll 400 in 8 ml of double-distilled water, bringing up the final volume to 10 ml with double-distilled water. Aliquots of 1 ml may be stored in 1.5 ml microcentrifuge tubes at -20°C for up to 1 year.
2. Prehybridization solution: 200 μl 1 M phosphate buffer, pH 7.4, 200 μl 50× Denhardt's solution, 1 g dextran sulfate, and 9.6 ml double-distilled water. Aliquots of 1.0 ml may be stored in 1.5 ml microcentrifuge tubes at −20°C for up to 1 year.
3. Hybridization solution (without probe): 200 μl 1 M phosphate buffer, pH 7.4, 200 μl 50× Denhardt's solution, 1 g dextran sulfate, 1.5 ml 20× saline sodium citrate (SSC), 100 μl 10 mg/ml salmon sperm DNA (sonicated or sheared), 50 μl 25 mg/ml yeast tRNA, 5 ml deionized formamide, and 3.075 ml double-distilled water. Aliquots of 975 μl may be stored in 1.5 ml microcentrifuge tubes at −20°C for up to 1 year.

2.4 Post-hybridization

1. 1% BSA in Tris-saline-brij solution: 10 ml of 1 M Tris–HCl, pH 7.5, 10 ml of 1 M NaCl, 0.5 ml 1 M $MgCl_2$, 1 g albumin, bovine fraction V (BSA), and 250 μl 35% brij stock solution in 100 ml of double-distilled water. Aliquots of 1 ml may be stored in 1.5 ml microcentrifuge tubes at −20°C for up to 1 year.
2. Streptavidin–alkaline phosphatase complex working solution: Mix fresh for each assay 2 μl streptavidin–alkaline phosphatase (Dako, Carpinteria, CA) (should be kept at 4°C) and 1 ml 1% BSA in Tris-saline-brij solution (see Note 1).
3. Tris-saline-Triton solution, pH 7.5: 100 ml 1 M Tris–HCl, 100 ml 1 M NaCl, 5 ml 1 M $MgCl_2$, and 670 ml 15% Triton

X-100 in 1 l double-distilled water. This may be stored at 2–8°C for up to 6 months.

4. Tris-saline, pH 9.5: 50 ml 1 M Tris–HCl, pH 9.5, 50 ml 1 M NaCl, and 25 ml 1 M $MgCl_2$ in 500 ml of double-distilled water. This may be stored at 2–8°C for up to 6 months.
5. 5-Bromo-4-chloro-3-indoyl phosphate-*p*-toluidine (BCIP) solution, 50 mg/ml: 50 mg BCIP in 1 ml *N*, *N*-dimethylformamide. This may be stored at 2–8°C for up to 2 months (see Note 1).
6. Nitroblue tetrazolium chloride (NBT), 50 mg/ml: 50 mg NBT chloride, 500 μl *N*,*N*-dimethylformamide, and 500 μl double-distilled water. This may be stored at room temperature in a light tight foil-wrapped vial for up to 2 months.
7. McGadey's Reagent (must be made fresh each time): 1.0 ml Tris-saline, pH 9.5, 3.3 ml 50 μg/ml BCIP, and 6.7 μl 50 mg/ml NBT, mixing gently. Discard after use.

3 Methods

In situ hybridization for EBER can be performed a number of ways. Some laboratories, particularly early on, chose to perform the procedure using isotopically labeled probes such as S35. However, since EBER is generally found in greater than 10^6 copies/EBV-infected cell, isotopic methods are not necessary and much more cumbersome than colorimetric procedures (8, 9). Some companies have automated the non-isotopic process, and, in general, these methodologies are perfectly adequate.

3.1 Preparation of Slides

1. Cut paraffin sections at a thickness of 4–5 μm onto charged slides (see Notes 2 and 3).
2. Bake sections at 65°C overnight prior to the hybridization procedure (see Note 4).
3. Deparaffinize tissue by placing slides in 100% xylene for 15 min at room temperature. Dip 3–4 times in the first 5 min.
4. Transfer slides to 100% absolute ethanol for 10 min.
5. Transfer slides to another 100% absolute ethanol for 10 min.
6. Prepare pronase E digestion buffer by adding 420 μl of pronase E stock to 2.5 ml of 50 mM Tris–HCl, pH 7.4, 5 mM EDTA. Discard any excess at the end of the procedure.
7. Digest proteins on slide by placing 50–150 μL (enough to cover tissue) of the pronase E digestion buffer on each tissue section. Incubate 10 min at room temperature.
8. Stop protein digestion by tilting the slides on edge and blot on paper towels.

9. Place slides back to back and insert into a slide staining rack and wash slides for 5 min using washing buffer. Repeat wash for 5 additional minutes.
10. Briefly dehydrate the slides in a series of increasing graded alcohols (3–4 dips in 30, 60, 95, and 100% ethanol).
11. Let slides air-dry at room temperature (see Note 5).

3.2 Preparation of Probes

1. Add 10 μl 5× TdT tailing buffer, 0.5 μg relevant oligonucleotide probe, 5–10 μl dUTP-biotin (11- or 21-dUTP-biotin), 2 μl 15 units/μl TdT, and 29.7 μl double-distilled water to a total volume of 50 μl (see Note 6).
2. Mix gently above mixture and incubate at 37°C for 30–60 min.
3. Add 1 μl yeast 25 mg/ml yeast tRNA and vortex.
4. Precipitate with 1:10 volume of 3 M sodium acetate and 2× volume 100% ethanol.
5. Place the microfuge tube at −70°C for 30–60 min.
6. Centrifuge in a microcentrifuge at 4°C for 30 min.
7. Carefully remove supernatant and rinse tube with cold 70% ethanol.
8. Vacuum dry the pellet for a short time and resuspend in 50 μl double-distilled water (final concentration of 10 ng/μl).

3.3 Hybridization

1. Place slides in a plastic slide folder lined in the middle with water-soaked strips of gauze.
2. Add 50–500 μl (enough to fully cover the tissue) of pre-hybridization solution to each tissue section (see Note 7). Place the slides in the plastic slide holder. Incubate in a moist chamber at 37°C for 30–60 min.
3. Blot off pre-hybridization solution and wipe off excess from around the tissue section.
4. Add probe to hybridization solution, adding 25 μl of probe to 975 μl of hybridization solution for each ml to be used (final probe concentration of 250 ng/ml) (see Note 8). The hybridization solution with EBER probe added is stable at −20°C for up to 1 year. However, the hybridization solution with polyT added should not be reused.
5. For EBER1, apply about 25 μl of hybridization solution with EBER probe added on the tissue section, and carefully place a glass coverslip on top, avoiding any air bubbles. Then use rubber cement to seal around the coverslip. After the cement has dried, place the slides in to a ThermoBrite (StatSpin Inc., Norwood, MA) to denature 10 min at 95°C. For polyT, apply 50–150 μl (enough to fully cover the tissue) of hybridization

solution containing polyT probe on each tissue section (approximately 1 ml/10 slides), but do not denature the slides.

6. Incubate the slides with hybridization solution containing probe at 37°C in the plastic slide holder in a moist chamber (such as a Tupperware container) overnight (see Note 9).

3.4 Post-hybridization

1. For EBER1, carefully remove the rubber cement and the coverslip. For polyT, blot the hybridization solution and wipe off excess from around the tissue section.
2. Place the slides in a glass staining rack containing 2× SSC, dip the slides 3–4 times, and incubate at room temperature for 10 min.
3. Repeat the above step 2 more times, each time changing the 2× SSC, for a total of three times.
4. Dry off the slides and wipe off excess solution around the tissue section.
5. Apply 50–150 μl (enough to fully cover the tissue) of the freshly prepared streptavidin–alkaline phosphatase complex working solution to each tissue section.
6. Place the slides back in the plastic slide folder and incubate at 37°C in a moist chamber for 2 h.
7. Blot the tissue sections and place the slides back to back in a glass rack.
8. Wash the slides with Tris-saline-Triton for 3 min.
9. Repeat two more times, each time changing the Tris-saline-Triton, for a total of three times.
10. Do a final wash with 3 min with Tris-saline, pH 9.5 on a shaker. Keep dipping the slides for the final minute.
11. Wipe off the slides and apply 50–150 μl of McGadey's reagent per tissue section (enough to fully cover the tissue). Incubate at 37°C for 1–2 h.
12. Briefly wash in distilled water (a few dips), and wipe off excess water.
13. To view slides, drop on 100% ethanol to cover the tissue, and temporarily coverslip (Fig. 1) (see Note 10). A positive signal is a blue–black color over the cell nucleus, highlighting the chromatin structure, and sometimes with exclusion of staining in the nucleolus (10). Variation in the intensity of the staining is virtually always due to the degree of RNA preservation rather than the copy number of EBER. If no positive signal is seen at all, one must ensure that there is at least some positivity (even if weak) with the polyT probe to demonstrate that there was adequate RNA preservation in the tissues. If both the EBER

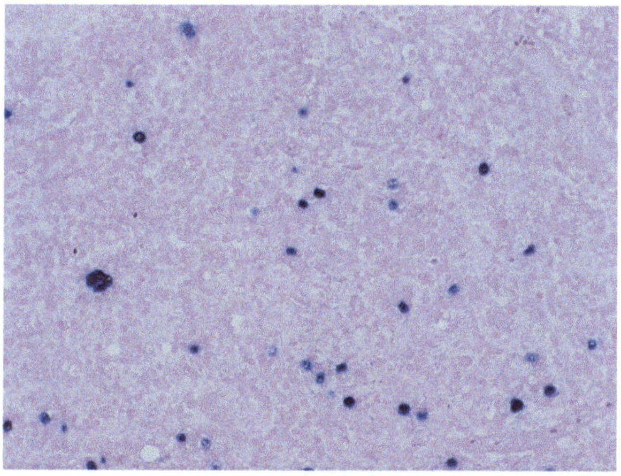

Fig. 1 This EBER in situ hybridization demonstrates scattered EBER-positive small and large lymphoid cells in a case of angioimmunoblastic T-cell lymphoma. No counterstain was used

and polyT slides are completely negative, one cannot rule out the possibility of degradation of the RNA in the tissue and therefore false negativity with the EBER stain.

4 Notes

1. In our experience, if there is a heavy background, it is most often due to the use of old or suboptimally refrigerated streptavidin–alkaline phosphatase complex or BCIP.
2. Formalin-fixed tissues work the best. B5-fixed tissues give inferior results, and require close attention to verifying RNA preservation by examination of the appropriate control slide. In addition, B5-fixed tissues often show a crystalline artifact that must be distinguished from a positive signal.
3. One may combine immunohistochemical studies with EBER in situ hybridization to determine the immunophenotype of any EBER-positive (or negative) cells. In this case, the immunohistochemical studies should be performed first, in general without any modifications necessary. In this case, the slides should be dried and in situ hybridization protocol can be started at step 6 above.
4. If time is a concern, one can microwave for 2 min instead of baking overnight. Another alternative is to bake the slides for at least 2 h, although one is taking a little bit of risk that the tissue may come off at some point in the procedure.

5. One may stop the procedure at the point.
6. In tissues with a high content of endogenous biotin, it may be advantageous to employ a digoxigenin-labeled probe. In this case, 11- or 21-dUTP-digoxigenin can be substituted in the labeling reaction.
7. The prehybridization step may be omitted, particularly if the slides have been denatured.
8. The polyT probe is necessary to ensure that there is adequate RNA preservation in the tissue being studied. Other laboratories utilize probes targeting cellular U6 RNA as a test for RNA preservation (10). The non-EBV probe may not be necessary, but can provide additional assurance as to the specificity of the EBER results.
9. One may shorten this time to 2–4 h.
10. One may counterstain the slides to view the context of the results, and one can permanently coverslip the slides. However, unless alcohol-based counterstains and coverslips are used, any positive signals will diffuse out as a crystalline precipitate over time and the results will be lost. Many laboratories use a methyl green counterstain as the blue–black staining stands out well against a light green background that stains chromatin.

References

1. Rickinson A (2002) Epstein-Barr virus. Virus Res 82:109–113
2. Swaminathan S (2008) Noncoding RNAs produced by oncogenic human herpesviruses. J Cell Physiol 216:321–326
3. Gan YJ, Razzouk BI, Su T, Sixbey JW (2002) A defective, rearranged Epstein-Barr virus genome in EBER-negative and EBER-positive Hodgkin's disease. Am J Pathol 160:781–786
4. Deamant FD, Albujar PF, Chen Y-Y, Weiss LM (1993) Epstein-Barr virus distribution in non-neoplastic lymph nodes. Mod Pathol 6: 729–732
5. Niedobitek G, Herbst H, Young LS, Brooks L, Masucci MG, Croker J et al (1992) Patterns of Epstein-Barr virus infection in non-neoplastic lymphoid tissue. Blood 15:2520–2526
6. Rezk RA, Weiss LM (2007) Epstein-Barr virus-associated lymphoproliferative disorders. Hum Pathol 38:1293–1304
7. Gulley ML, Tang W (2008) Laboratory assays for Epstein-Barr virus-related disease. J Mol Diagn 10:279–292
8. Chang KL, Weiss LM (1992) Description of an in situ hybridization methodology for detection of Epstein-Barr virus RNA in paraffin-embedded tissues, with a survey of normal and neoplastic tissues. Diagn Mol Pathol 1:246–255
9. Hamilton-Dutoit SJ, Pallesen G (1994) Detection of Epstein-Barr virus small RNAs in routine paraffin sctions using non-isotopic RNA/RNA in situ hybridization. Histopathology 25:101–111
10. Gulley ML, Glaser SL, Craig FE, Borowitz M, Mann RB, Shema SJ, Ambinder RF (2002) Guidelines for interpreting EBER in situ hybridization and LMP1 immunohistochemical tests for detecting Epstein-Barr virus in Hodgkin lymphoma. Am J Clin Pathol 117: 259–267

Chapter 17

Epstein–Barr Virus (EBV) Load Determination Using Real-Time Quantitative Polymerase Chain Reaction

Hongxin Fan and Ryan S. Robetorye

Abstract

Epstein–Barr virus (EBV) infects virtually the entire human population and infection persists throughout the lifetime of its host. EBV has been associated with the development of a wide variety of neoplasms, including lymphoma, carcinoma, and sarcoma. In addition, EBV-associated lymphoproliferative disorders are particularly prevalent in immunosuppressed individuals, including AIDS patients, transplant recipients, and patients with congenital immunodeficiencies. In recent years, EBV viral load assessment has been extensively implemented in clinical practice for the diagnosis and monitoring of EBV-associated malignancies and lymphoproliferative disorders. The real-time quantitative polymerase chain reaction (RQ-PCR) has become the method of choice for quantification of specific EBV nucleic acid sequences. This method is fast, extremely sensitive, and accurate, requires only very small amounts of input nucleic acid, and is relatively simple to perform. These characteristics have made it the method of choice for EBV viral load determination. This chapter describes the use of a laboratory-developed RQ-PCR EBV viral load assay for the detection of EBV DNA in cell-free plasma and cerebrospinal fluid samples.

Key words Epstein–Barr virus, Viral load, Quantitative real-time PCR

1 Introduction

The Epstein–Barr virus (EBV) has been implicated in the development of a wide variety of neoplasms, including lymphomas such as Burkitt lymphoma, Hodgkin lymphoma, extranodal NK/T-cell lymphoma (nasal type), EBV-positive diffuse large B-cell lymphoma of the elderly, EBV-positive T-cell lymphoproliferative disorders of childhood, plasmablastic lymphoma, primary effusion lymphoma, angioimmunoblastic T-cell lymphoma, and lymphomatoid granulomatosis, carcinomas such as nasopharyngeal carcinoma, and gastric adenocarcinoma, and leiomyosarcomas (1). In addition, EBV-associated lymphoproliferative disorders are observed in patients with AIDS, immunosuppressed transplant recipients (post-transplant lymphoproliferative disorders), and in patients with primary immune disorders such as severe combined

Magdalena Czader (ed.), *Hematological Malignancies*, Methods in Molecular Biology, vol. 999,
DOI 10.1007/978-1-62703-357-2_17, © Springer Science+Business Media New York 2013

immunodeficiency, CD40 and CD40 ligand deficiencies, common variable immunodeficiency, Wiskott-Aldrich syndrome, and X-linked lymphoproliferative syndrome (1, 2).

In recent years, EBV viral load assessment has become a valuable tool in clinical practice for the diagnosis and monitoring of EBV-associated malignancies and lymphoproliferative disorders (1, 3). Commercially developed kits are now available for EBV viral load determination, such as the LightCycler EBV Quantification Kit (Roche Molecular Diagnostics, Pleasanton, CA) and the Artus EBV Kit (Qiagen, Valencia, CA). However, in this chapter, we describe a relatively inexpensive and easy to perform laboratory-developed EBV viral load assay (4) that utilizes real-time quantitative PCR (RQ-PCR) and an Applied Biosystems (ABI) 7900HT Sequence Detection System (see Note 1). Although various sample types (see Note 2) can be analyzed for different EBV-associated disorders (6), this chapter confines discussion to use of a RQ-PCR EBV viral load assay for cell-free plasma and cerebrospinal fluid (CSF) specimens only. Briefly, viral DNA is extracted from plasma or CSF samples and is amplified with specific primers and hybridization probes targeting EBV BamH1 W region by RQ-PCR on an ABI 7900HT instrument (Applied Biosystems). This approach uses a dual-labeled fluorogenic probe known as a TaqMan hybridization probe to measure the accumulation of PCR product by measuring the amount of the fluorophore during the exponential stages of the PCR. The TaqMan probe is a single-stranded oligonucleotide that is complementary to a segment of 20–60 nucleotides within the DNA template and is located between the two PCR primers. One fluorescent dye on the 5′ end of the probe serves as a reporter (i.e., 6-carboxyfluorescein, or FAM), and its emission spectrum is quenched by a second fluorescent dye at the 3′ end of the probe (i.e., 6-carboxy-tetramethyl-rhodamine, or TAMRA). During each PCR extension cycle, the 5′–3′ exonuclease activity of *Taq* polymerase degrades the 5′ portion of the probe and releases the reporter dye, resulting in an increase in the fluorescence reporter signal. The fluorescence detected is directly proportional to the amount of the fluorophore released, and therefore, proportional to the amount of EBV DNA template present in the PCR. The exponential phase of the PCR is used to determine the threshold cycle, or C_T, which is the number of PCR cycles at which a significant increase in fluorescence is detected above background levels. The C_T is directly proportional to the number of copies of EBV DNA template present in the reaction. The quantity of EBV viral load is determined by interpolation from a standard curve obtained from serially diluted EBV DNA standards of known copy number run along with the test samples in each PCR plate. The addition of small amounts of Exogenous Internal Positive Control (IPC) DNA to the PCR is used to monitor the efficacy of the DNA extraction and amplification steps. The EBV viral load assay described in this chapter is accurate and precise within a wide dynamic range for measuring targeted EBV sequences.

2 Materials

2.1 Samples and DNA Extraction

1. Cell-free plasma and CSF samples.
2. EZ1 Virus Mini Kit V2.0 (Qiagen, Valencia, CA).
3. EZ1 Virus Card V2.0 (Qiagen, Valencia, CA).
4. TaqMan Exogenous Internal Positive Control (IPC) DNA (Applied Biosystems, Carlsbad, CA).
5. BioRobot® EZ1 workstation (Qiagen, Valencia, CA).
6. EBV B95-8 (Type 1) Quantitated Viral DNA (Advanced Biotechnologies Inc., Columbia, MD) (see Note 3).
7. OptiQuant EBV DNA quantification panel (Acrometrix, Benicia, CA).
8. Pipettes and pipette tips.
9. General laboratory equipment, including vortex mixer, desktop centrifuge, microcentrifuge, spectrophotometer, and incubators.

2.2 Quantitative Real-Time PCR

1. Real-time PCR thermal cycler (ABI Prism 7900HT Sequence Detection System, Applied Biosystems, Carlsbad, CA).
2. MicroAmp Optical 96-well Reaction Plate (Applied Biosystems, Carlsbad, CA).
3. TaqMan Universal PCR Master Mix (Applied Biosystems, Carlsbad, CA).
4. TaqMan Exogenous Internal Positive Control Reagents (with TaqMan VIC reporter Dye; Applied Biosystems, Carlsbad, CA).
5. Optical Adhesive Film (Applied Biosystems, Carlsbad, CA).
6. Nuclease-free H_2O.
7. Forward and reverse EBV BamH1 W primers (see Note 4).
8. TaqMan EBV BamH1 W probe (see Note 5).

3 Methods

3.1 DNA Extraction from CSF and Plasma Samples

DNA can be extracted using either manual or automated methods based on the resources available in individual laboratories. Here, we describe an automated DNA extraction method for CSF and plasma samples using the Qiagen EZ1 workstation and EZ1 DNA

Virus Mini Kit (see Note 6), with the additional modification of adding Exogenous Internal Positive Control (IPC) DNA to the samples before DNA extraction.

1. Collect peripheral blood samples (3–5 ml) in EDTA (purple top) tubes. Separate plasma from the cellular portion of blood samples by centrifugation of EDTA blood at 1,500×*g* for 10 min. Transfer the plasma (supernatant) to a new tube (see Note 7) and proceed immediately to DNA extraction step, or freeze plasma at −20°C until ready to extract.
2. Fresh CSF samples should be sent to the laboratory for immediate processing, or the samples may be refrigerated at 4°C and processed by the laboratory within 24 h. Prepare the CSF sample by centrifugation at 1,500×*g* for 10 min to remove possible cells. Transfer the CSF supernatant to a new tube for immediate DNA extraction, or freeze at −20°C until ready for extraction.
3. Extract viral DNA from plasma or CSF samples using the EZ1 Virus Mini Kit with the minor modification of adding IPC DNA before extraction. Briefly, add 2 μl of IPC DNA to each plasma or CSF sample and extract viral DNA on the BioRobot® EZ1 Workstation by using the EZ1 Virus Mini Kit along with the EZ1 Virus Card according to the manufacturer's instructions (7). Use a starting sample volume of 400 μl, and a final elution volume of 90 μl.
4. After extraction, DNA samples may be stored temporarily at 4°C or at −20°C until ready to proceed to RQ-PCR.

3.2 Standards

1. Use commercially available EBV B95-8 (Type 1) Quantitated Viral DNA (Advanced Biotechnologies Inc.) to prepare standard curve dilutions (see Note 3).
2. Before each RQ-PCR run, freshly prepare all standard curve dilutions for one-time and immediate use. Prepare standard dilutions in a range from 10^0 to 10^4 copies per RQ-PCR (e.g., 5–50,000 copies per RQ-PCR, or use another dynamic range of choice) by tenfold serial dilutions of one volume of EBV standard DNA into nine volumes of H_2O. For example, adding 5 μl of original EBV standard DNA into 45 μl of nuclease-free H_2O produces the first tube of 50 μl standard, and subsequent tenfold serial dilutions are performed from this tube. Use these tenfold serially diluted DNA samples to produce the EBV standard curve and include a standard curve in each RQ-PCR run plate (see Subheading 3.4, step 3).

3.3 Controls

1. Include blank or no template controls, consisting of nuclease free-H_2O, in each RQ-PCR run to ensure that the samples are not contaminated with DNA or PCR amplicon from previous runs.

2. An EBV-negative control sample (e.g., DNA from an EBV-negative cell line) should be included in each RQ-PCR run to monitor assay performance.
3. EBV DNA samples containing high and low EBV viral loads (high EBV copy number and low EBV copy number positive controls) should be included in each RQ-PCR run to monitor assay accuracy, maintenance of linearity, stability of standards, and success of the RQ-PCR.

3.4 Real-Time Quantitative PCR Set-Up

1. Remove all reagents and patient samples from storage. Keep all thawed reagents and patient samples cool on wet ice prior to use. TaqMan probe aliquots should also be protected from light and should not be thawed until immediately prior to use.
2. Prepare the RQ-PCR master mix tube. The final volume of master mix is based on the total number of reactions required for each RQ-PCR. Each RQ-PCR reaction well should contain a total of 20 μl of master mix (see Note 8) that includes the following: 0.4 μl of nuclease-free H_2O, 15 μl of 2× Taqman Universal PCR Master Mix, 0.2 μl of each EBV BamH1 W forward and reverse primer (see Note 4; the final concentration of each primer should be 300 nM), 1.2 μl of EBV BamH1 W TaqMan probe (see Note 5; the final concentration of probe should be 200 nM), and 3 μl of TaqMan Exogenous Internal Positive Control Reagent.
3. Set up the RQ-PCR in a 96-well plate by adding 20 μl of master mix per well along with 10 μl of patient test DNA, EBV standard DNA, or EBV positive and negative control DNA samples to appropriate wells (or 10 μl of nuclease-free H_2O to no template control wells) (see Notes 8 and 9). Each RQ-PCR plate should include standard curve samples, no template controls, patient test samples in duplicate or triplicate, and EBV-negative and -positive controls (including high and low EBV viral load samples). It includes two wells of no template control, two wells of EBV-negative DNA control, ten wells of standard curve samples (5 tenfold serial dilutions of EBV standard DNA in duplicate), high and low EBV viral load controls in duplicate, and six patient DNA test samples in duplicate. When finished pipetting samples in the 96-well reaction plate, seal the reaction plate with an optical adhesive film.
4. Centrifuge the reaction plate at low speed for 2 min and then load the plate onto the Applied Biosystems 7900HT real-time PCR instrument. Use Applied Biosystems Sequence Detection Software (SDS) to document and run the assay (see Subheading 3.5, steps 1 and 2).
5. Run the RQ-PCR using modified universal thermal cycling conditions: 50°C for 2 min, 95°C for 10 min, 40 cycles of 95°C for 15 s, and 60°C for 1 min.

3.5 Program and Run Applied Biosystems 7900HT Instrument

1. Operate the Applied Biosystems 7900HT instrument and the SDS software according to the manufacturer's recommendations (8, 9).
2. Launch the SDS software and open a new plate template window to denote well locations on the 96-well plate for the standard dilutions, controls, and testing samples. Record EBV standard copy number values (e.g., 5, 50, 500, 5,000, 50,000 copies of EBV DNA) for wells containing standards and also denote replicate samples for duplicate or triplicate testing. Make sure that all wells are checked for both FAM and VIC TaqMan reporter dye detection and data collection (EBV-FAM and IPC-VIC). Save the template window with the recorded data as a SDS run file.
3. Select the connect button and load the 96-well plate into the ABI 7900HT instrument. Select the start button to begin the actual run.

3.6 Data Collection and Analysis

1. After the run is completed, remove the reaction plate from the instrument and save the results of the run. When the analysis button is selected in the SDS software, the results will be analyzed automatically if the standards and testing sample information was recorded as noted above (see Subheading 3.5, step 2).
2. View the standard curve results in the amplification plot and standard curve plot views in the SDS software. Determine the crossing threshold cycles (C_T) for the standard curves of the EBV standard DNAs (FAM reporter dye) in the exponential phase of the reactions, either manually or automatically (see Note 10). Select the fluorescence threshold at which the C_T is determined for IPC amplification (VIC reporter dye) as a fixed value (e.g., 0.20) for different runs (see Note 11 and Fig. 1).
3. If the standard curves are deemed to have acceptable slopes and correlation coefficients (see Note 10), export the results from the SDS software as a text file.

3.7 Calculations

1. The ABI SDS software automatically calculates the EBV copy number per RQ-PCR based on the EBV DNA standard curve results from each run plate. However, the actual reported EBV viral load must take into account any dilutions made during the pre-amplification process. For example, the DNA extraction step has a starting sample volume of 400 μl of plasma or CSF and a final elution volume of 90 μl, and 10 μl of the eluted DNA is subsequently used for the RQ-PCR. Therefore, the actual DNA copy number in the equivalent of 1 ml of starting sample (EBV copies/ml) is obtained by multiplying the dilution factor of the sample by the RQ-PCR determined EBV copy number as follows:

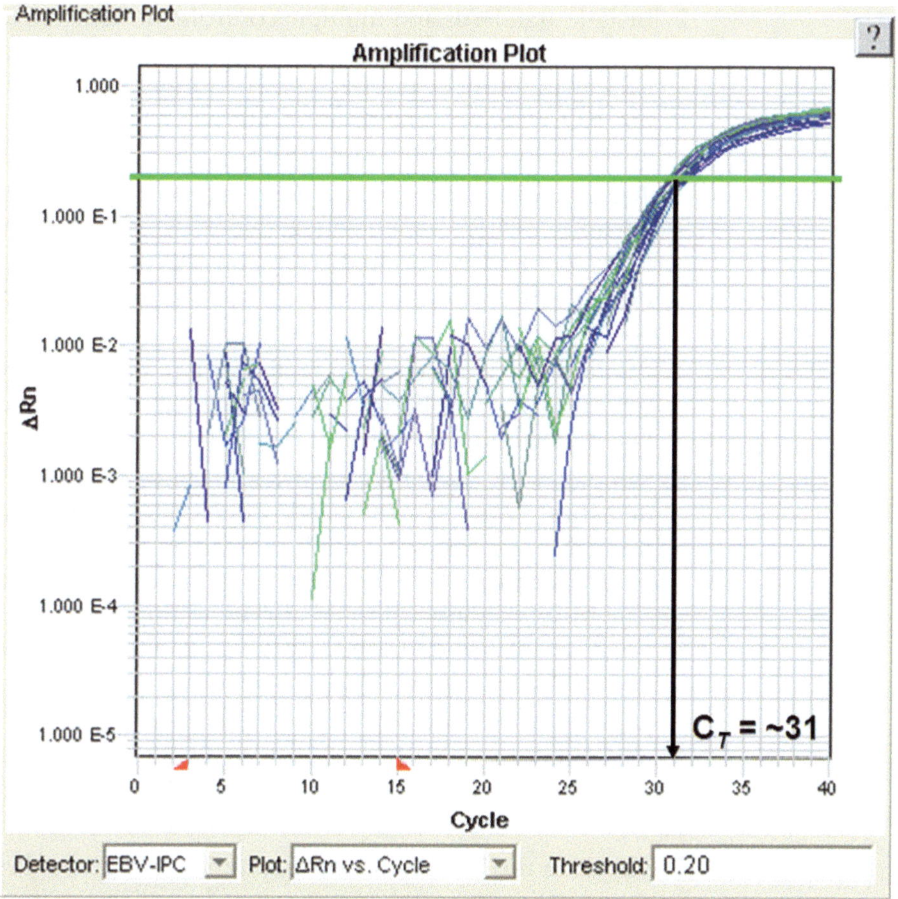

Fig. 1 EBV IPC DNA Amplification Plot. Change in relative fluorescence (Rn) is plotted versus PCR cycle number. Rn is the fluorescence of the VIC reporter dye divided by the fluorescence of a passive reference dye. The C_T (threshold cycle) is the intersection between the amplification curve and the fluorescence threshold line (*heavy green horizontal line*) set at 0.20. If the fluorescence threshold is set at 0.20 after RQ-PCR amplification, the resulting C_T value of IPC samples should be in the range from 30 to 32 cycles (see Note 11). In this particular run, the C_T is approximately 31

$$\text{EBV copies/ml} = \text{EBV copies/RQ-PCR} \times 22.5.$$

The 22.5× dilution factor is obtained from the combination of a 9× dilution (90 μl eluted EBV DNA and subsequent use of 10 μl in the RQ-PCR), and a 2.5× dilution (conversion of 400 μl starting sample volume to a 1 ml equivalent; 1 ml/400 μl = 2.5 × dilution). Final dilution factor = 9 × 2.5 = 22.5 (see Note 12).

2. Report EBV viral load as EBV copies per ml or, or if desired, EBV viral load can be converted to logarithm base 10 ($\log_{10}$) EBV copies per ml.

3.8 Quality Control of the Assay

1. Use fixed amounts of IPC DNA added to each patient sample (plasma or CSF) before DNA extraction to monitor the assay for DNA extraction failure and/or to detect PCR inhibitors.

2. Include standards and multiple controls (no template control, EBV-negative control, and high EBV copy number and low EBV copy number positive controls) in each run to monitor the RQ-PCR for amplification efficiency, assay accuracy and linearity, and contamination issues.
3. The integrity of the standard curve is crucial for accurate determination of EBV viral load (see Note 13). When a new lot of EBV standard is required, compare the performance of the new lot with the current lot before using the new material in a clinical test run.
4. Run each patient sample in replicate. Use identical DNA concentrations for replicates, and average the resulting values for final reporting.
5. Samples with high EBV viral loads above the assay limit of detection (e.g., >50,000 EBV copies/RQ-PCR) should be diluted (e.g., 1:5 or 1:10 dilution) in an EBV-negative sample (plasma or CSF) and then re-extracted and re-amplified. The results obtained should also be multiplied by the appropriate additional dilution factor (e.g., multiply by 5 or 10) to obtain the final EBV viral load value.
6. Samples with a low EBV viral load below the lower limit of detection (e.g., <5 EBV copies/RQ-PCR) should be reported with appropriate comments (e.g., EBV DNA detected, but below the lower limit of accurate quantitation).
7. Calibrate the EBV viral load assay every 6 months. Previously tested patient samples or commercially available materials with known EBV viral load should be used for this purpose (see Note 14).
8. Participate in regularly scheduled and graded laboratory proficiency assessments. For example, the College of American Pathologists (CAP) offers a viral load assay (VLS) survey program for EBV viral load testing.

3.9 Result Interpretation

1. At the end of each RQ-PCR, examine the standard curve to confirm that the slope of the curve is within the range of -3.3 ± 0.3. The standard curve should also be linear with a R^2 value close to 0.99. See Fig. 2 for an example of an EBV DNA standard curve.
2. Check the no template controls and EBV negative controls at the completion of each RQ-PCR to confirm that these controls show no evidence of assay contamination. Detection of EBV in these samples indicates assay contamination, and the assay should be repeated. High and low EBV DNA control results should also be within expected ranges.
3. Check each assay for evidence of DNA extraction failure and/or the presence of PCR inhibitors. Since an equal amount of IPC DNA is added to each patient sample, similar

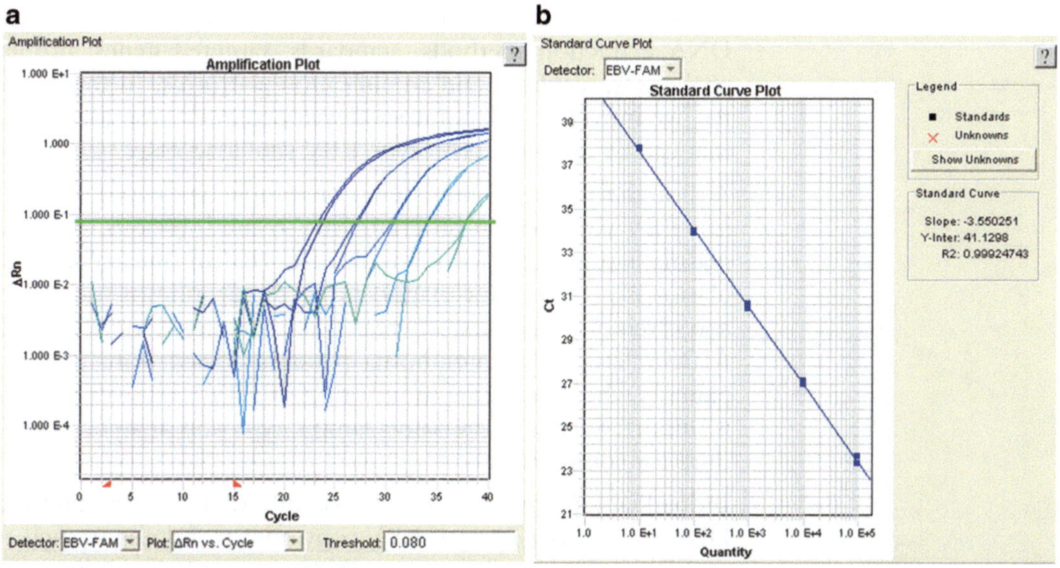

Fig. 2 EBV DNA Standards Amplification Plot and Standard Curve Plot. (**a**) Serially diluted EBV standard DNA amplification plot with duplicate samples. The change in relative fluorescence (Rn) is plotted versus PCR cycle number. Rn is the fluorescence of the FAM reporter dye divided by the fluorescence of a passive reference dye. The fluorescence threshold line (*heavy green horizontal line*) is selected in the exponential phase of the amplification plot to achieve the best slopes and correlation coefficients (R^2) and to minimize the variability of replicate samples (see Note 10). (**b**) Standard curve plot obtained from serially diluted EBV DNA standards in duplicate. The ABI SDS software automatically plots a standard curve based on the C_T results for each standard from each run plate. The C_T of each the standards is plotted versus the respective EBV DNA copy number of the standard. The slope of each standard curve should ideally be close to −3.3, but a range of −3.3 ± 0.3 cycles is acceptable. The standard curve should also be linear with a R^2 value close to 0.99. This particular run showed a slope of −3.55 and a R^2 value of 0.999 (see Note 10)

IPC amplification efficiency should be achieved among all patient samples if DNA extraction was successful and no PCR inhibitors are present (see Fig. 1).

4. Check replicate samples to make sure that EBV viral load is similar among the replicates of each sample (see Note 15). However, very low EBV viral load samples may show variability in viral load results (see Note 16). In low EBV load samples, the coefficient of variation (CV) among replicate samples may be as high as 50% (see Note 17).
5. Correlate EBV viral load levels with clinical status and prior EBV levels for appropriate test interpretation (see Note 18).

4 Notes

1. Currently, there is no consensus method for determining EBV viral load (5). Lack of a standard EBV viral load protocol can be problematic when comparing EBV load results obtained from different laboratories, since many pre-analytic and post-analytic

factors can affect EBV load results, including use of different DNA extraction methods, standards, targeted genes, primer probe sets, reagents, and amplification platforms. In this chapter, we introduce a laboratory-developed EBV viral load assay that can be used as a prototype EBV viral load assay (4).

2. Although there is no consistency on sample types used to monitor EBV viral load in different EBV-related diseases, cell-free plasma is preferable for many diseases (6). In our experience, plasma is preferred for diagnostic or monitoring of transplant and carcinoma patients, whereas CSF is preferred for suspected AIDS-related CNS lymphoma patients. Please note that for patients who need serial monitoring of EBV load over time, it is important to use the same sample type and analytic procedure for comparison.

3. Individual laboratories may choose different sources for EBV DNA standards as long as EBV copy number is known, such as an EBV-infected cell line (e.g., Namalwa or Raji cell line), or plasmid DNA that contains EBV sequences. Our laboratory chooses to use a commercial source for EBV DNA (Advanced Biotechnologies Inc.) that is obtained from the EBV B95-8 cell line. EBV copy number is quantitated by the vendor (EBV copy number approximately $1–2 \times 10^4$ copies/μl), and although EBV quantity varies in different lots, EBV copy number is indicated in the vendor's product information sheet that accompanies each product shipment. Note that total EBV copy number depends on the volume of the standard added to each PCR. For example, adding 5 μl of standard that contains 10,000 EBV copies per μl is equivalent to a total of 50,000 copies of EBV DNA. New batches of EBV standard should be aliquoted into small volumes for one time use and stored at –20°C. Aliquots should not be subjected to repeated freeze–thaw cycles, and the aliquots should be used before the expiration date recommended by the vendor for each lot of the product.

4. The EBV viral load assay discussed in this chapter utilizes EBV BamH1 W primers (4). Primer sequences used for the assay are as follows: EBV W1 forward primer sequence: 5′-GCAGCCGCC CAGTCTCT-3′; EBV W2 reverse primer sequence: 5′-ACAGACAGTGCACAGGAGCCT-3′. Prior to performing RQ-PCR, primer working solutions should be prepared by diluting the primers in nuclease-free H_2O to achieve the desired primer concentration (e.g., 45 pmol/μl).

5. The EBV viral load assay described in this chapter utilizes a TaqMan EBV BamH1 W probe (4). The TaqMan probe sequence is as follows: 6-FAM-5′-AAAAGCTGGCGCCCT TGCCTG-TAMRA-3′. Prior to performing RQ-PCR, a probe working solution should be prepared by diluting probe in nuclease-free H_2O to achieve the desired probe concentration

(e.g., 5 pmol/μl). New batches of probe should be aliquoted into small volumes for one-time use, and stored at −20°C. Aliquots should not be subjected to repeated freeze–thaw cycles, and the aliquots should be protected from light to avoid degradation of the probe fluorophores.

6. DNA extraction protocols other than the EZ1 Virus Mini Kit method may also be used as long as DNA quality and quantity is ensured. In our experience, using relatively large starting plasma volumes (~400 μl) and adding carrier RNA can increase viral DNA yield and assay sensitivity.
7. At this step, the plasma supernatant layer should be carefully aspirated so that the buffy coat layer is not disturbed. Normal B-cells carry low levels of EBV, and B-cell contamination of the plasma sample may cause a false positive EBV viral load result.
8. Our laboratory uses the ABI 7900HT Fast Real-Time PCR System with a standard 96-well block module and a maximum PCR volume of 30 μl. We have found that adding 10 μl of DNA to 20 μl of master mix (for a 30 μl total PCR volume) produces the most consistent results.
9. Add 10 μl of DNA or 10 μl of nuclease-free H_2O to appropriate reaction plate wells as follows: to no template control wells, add 10 μl of nuclease-free H_2O; to standard curve wells, add 10 μl of serially diluted EBV standard DNA; to patient test sample wells, add 10 μl of patient DNA.
10. When the threshold cycle is determined manually, it should be selected in the exponential phase of the amplification plot to achieve the best slopes and correlation coefficients (R^2) and to minimize the variability of replicate samples. The slope of each standard curve should ideally be close to −3.3, but a range of −3.3 ± 0.3 cycles is acceptable. The standard curve should also be linear with a R^2 value close to 0.99.
11. In this EBV viral load assay, we use the C_T value obtained from the IPC amplification plot to monitor the DNA extraction and PCR amplification steps. 2 μl of IPC DNA is added to each plasma or CSF sample before extraction, and 10 μl of the 90 μl total volume of eluted DNA from the Qiagen EZ1 workstation is subsequently used for the RQ-PCR. If the fluorescence threshold is set at 0.20 after RQ-PCR amplification, the resulting C_T value of IPC samples should be in the range from 30 to 32 cycles (see Fig. 1). However, each individual laboratory should determine acceptable IPC C_T values for their specific assay. Note that there may be C_T value variation in different lots of IPC DNA. If the IPC C_T is higher than expected, this may be due to either DNA extraction failure or the presence of PCR inhibitors in the sample. Very high EBV load samples

may competitively inhibit IPC PCR amplification. If EBV viral load is above the assay's upper limit of detection, the patient sample should be appropriately diluted using an EBV-negative sample (plasma or CSF) and then re-extracted and re-amplified (see Subheading 3.8, step 5).

12. Note that no dilution of sample occurs during the DNA purification step as the EBV in the 400 μl sample is simply concentrated into a 90 μl volume. The final calculated dilution factor will vary from laboratory to laboratory depending on actual starting sample volume, elution volume, and the volume of DNA used per RQ-PCR.
13. To ensure assay accuracy, the same lot of EBV DNA standard should be used for each individual EBV viral load test run.
14. Long-term monitoring of the EBV viral load assay's results and comparison of previous trends is recommended. We use commercially available materials to calibrate our EBV viral load assay every 6 months (OptiQuant EBV DNA panel, Acrometrix). The calibration panel is processed starting from the DNA extraction step, so that it can be used to monitor our entire EBV load assay from start to finish. The manufacturer's expected results should be obtained (see OptiQuant EBV DNA panel product insert sheet for further details).
15. Run test samples in duplicate or triplicate according to individual laboratory statistical needs. Our laboratory runs patient sample replicates only in the RQ-PCR step, since the automated EZ1 DNA extraction system produces consistent DNA yield with low variation for each sample.
16. For very low EBV viral load samples, inconsistent results may be obtained from replicate samples (e.g., one well positive with low EBV load, and one well completely negative for EBV). It is important to exclude the possibility of sample contamination in such cases by repeating the analysis. Very low EBV viral load results should be reported with caution and additional replicates may be required to confirm the low EBV load in such patients.
17. Individual molecular diagnostics laboratories must validate EBV viral load assays (analytic and clinical validation) in their own specific patient population before offering the test for clinical sample testing. This validation should include verification of assay specificity, accuracy, sensitivity, linearity, intra-assay precision and inter-assay reproducibility. We consider a threefold EBV viral load change as clinically significant based on our reproducibility study, with a highest coefficient of variation of approximately 50%.
18. Keep in mind that monitoring EBV viral load at multiple time points in each patient is more important than a single EBV viral load value for the clinical management of patients.

Acknowledgment

The authors would like to thank Yao Wang for her excellent technical assistance.

References

1. Gulley ML, Tang W (2008) Laboratory assays for Epstein–Barr virus-related disease. J Mol Diagn 10:279–292
2. Van Krieken JH, Onciu M, Elenitoba-Johnson KSJ, Jaffe ES (2008) Lymphoproliferative diseases associated with primary immune disorders. In: Swerdlow SH et al (eds) WHO classification of tumours of haematopoietic and lymphoid tissues, 4th edn. International Agency for Research on Cancer, Lyon, France
3. Navarro WH, Kaplan LD (2006) AIDS-related lymphoproliferative disease. Blood 107:13–20, Review
4. Ryan JL, Fan H, Glaser SL, Schichman SA, Raab-Traub N, Gulley ML (2004) Epstein–Barr virus quantitation by real-time PCR targeting multiple gene segments: a novel approach to screen for the virus in paraffin-embedded tissue and plasma. J Mol Diagn 6:378–385
5. Hayden RT, Yan X, Wick MT, Rodriguez AB, Xiong X, Ginocchio CC et al for the College of American Pathologists Microbiology Resource Committee (2012) Factors contributing to variability of quantitative viral PCR results in proficiency testing samples: a multivariate analysis. J Clin Microbiol 50(2):337–345
6. Kimura H, Ito Y, Suzuki R, Nishiyama Y (2008) Measuring Epstein–Barr virus (EBV) load: the significance and application for each EBV-associated disease. Rev Med Virol 18: 305–319, Review
7. Qiagen (October 2010) EZ1® Virus handbook. For automated, simultaneous purification of viral DNA and RNA from 1–14 serum, plasma, and CSF, urine, whole blood, and stool, transport media, respiratory samples, and dried swab samples using EZ1 instruments. Third Edition. http://www.qiagen.com/literature
8. Applied Biosystems (2003) ABI PRISM® 7900HT sequence detection system and SDS enterprise database user guide basic operation and maintenance Rec C. http://www3.appliedbiosystems.com
9. Applied Biosystems (2001) ABI PRISM® 7900HT sequence detection system user guide basic operation and maintenance Rev A4. http://www3.appliedbiosystems.com

Chapter 18

Molecular and Immunohistochemical Detection of Kaposi Sarcoma Herpesvirus/Human Herpesvirus-8

Amy Chadburn, Janet Wilson, and Y. Lynn Wang

Abstract

Kaposi sarcoma herpesvirus/human herpesvirus-8 (KSHV/HHV-8) is etiologically related to the development of several human diseases, including Kaposi sarcoma, primary effusion lymphoma (PEL)/extra-cavitary (EC) PEL, multicentric Castleman disease (MCD), and large B-cell lymphoma arising in KSHV/HHV-8-associated multicentric Castleman disease. Although serologic studies can identify persons infected with this virus, molecular genetics, specifically PCR (polymerase chain reaction) and immunohistochemical techniques, are rapid, sensitive, and specific, and are able to more closely link KSHV/HHV-8 to a given disease process. As these KSHV/HHV-8-related diseases cause significant morbidity and mortality in affected individuals, the identification of the virus within lesional tissue will allow for more targeted therapy.

Key words Kaposi sarcoma herpesvirus, Human herpesvirus-8, Polymerase chain reaction, Immunohistochemistry (IHC), ORFK9-3, ORF73, LANA/LNA-1

1 Introduction

Since its discovery in 1994, the Kaposi sarcoma herpesvirus (KSHV), also known as human herpesvirus 8 (HHV-8), has been etiologically associated with the development of Kaposi sarcoma (KS), primary effusion lymphoma (PEL)/extra-cavitary (EC) PEL, multicentric Castleman disease (MCD), and large B-cell lymphoma arising in KSHV/HHV-8-associated multicentric Castleman disease (MCD) (1–3). These KSHV/HHV-8-associated lesions tend to occur preferentially in immunocompromised patients, particularly those infected by HIV; however, they can also occur in other patient populations, including immunocompetent individuals. For example, Kaposi sarcoma (KS) not only occurs in the setting of HIV infection (epidemic KS), but can also be seen in patients who are therapeutically immunosuppressed (iatrogenic KS), who live in high-incidence areas such as Africa (endemic KS), or who develop the "classic" form (sporadic KS) (4–6).

Magdalena Czader (ed.), *Hematological Malignancies*, Methods in Molecular Biology, vol. 999,
DOI 10.1007/978-1-62703-357-2_18, © Springer Science+Business Media New York 2013

Although the KSHV/HHV-8-associated lesions have been recognized for nearly 15 years, they can still present as diagnostic dilemmas. The KS lesions may be difficult to separate from other spindle cell or vascular tumors such as angiosarcoma. Primary effusion lymphomas/EC-PELs usually lack expression of B-cell-associated antigens and may express epithelial markers such as epithelial membrane antigen (EMA) and, thus, can be misdiagnosed as a poorly differentiated carcinoma. The morphologic features seen in MCD are not disease specific and can be seen in other settings not associated with KSHV/HHV-8 infection. Hence, it is helpful to have molecular and immunophenotypic studies to aid in the identification of this virus.

KSHV/HHV-8 was initially identified by molecular means in contrast to most other viruses. In 1994, Chang et al., used a relatively new molecular technique, representational difference analysis (RDA), to isolate unique sequences of KSHV/HHV-8 present in KS tissues from a patient with AIDS (7). From this analysis four distinct amino acid sequences were identified, two of which, designated KS330Bam and KS631Bam, were found to be specific for AIDS-KS tissues based on Southern blot hybridization studies. These studies were confirmed and extended by PCR (polymerase chain reaction) analysis with primers designed from KS330Bam that amplified a 233 bp fragment of KS330Bam, designated $KS330_{233}$. Thus, the first set of primers was developed for the identification of the-then-new virus, KSHV/HHV-8.

Of the molecular tests available for the detection of KSHV/HHV-8, the polymerase chain reaction (PCR) is the easiest and the most commonly used method. However, as with all PCR tests, extreme care must be exercised to prevent contamination. In the past, several studies identified KSHV/HHV-8 in a variety of tissue types and disease entities that could not be consistently confirmed by other laboratories (8–12). In most instances, these unconfirmed studies used techniques that greatly increased the sensitivity of detection, such as nested PCR, raising the possibility that some of these findings were falsely positive. However, most of the time, this is unnecessary as a single-step PCR will allow for the detection of as little as 1–10 copies of KSHV/HHV-8 in 100 ng of DNA (13). A wide variety of primers are currently available which can be used for PCR in the detection of KSHV/HHV-8 (see Table 1). PCR analysis for KSHV/HHV-8 can be done on a variety of materials including fresh/frozen tissues, cell suspensions, and formalin-fixed routinely processed tissues.

KSHV/HHV-8 can also be identified by Southern blot analysis using genomic DNA. This, of course, requires fresh or frozen tissue or cells. Southern blot hybridization, particularly in PEL/EC-PELs, is useful as it can indicate a specific association of the virus with the tumor whereas PCR will be positive whether the KSHV/HHV-8 is within the tumor cells or in some bystander cells

Table 1
Oligonucleotide sequences for the PCR detection of KSHV/HHV-8

Region	Size of amplicon (bp)	Primer	Primer sequence
ORF26	233	Forward	5′-AGCCGAAAGGATTCCACCAT-3′
		Reverse	5′-TCCGTGTTGTCTACGTCCAG-3
ORF72	138	Forward	5′-CGCCTGTAGAACGGAAACAT-3′
		Reverse	5′-TTGCCCGCCTCTATTATCAG-3′
ORFK2	196	Forward	5′-AGAAGCTCCATGACGTCCAC-3′
		Reverse	5′-TTCTAGAGCCCGCTGCTATT-3′
ORFK9-3	184	Forward	5′-CCCTTTCGCGGATATACACA-3′
		Reverse	5′-AGTGAGGGGAAAGCGTCAAT-3′
β-globin	251	Forward	5′-ACACAACTGTGTTCACTAGC-3′
		Reverse	5′-GGAAAATAGACCAATAGGCTG-3′

that are not part of the neoplastic process. As PELs/EC-PELs contain a large number of KSHV/HHV-8 copies (up to 200) within each tumor cell (14), detection of the virus by Southern blot is not particularly difficult. However, it involves radioisotope in most cases and is time consuming and labor intensive. With the improved sensitivity of PCR and the specificity of immunohistochemistry (see below), Southern blotting is no longer necessary in most instances for the identification of KSHV/HHV-8.

Although molecular methods can relatively easily identify the presence of the virus within a specimen, many laboratories are now using immunohistochemistry to identify individual KSHV/HHV-8-infected cells (see Note 1). Monoclonal antibodies directed to the gene products of viral open reading frames, such as LANA, are highly specific for the virus. The LANA antibody can be used on routinely processed tissues and the punctate nuclear pattern of immunoreactivity is highly specific and sensitive for the virus (15). The advantage of immunostaining is that it allows for identification of individual infected cells and is extremely useful in cases of KS and MCD as well as in KSHV/HHV-8-positive lymphomas. Additional antibodies for other KSHV/HHV-8 gene products are available, but most others are expressed only during specific periods of latency or lytic replication or in specific settings (16). Since LANA-1 tethers the virus to the human genome (16), and is expressed throughout latency in KSHV/HHV-8-infected cells in KS, PEL/EC-PEL, MCD, and large B-cell lymphoma arising in KSHV/HHV-8-associated MCD, the antibody against this viral protein is the most useful for identifying the virus (15–17). Because of the complementary nature of this technique to PCR analysis, detection of KSHV/HHV-8 by this method will also be outlined.

2 Materials

2.1 PCR Analysis

PCR amplification can be done on DNA extracted from fresh, frozen, or routinely processed paraffin-embedded tissue using standard methods (see Note 2) (18, 19). The following text describes the materials and conditions that may be used when employing primers to the ORFK9-3 region (Table 1). Primers to the ORF26, ORF72, and ORFK2 regions are also listed in Table 1. The PCR conditions for the latter primer sets have been previously described (7, 13, 20, 21). Each assay is run with positive and negative controls (see Note 3).

1. Oligonucleotide primers and probes: The sequences for primers for ORF26 (capsid protein), ORF72 (viral cyclin), ORFK2 (viral interleukin-6), and ORFK9-3 (vIRF, viral interferon regulatory factor) are listed in Table 1. Any "housekeeping" primer set can be used as an internal control for integrity of the DNA and for the absence of inhibitors. One of these "housekeeping" primer sets is β-globin; the primer set for β-globin is included in Table 1.
2. PCR thermocycler.
3. Reagents for DNA extraction from blank paraffin-embedded tissue sections.
   (a) Xylene.
   (b) Proteinase K solution (500 μg/ml; Invitrogen, Carlsbad, CA).
4. Reagents for the polymerase chain reaction mixture (ORFK9-3 region):
   (a) PCR reaction buffer, 10×, with $MgCl_2$ (Roche Diagnostics Corporation, Indianapolis, IN).
   (b) GoTaq Flexi DNA polymerase (5 U/μl, Promega; Madison, WI).
   (c) Forward and reverse primers (synthesized by Invitrogen; Carlsbad, CA, Table 1).
   (d) dNTP mix (10 mM, Promega; Madison, WI). Dilute with dH_2O to 2.5 mM, aliquot and store at −20°C.
   (e) 50–100 ng high-molecular-weight DNA from fresh/frozen tissues or 2 and 4 μl of paraffin-embedded tissue extract.
5. Reagents for the analysis of the PCR products.
   (a) 10% polyacrylamide gel.
   (b) 10× Tris–Borate–EDTA buffer (TBE; VWR, West Chester, PA).
   (c) 25 bp DNA molecular marker (Invitrogen, Carlsbad, CA).

2.2 Immunohistochemistry

Immunohistochemical staining procedures for antigens change based on a large number of variables including, but not limited to, the automated immunostaining system employed, the type of tissue fixation, retrieval methods available, and the primary antibody clone. In addition, immunostaining can be done on a variety of tissue sample types including smears, cytospins, frozen tissue sections, and routinely processed tissues; for each tissue type there is a potential need to modify the immmunostaining procedure. However, although each of these variables may dictate differences in specific steps in the staining procedure, the basic principles are the same and each staining should be accompanied by controls (see Note 4). Below is one example of the materials that would be required for immunohistochemical detection of the gene product of ORF 73 (LANA-1; LNA-1) in formalin-fixed paraffin-embedded tissue sections using a DAKO Autostainer Plus (DAKO Corporation North America, Carpinteria, CA).

1. Antibody: HHV-8 (LANA; Advanced Biotechnologies, Columbia, MD).
2. Detection system: Vector Rat Elite Kit (Vector Laboratories, Inc., Burlingame, CA).
3. Chromogen: Diaminobenzidine (DAB; DAKO North America).
4. Buffer: 10× Citra pH 6.0 (Biogenex, San Ramon, CA).
5. Xylene and ethanol series (100% ethanol, 95% ethanol, 70% ethanol).
6. Hematoxylin.
7. Dual endogenous enzyme blocking solution (Dako, Carpinteria, CA).
8. Rat IgG (Vector Laboratories, Inc., Burlingame, CA).
9. Tris buffer (0.05 mol/l Tris–HCl, 0.15 mol/l NaCl, 0.05% Tween 20 and preservative, pH 7.6, Dako, Carpinteria, CA).
10. Dako Autostainer Plus (Dako, Carpinteria, CA).
11. Oven (60°C).
12. Microtome.
13. Decloaking Chamber (Biocare Medical, Concord, CA).
14. Miscellaneous: Charged glass slides, coverslips, permount.

3 Methods

3.1 Isolation of Nucleic Acid

DNA for PCR can be extracted from fresh, frozen, or routinely processed paraffin-embedded tissues (see Note 5) (18, 19). Paraffin tissue on blank slides or as sections in a tube (see Note 6) may be used for PCR.

1. Place slide(s) in a 50 ml Falcon tube. Cover section(s) completely with xylene. Leave at room temperature for 10 min.
2. Discard xylene and repeat step 1.
3. Discard xylene and replace with 100% ethanol covering the section(s) completely.
4. Discard ethanol and repeat step 3.
5. Discard ethanol and remove slide(s) from the 50 ml Falcon tube.
6. Air-dry the section completely.
7. Pipette 100–300 μl of Proteinase K solution (500 μg/ml; Invitrogen, Carlsbad, CA) onto the slide (see Note 7).
8. Using a clean disposable scalpel, carefully scrape the section off the slide. Once removed, use a Pipetman to aspirate the section and solution and transfer into a clean 1.5 ml microcentrifuge tube.
9. Digest overnight at 37°C or for 3 h at 55°C.
10. Heat tubes to 95°C for 10 min to inactivate the Proteinase K activity.
11. Briefly spin down samples in a microcentrifuge.
12. The tissue extract of DNA from the paraffin section(s) can now be used for PCR or stored at –20°C.

3.2 Polymerase Chain Reaction

All samples should be run in duplicate with different amounts of the sample DNA extracted from paraffin tissue sections (2 and 4 μl). DNA extracted from fresh or frozen material should be diluted so that the final concentration is between 25 and 50 ng/μl. Two and four (2 and 4) μl of DNA is added to each tube. For samples from formalin-fixed paraffin-embedded material 2–4 μl of tissue extract should be used. Each test reaction should be accompanied by a positive control, negative control, and a "no-template" control reactions (see Note 3). The total PCR reaction volume (including DNA) per reaction is 25 μl.

1. Prepare the *master mix* within a plastic 1.5 ml microfuge tube. The mix should be prepared in an area that is physically separate from areas for DNA extraction, PCR amplification, and electrophoresis. The total amount of master mix needed is obtained by multiplying the number of samples to be analyzed plus one (see Table 2 using five reactions as an example). Mix well.
2. Add 23 μl master mix to each 0.2 ml PCR reaction tube.
3. Add 2–4 μl sample DNA in the following order (patient DNA positive control, negative control, and no template (i.e., dH_2O, added last; see Note 7).

Table 2
Example of the preparation of the *master mix* for five samples for KSHV/HHV-8 PCR using primers to ORFK9-3

	Per tube (μl)	For six tubes (μl)	Final concentration
10× buffer (+$MgCl_2$)	2.5	15	1×
dNTP (2.5 mM)	1.0	6	100 μM
K9-3F primer (250 ng/μl)	0.5	3	125 ng
K9-3R primer (250 ng/μl)	0.5	3	125 ng
Taq pol (5 U/μl)	0.15	0.9	0.75 U
dH_2O	18.35	138	
Total	23	138	
DNA	2 and 4 μl		

Table 3
PCR thermocycler protocol for the amplification of KSHV/HHV-8 using primers to the ORFK9-3 region

94°C 62 (61–60–59–58)°C 72°C	30 s 30 s 45 s	1°C decrease in each subsequent cycle, five cycles total
94°C 57°C 72°C 4°C	30 s 30 s 45 s Hold	31 cycles

4. Place the PCR reaction tubes in the PCR thermocycler—perform the touchdown program (Table 3).
5. Load the PCR products on the 10% PAGE in 1× TBE buffer with a 25 bp molecular weight DNA ladder.
6. Run the gel at 150 V for 60 min.
7. Visualize with ethidium bromide staining and UV illumination.
8. Interpretation of PCR results (see Notes 7 and 8): The presence of a 184 bp PCR amplification product in a test sample is indicative of the presence of the KSHV/HHV-8 genome. Negative and "no-template" controls should NOT contain any band while the positive control should show the 184 bp band (Fig. 1).

3.3 Immunohistochemistry

1. Cut two 3–4 μm tissue sections (test section and negative control section) from the paraffin block of the test tissues and one section from the positive control block.

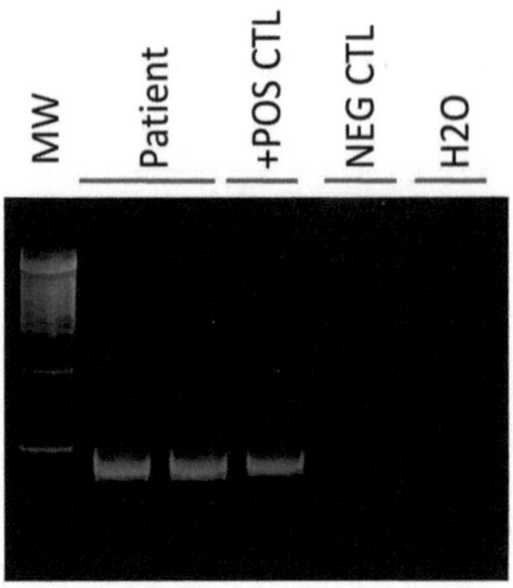

Fig. 1 PCR analysis shows the presence of a 184 bp amplification product in both patient samples (*lanes 1* and *2*) as well as in the positive control (*lane 3*). Note that the negative control and "no-template" (i.e., H_2O) control lanes have no bands

2. Place tissue sections on charged slides.
3. Bake slides in a 60°C oven for at least 30 min.
4. Deparaffinize by sequentially placing the slides in three changes of xylene for 5 min each; the xylene is removed with two changes of 100% ethanol.
5. Rehydrate slides with ten dips through each of two changes of 95% ethanol and two changes of 70% ethanol; the slides are then rinsed in distilled H_2O.
6. Slides are placed in the Decloaker containing the Citra buffer (50 ml consisting of 5 ml of concentrated buffer + 45 ml of distilled H_2O); when the temperature has reached 90°C and 24 psi, the Decloaker will beep and begin cooling.
7. When the Decloaker beeps again, the slides may be removed.
8. The slides are placed on the DAKO Autostainer Plus with the following protocol:
   (a) Dual-endogenous enzyme blocking: 10 min.
   (b) Vector blocking serum (Vector Elite Kit): 30 min.
   (c) HHV-8 (LANA) antibody diluted 1:1,000 in Tris buffer (test case and positive control) OR rat IgG diluted 1:1,000 in Tris buffer (negative control): 45 min.
   (d) Anti-rat biotinylated solution (Vector Elite Kit): 30 min.
   (e) Anti-rat ABC reagent (Vector Elite Kit): 30 min.
   (f) DAB: 10 min.
9. Remove the slides from the autostainer.
10. Counterstain in hematoxylin for one min.

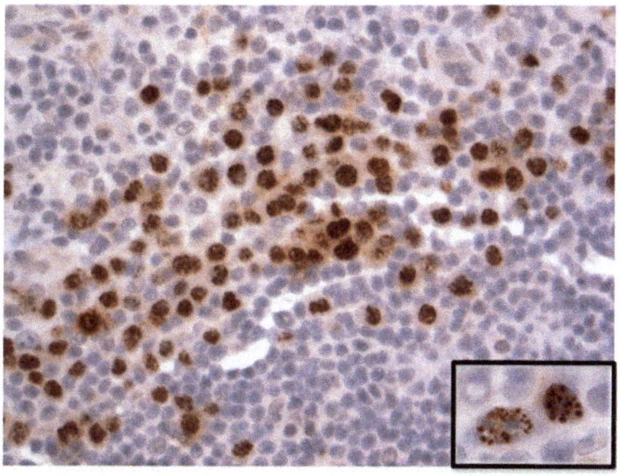

Fig. 2 Immunoperoxidase staining for ORF73 (LANA; LNA-1): Immunostaining shows the punctate pattern nuclear immunoreactivity in a case of KSHV/HHV-8-associated multicentric Castleman disease (immunoperoxidase staining 40× original magnification; insert 100× original magnification)

11. Dehydrate through graded ethanols to xylene.
12. Coverslip.
13. *Analysis and interpretation of results* (see Notes 9 and 10): Slides are reviewed under a light microscope. Identification of the characteristic punctate pattern in the nucleus of the appropriate cells is considered positive (Fig. 2), but only if the positive control also exhibits the same pattern of immunoreactivity and the negative control is negative.

4 Notes

1. Choice of test depends on the question that is to be answered. Although PCR is fast and very sensitive, it may be more important to identify individual KSHV/HHV-8-infected cells by immunohistochemistry. Alternatively, when the entire specimen is composed of the lesion, PCR may be more appropriate.
2. Fresh, frozen, and formalin-fixed tissues are usually amplifiable by PCR. It is important with respect to routinely processed tissue to use samples that have been fixed in a fixative that allows the DNA to be amplified. One of the more "amplifiable" fixatives is formalin. Tissue fixed in fixatives such a Bouin's and B5 are poorly amplifiable; decalcification also decreases the ability of Taq polymerase to successfully amplify viral DNA sequences.
3. Any PEL cell line can be used as a positive control for PCR analysis; at least four KSHV/HHV-8-positive cell lines are

available through the American Type Culture Collection (ATCC; Rockville, MD; http://www.atcc.org) and include the BC-3 cell line which is KSHV/HHV-8 positive, but Epstein–Barr virus (EBV) negative (ATCC designation CRL-2277). The BC-3 cell line contains approximately 30 copies of the viral genome per cell and thus can be diluted up to 1,000-fold and still retain functionality as a PCR positive control. As opposed to PEL cell lines, DNA from KS cell lines, however, should not be used as positive controls since the virus is often "lost" after a few passages in culture. The negative control can be any KSHV/HHV-8-negative cell line such as HL60 or Nalmalva both of which are available from the ATCC. The "no-template" control reaction uses dH_2O instead of DNA.

4. For immunohistochemistry, any case previously shown to contain KSHV/HHV-8-positive cells will suffice as a positive control. A cell block generated from cell line cells, such as the BC-3 cell line described above, is an excellent source of positive control slides. The cell block can be processed in the same manner as any other tissue specimen (including the KSHV/HHV-8 case tissues) in the laboratory. The negative control consists of a slide of the test case immunostained in an identical manner as the true test slide except it receives in the primary step rat IgG instead of the LANA antibody.
5. PCR is very sensitive and there is always the risk of contamination. Thus, extreme care must be taken at all steps of the procedure. It is important to extract the DNA in an area that is physically separate from that used for amplification and manipulation of the PCR products to minimize the chance of cross-contamination. In order to maximize detection of contamination, set up the PCR reactions in the following order: patients' samples, positive control, negative control, "no template" (i.e., dH_2O).
6. Procedure for extraction of DNA from paraffin tissue sections in a tube:
   (a) Place the tissue sections (1–3 depending on the tissue size) into a microcentrifuge tube.
   (b) Add 1 ml of xylene to the tube and sections.
   (c) Mix the sections and xylene with a pipette then spin the mixture in a microfuge for 10 min at room temperature.
   (d) Carefully remove the supernatant, then repeat steps b and c.
   (e) Carefully remove the supernatant, add 1 ml of ethanol, and gently pipette the mixture.
   (f) Spin the mixture at full speed for 10 min at room temperature.
   (g) Carefully remove the supernatant, then repeat step e.

(h) Carefully remove the supernatant; then allow the DNA pellet to air-dry completely.

(i) Resuspend the cell pellet in 50–300 μl of Proteinase K solution (500 μg/ml) according to the size of the DNA pellet.

(j) Proteinase K digestion is carried out at 37°C overnight, or for 3 h at 55°C after which the tubes are heated at 95°C for 10 min to inactivate Proteinase K activity.

(k) Briefly spin down samples. Sample is ready for PCR or can be stored at −20°C.

7. PCR controls are crucial: Positive, negative, "no template," and "housekeeping" should be evaluated before patients' results are interpreted.
8. PCR products can be visualized without hybridization even with only very low copy numbers (<5–100) present. However, hybridization is useful to confirm the specificity of the amplified products, if deemed necessary (13).
9. Like PCR, immunohistochemistry is dependent on tissue properties and is more sensitive than PCR to proper fixation. While poorly fixed tissues usually may still amplify, immunohistochemistry is more likely to fail.
10. There are multiple variables that can alter the immunostaining procedure. If the immunostaining procedure fails to show a positive signal in the positive control slide, first check the antibody (lot, expiration date, etc.), the type of tissue fixation (formalin, Bouin's, B5, etc.), and the "degree" of fixation (i.e., is it properly fixed); alterations may be in order. If all seems correct, repeat the staining once; if there is again no positive signal change one variable at a time to solve the problem.

References

1. Carbone A, Cesarman E, Spina M, Gloghini A, Schulz TF (2009) HIV-associated lymphomas and gamma-herpesviruses. Blood 113:1213–1224
2. Mesri EA, Cesarman E, Boshoff C (2010) Kaposi's sarcoma and its associated herpesvirus. Nat Rev Cancer 10:707–719
3. Chadburn A, Hyjek E, Mathew S, Cesarman E, Said J, Knowles DM (2004) KSHV-positive solid lymphomas represent an extra-cavitary variant of primary effusion lymphoma. Am J Surg Pathol 28:1401–1416
4. Cesarman E, Knowles DM (1997) Kaposi's sarcoma-associated herpesvirus: a lymphotropic human herpesvirus associated with Kaposi's sarcoma, primary effusion lymphoma, and multicentric Castleman's disease. Semin Diagn Pathol 14:54–66
5. Kalt I, Masa SR, Sarid R (2009) Linking the Kaposi's sarcoma-associated herpesvirus (KSHV/HHV-8) to human malignancies. Methods Mol Biol 471:387–407
6. Ganem D (1997) KSHV and Kaposi's sarcoma: the end of the beginning? Cell 91:157–160
7. Chang Y, Cesarman E, Pessin MS, Lee F, Culpepper J, Knowles DM et al (1994) Identification of herpesvirus-like DNA sequences in AIDS-associated Kaposi's sarcoma. Science 266:1865–1869
8. Monini P, de Lellis L, Fabris M, Rigolin F, Cassai E (1996) Kaposi's sarcoma-associated herpesvirus DNA sequences in prostate tissue and human semen. N Engl J Med 334:1168–1172
9. Parravicini C, Lauri E, Baldini L, Neri A, Poli F, Sirchia G et al (1997) Kaposi's sarcoma-associated herpesvirus infection and multiple

myeloma. Science 278:1969–1970, author reply 1972–1963
10. Rettig MB, Ma HJ, Vescio RA, Pold M, Schiller G, Belson D et al (1997) Kaposi's sarcoma-associated herpesvirus infection of bone marrow dendritic cells from multiple myeloma patients. Science 276:1851–1854
11. Tasaka T, Said JW, Morosetti R, Park D, Verbeek W, Nagai M et al (1997) Is Kaposi's sarcoma–associated herpesvirus ubiquitous in urogenital and prostate tissues? Blood 89:1686–1689
12. Whitby D, Boshoff C, Luppi M, Torelli G (1997) Kaposi's sarcoma-associated herpesvirus infection and multiple myeloma. Science 278:1971–1972, author reply 1972–1973
13. Cesarman E (2001) Molecular detection of Kaposi's sarcoma-associated herpesvirus/human herpesvirus-8. In: Killeen AA (ed) Methods in molecular medicine: molecular pathology protocols. Humana, Totowa, NJ, pp 331–336
14. Lacoste V, Judde JG, Bestett G, Cadranel J, Antoine M, Valensi F et al (2000) Virological and molecular characterisation of a new B lymphoid cell line, established from an AIDS patient with primary effusion lymphoma, harbouring both KSHV/HHV8 and EBV viruses. Leuk Lymphoma 38:401–409
15. Kellam P, Bourboulia D, Dupin N, Shotton C, Fisher C, Talbot S et al (1999) Characterization of monoclonal antibodies raised against the latent nuclear antigen of human herpesvirus 8. J Virol 73:5149–5155
16. Jenner RG, Boshoff C (2002) The molecular pathology of Kaposi's sarcoma-associated herpesvirus. Biochim Biophys Acta 1602:1–22
17. Dupin N, Fisher C, Kellam P, Ariad S, Tulliez M, Franck N et al (1999) Distribution of human herpesvirus-8 latently infected cells in Kaposi's sarcoma, multicentric Castleman's disease, and primary effusion lymphoma. Proc Natl Acad Sci USA 96:4546–4551
18. Miller SA, Dykes DD, Polesky HF (1988) A simple salting out procedure for extracting DNA from human nucleated cells. Nucleic Acids Res 16:1215
19. Wright DK, Manos MM (1990) Sample preparation from paraffin-embedded tissues. In: Innis MA, Gelfand DH, Sninsky JF, White TF (eds) PCR protocols: a guide to methods and applications. Academic, San Diego, CA, pp 153–158
20. Pan L, Milligan L, Michaeli J, Cesarman E, Knowles DM (2001) Polymerase chain reaction detection of Kaposi's sarcoma-associated herpesvirus-optimized protocols and their application to myeloma. J Mol Diagn 3:32–38
21. Cesarman E, Nador RG, Bai F, Bohenzky RA, Russo JJ, Moore PS et al (1996) Kaposi's sarcoma-associated herpesvirus contains G protein-coupled receptor and cyclin D homologs which are expressed in Kaposi's sarcoma and malignant lymphoma. J Virol 70:8218–8223

Chapter 19

Detection of Cytomegalovirus Infection by Quantitative Polymerase Chain Reaction

Magdalena Czader, Kristin Post, and Liang Cheng

Abstract

Human cytomegalovirus (CMV), also known as human herpes virus-5 (HHV-5), is a common human pathogen acquired early in life in the majority of immunocompetent individuals. Primary infection establishes a state of latency and the virus can be reactivated during immunosuppression. CMV is a significant cause of morbidity and mortality in newborns and patients with impaired immune system. Prenatal infection can result in intrauterine growth retardation, hepatitis, myocarditis, pneumonitis, and neurologic abnormalities. Individuals with congenital or acquired immunosuppression can develop a primary CMV infection, infection with another CMV strain or experience reactivation of the latent virus. The hematopoietic stem cell and solid organ transplant recipients are at high risk of developing CMV infection, especially early in a post-transplant period. The definition of CMV disease includes the evidence of end-organ involvement in the presence of CMV detected by a validated laboratory assay. The selection of a laboratory method is highly dependent on the type of sample to be tested and the clinical presentation. In the clinical practice, the quantitative PCR-based assays are most helpful, since they can measure the level of CMV DNA in whole blood, plasma, cerebrospinal fluid, amniotic fluid, tissue, and urine, and follow the kinetics of infection. In this chapter we describe the PCR assay designed to quantify CMV DNA in human plasma by amplifying a 105 base-pair (bp) fragment of the CMV immediate-early DNA polymerase gene.

Key words CMV, Quantitative PCR, Molecular viral load, CMV immediate-early DNA polymerase gene

1 Introduction

Human cytomegalovirus (CMV), also known as human herpes virus-5 (HHV-5), a member of family Herpesviridae and subfamily Betaherpesvirinae, is a common human pathogen. In the majority of immunocompetent individuals, CMV is acquired early in life during an asymptomatic infection. A proportion of young patients present with primary infection similar to infectious mononucleosis including fever, atypical lymphocytosis, and malaise. The infected cells include lymphocytes, neutrophils, monocytes, endothelial cells, epithelial cells, and smooth muscle cells (1). Primary infection

Magdalena Czader (ed.), *Hematological Malignancies*, Methods in Molecular Biology, vol. 999,
DOI 10.1007/978-1-62703-357-2_19, © Springer Science+Business Media New York 2013

establishes a state of latency with virus residing in granulocytes and monocytes (2–4). The reactivation of the infection can occur during immunosuppression and infected individuals can transmit CMV through blood or organ transplantation. In newborns and in patients with impaired immune system, CMV is a significant cause of morbidity and mortality. When the infection is acquired during prenatal period, it can result in intrauterine growth retardation, hepatitis, myocarditis, pneumonitis, and neurologic abnormalities including hearing loss and chorioretinitis. Individuals immunocompromised due to congenital or acquired immunodeficiency, or due to iatrogenic immunosuppression, can develop a primary CMV infection, infection with another CMV strain or experience reactivation of the latent virus. Both hematopoietic stem cell (HSC) and solid organ transplant recipients are at risk of developing CMV infection, especially early in a post-transplant period (5–7). The severity of the disease depends on the extent of immunosuppression, type of transplant, and immune status of the recipient (primary vs. secondary infection/reactivation). The definition of CMV disease includes the evidence of end-organ involvement in the presence of CMV detected by a validated laboratory assay. Patients usually present with fevers, malaise, and cytopenias. The end-organ manifestations can be severe and include CMV pneumonia, gastrointestinal tract involvement (ulcerations, diarrhea), and in rare instances hepatitis, retinitis, and encephalitis. The rejection or delayed engraftment of transplanted organ has also been described. In HIV-positive patients, CMV infection is associated with fevers, gastrointestinal involvement, retinitis, and encephalitis.

Numerous laboratory methods have been developed to detect CMV infection. Their selection is highly dependent on the type of sample to be tested and the clinical presentation. Direct demonstration of the virus can be accomplished in tissues (H&E, Wright-Giemsa, or Papanicolaou stains) or blood samples (pp65 antigenemia assay in isolated leukocytes). The latter assay has been particularly useful due to its high sensitivity and is relatively quick and easy to perform. It also correlates well to real-time polymerase chain reaction (PCR) assays.

The qualitative PCR-based assays are available, however, are not commonly used due to their limited clinical usefulness. In clinical practice, the quantitative assays are most helpful, since they can measure the level of CMV DNA in whole blood, plasma, cerebrospinal fluid, amniotic fluid, tissue, and urine and follow the infection kinetics (8–15). Various DNA extraction methods, amplification targets, calibrators, and detection system are used across different laboratories contributing to significant differences in reported CMV viral loads as evidenced by the results of comparison studies and proficiency testing (16, 17). The recent development of the World Health Organization quantitative DNA standards may help in standardizing CMV testing (18, 19).

The DNA CMV reporting in international units per mL allows for the comparison across methods. Additionally, standard reporting may facilitate establishing the threshold levels for preemptive therapy.

In the following paragraphs, we describe the PCR assay designed to quantify CMV DNA in human plasma by amplifying a 105 base-pair (bp) fragment of the CMV immediate-early DNA polymerase gene. Detection occurs by specific probe hybridization/dual probe FRET. In this system a signal is detected only when both the fluorescein and the LightCycler—Red dye labeled probe bind simultaneously to adjacent sequences on the single stranded target strand. The FRET can occur and maximum signal can be detected when both HybProbe probes are bound quantitatively at the end of the annealing phase. The performance characteristics of the assay in our laboratory are listed in Note 1.

2 Materials

2.1 Sample Preparation and DNA Extraction

1. Peripheral blood drawn in a 6 mL EDTA tube (lavender or pearl top tube) (see Note 2).
2. QIAamp DNA Blood Mini Kit for manual DNA extraction (Qiagen, Valencia, CA). Store at room temperature (RT).
3. Maxwell®16 Viral Total Nucleic Acid Purification for automated DNA extraction (Promega, Madison, WI). Store at RT.
4. Promega Maxwell®16 instrument for Automated DNA extraction (Promega, Madison, WI).

2.2 PCR Procedure

1. Artus CMV LightCycler (LC) PCR kit, which contains the CMV LC master mix vial (Qiagen, Valencia, CA) (20, 21). Store at −20 °C (see Notes 3 and 4).
2. CMV LC PCR Supplement Kit, which includes the following components: CMV LC/RG/TM Magnesium solution (Mg-Sol) (yellow cap tube), PCR Grade Water (white cap tube), CMV/LC/RG/TM Quantitation Standard (QS)1 (1×10^4 copies/μL = 2.5×10^6 copies/mL), CMV/LC/RG/TM QS 2 (1×10^3 copies/μL = 2.5×10^5 copies/mL), CMV/LC/RG/TM QS 3 (1×10^2 copies/μL = 2.5×10^4 copies/mL), CMV/LC/RG/TM QS 4 (1×10^1 copies/μL = 2.5×10^3 copies/mL), and CMV LC/RG/TM Internal Control (IC) (green cap tube). Store at −20 °C (see Notes 3 and 4).
3. Acrometrix Optiqual CMV negative control; AcroMetrix CMV Low Positive Control and High Positive Control (AcroMetrix® by Life Technologies™, Carlsbad, CA).
4. Tabletop centrifuge for 2 mL tubes.

5. Roche LightCycler® 2.0 with Software version 4.0 (Roche Diagnostics, Indianapolis, IN) (see Note 5).
6. Roche Color Compensation Kit (Roche Diagnostics, Indianapolis, IN).
7. LightCycler Centrifuge.
8. LightCycler 20 μL capillaries (Roche Diagnostics, Indianapolis, IN).
9. LightCycler Cooling Block.
10. LightCycler capping tool.

3 Method

3.1 Preparation of Plasma

1. Centrifuge at 1,600 × *g* for 20 min within 6 h of collection (see Notes 6 and 7).
2. Take off plasma with a sterile pipette and store in a 4 mL cryovial frozen at −80 °C until testing.

3.2 Manual DNA Extraction Using QIAamp DNA Mini Kit (See Notes 8 and 9)

1. Pipet 20 μL Protease into the bottom of a 1.5 mL microcentrifuge tube.
2. Add 200 μL of the plasma to the microcentrifuge tube.
3. Add 6 μL of the internal control.
4. Add 200 μL Buffer AL to the sample. Do not add Protease directly to the Buffer AL. It is important to add the sample between them.
5. Pulse-vortex briefly and incubate at 56 °C for 10 min.
6. Add 200 μL of absolute ethanol to the sample-buffer AL and pulse-vortex briefly.
7. Transfer the mixture from step 6 to the QIAamp Spin Column set in a 2 mL collection tube. Take care not to wet the rim.
8. Close the cap, and centrifuge at least 20,000 × *g* for 1 min.
9. Transfer the QIAamp Spin Column into a new clean 2 mL collection tube. Discard the collection tube containing the filtrate.
10. Carefully open the cap and add 500 μL Buffer AW1. Take care not to wet the rim.
11. Close the cap and centrifuge at least 20,000 × *g* for 1 min.
12. Transfer the QIAamp spin column into a new clean 2 mL collection tube. Discard the used collection tube with the filtrate.
13. Open the cap of the QIAamp Spin Column and add 500 μL Buffer AW2. Take care not to wet the rim.
14. Close the cap and centrifuge at least 20,000 × *g* for 3 min.

15. All buffer AW2 has to be removed before the next steps. To ensure that buffer AW2 is removed repeat the centrifugation of QIAamp Spin Column in a clean 2 mL collection tube at 20,000 × *g* for 1 min.
16. Place the QIAamp Spin Column into a clean 1.5 mL microcentrifuge tube, and discard the collection tube containing the filtrate.
17. Add 50 μL Buffer AE to the QIAamp Spin Column.
18. Allow the Buffer AE to incubate on the spin column membrane for at least 5 min at room temperature. Keep the spin column up-right during the incubation period.
19. Centrifuge at least 20,000 × *g* for 1 min and 30 s.
20. Discard the spin column and label the microcentrifuge tube of DNA with the appropriate identification (see Note 10).

3.3 Automated DNA Extraction Using Maxwell® 16 Viral Total Nucleic Acid Purification Kit (See Notes 8 and 9)

1. Run preparation
   (a) Label 1.5 mL microcentrifuge tubes with the identification of samples in a run.
   (b) Make up the Lysis and Proteinase K solution mixing 200 μL of Lysis Buffer and 20 μL of Proteinase K Solution for each sample (multiply the volumes dependent on the number of samples in the run).
   (c) Pipet 200 μL of plasma into appropriate 1.7 mL microcentrifuge tube after vortexing the plasma. Add 6 μL of Internal Control.
   (d) Add 220 μL of Lysis solution as prepared above to each tube.
   (e) Close tubes and vortex for few seconds.
   (f) Incubate at 56 °C for 10 min. During the incubation process prepare the cartridges.
2. Preparing the Cartridge.
   (a) Place each cartridge to be used into the LEV cartridge preparation rack with the label side facing away from the Elution Tubes. Press down on the cartridge to snap it into position.
   (b) Remove the seal from the top of each cartridge.
   (c) If processing fewer than 16 samples center the cartridges on the platform.
   (d) Place one plunger into well 8 of each cartridge, so that the bottom of the plunger is at the bottom of the cartridge. The plunger will fit loosely in the cartridge.
   (e) Elution Tubes should be placed in front holes of the platform.

(f) Place 50 μL of nuclease free water in the Elution Tubes. Make sure it is added to the bottom of tube. Make sure caps are facing outwards.

(g) After the incubation is complete transfer the sample lysate to well #1 of the cartridge.

3. Setting up the Maxwell® 16 instrument.

(a) Turn the Maxwell® 16 instrument on.

(b) Once the machine powers up, verify that "Rsch" is displayed in the lower right corner of the LCD and "LEV" in lower left corner.

(c) The next screen displayed is the "Menu" screen. Using the scroll buttons move the cursor to "Run." Press the "Run/Stop" button to select this option.

(d) On the next screen, using the scroll buttons move the cursor to "Viral." Press "Run/Stop" to select this option.

(e) Open the door when prompted to do so on the LCD display. Press the "Run/Stop" button to extend the platform out of the instrument.

(f) Place the LEV cartridge rack containing samples and plungers onto the Maxwell® 16 instrument platform.

(g) Press the "Run/Stop" button. The platform will retract. Close the door.

(h) The Maxwell® 16 Instrument will begin the purification run. The LCD screen displays the steps performed and the approximate time remaining in the run.

(i) Pressing the "Run/Stop" button or opening the door during the purification process will pause the run. Close the door if open and select whether to "continue" or "terminate" the run.

(j) When the purification is complete, the LCD screen will display a message that the run has ended and a prompt to "Open the Door."

(k) Open the instrument door and verify that all the plungers have been removed from the magnetic rod assembly. If the plungers have not been removed, push them down gently by hand to remove them.

(l) Press the "Run/Stop" button to pull out the platform from inside the instrument.

(m) Remove the elution tubes.

(n) Remove cartridges and plungers from the instrument platform and discard them.

(o) Choose "No" when asked if the tests are to be run again and press the "Run/Stop" button.

(p) The platform will retract. Close the door at the prompt and turn the machine off.

3.4 Preparing PCR Reaction

1. Generate a PCR worksheet for the CMV assay run (see Note 11).
2. Obtain the LightCycler cooling block stored at 4 °C in the clean area refrigerator.
3. Place the appropriate capillary tubes in the cooling block. Do not touch the surface of the capillary tubes; always use gloves when handling the capillaries.
4. Place the cooling block in one of the clean area hoods.
5. Remove the correct number of Master vials to test all patient samples plus 5 controls (each Master Vial contains enough reagents for 12 tests) (see Note 12).
6. Let the Master vials, Mg solution, and PCR grade water thaw in the cooling block.
7. Gently vortex and quick-spin the Master vials in the centrifuge.
8. Combine the contents of each Master vials into one vial and gently vortex again.
9. Prepare PCR reaction containing the following reagents in a single sterile Eppendorf tube. The reagents are multiplied dependent on the number of samples and controls (see Note 11).

Reagent	Amount per Sample
CMV LC Master Mix (blue vial)	12.5 μL
Mg Solution (yellow vial)	2.5 μL
Total volume	15.0 μL

10. Mix gently and aliquot 15 μL of master mix into each capillary tube (controls and patient sample capillaries) except the capillary in position 5.
11. Move LightCycler cooling block containing the capillary tubes and master mix from the clean hood to the processing hood.
12. Add 2 μL of Internal Control to the remaining master mix and aliquot 15 μL into the capillary in position 5.
13. Pipette 10 μL of water, control DNA, or sample DNA into the appropriate capillary tubes (for pipetting order see Note 12).
14. Cap the capillary tubes using the capping tool as each sample is added to help prevent contamination.
15. Take cooling block with samples to the LightCycler 2.0 located in the post-PCR area.

Table 1
LightCycler 2.0 setup

Target (°C)	Hold hh:mm:ss	Ramp rate	Sec target	Step size	Step delay	Acquisition mode
Initial activation of the hot start enzyme, 1 cycle						
95	00:10:00	20	0	0	0	None
Touch down step, 10 cycles						
95	00:00:05	20	0	0	0	None
65	00:00:20	20	55	1	1	None
72	00:00:15	20	0	0	0	None
Amplification of the DNA, 40 cycles, analysis mode-quantitation						
95	00:00:05	20	0	0	0	None
55	00:00:20	20	0	0	0	Single
72	00:00:15	10	0	0	0	None
Cooling, 1 cycle						
40	00:00:30	20	0	0	0	None

3.5 Programming the LightCycler Instrument to Create a Macro

1. Setup the instrument with the following parameters:

   Default Channel: 530

   Seek temperature: 30

   Max Seek Pos: 12

   Instrument type: 6 channel

   Capillary size: 20 μL
2. Create the Temperate Profile on the LightCycler 2.0 as listed in Table 1.

3.6 Amplification and Detection Performed on the LightCycler 2.0 Instrument

1. Log on the computer.
2. Double click on the LightCycler icon and log into the LightCycler software.
3. Turn on the LightCycler 2.0 instrument.
4. Click on "CMV/EBV" from the front screen.
5. Follow the prompts of the macro wizard to perform Self Test. A self test must be performed once each day the LightCycler is in use. Click on the box to run self test.
6. Save the results from the self test using CNTRL and Print SCN keys simultaneously to take a picture of the screen, and pasting the results in the Wordpad as Quality Control file.

7. Name the run and save it in the "Experiments" folder.
8. Adjust the sample count located in the upper left corner of the page to the sum of controls and patients included in the run.
9. Enter the accession numbers of each patient sample.
10. Click on the "Abs Quant" tab.
11. Under "Sample type" assign the appropriate sample type for the standard.
12. Type in the expected concentrations for the Quantitation standard.
13. Remove the capillary tubes from the cooler block and place them into the corresponding position in the carousel (cooling block sample #1 should be placed in position #1 on the carousel etc.).
14. Place the carousel into LightCycler centrifuge and press start.
15. Move the carousel into the LightCycler 2.0 instrument, close the lid and press "Start Run."
16. The LightCycler 2.0 instrument will check each position for a sample. Do not walk away from the instrument until this check has been completed especially if one of the capillaries is not in the carousel. The instrument will note this and ask if you want to continue the run. Answer yes before leaving.
17. Once the run is complete, close the report that was generated.
18. Perform "Absolute Quantitation."
19. Click on the arrow next to Color Compensation and "Select Color Compensation" from the drop-down box.
20. Choose the most current color compensation and select OK.
21. Click on the arrow by Standard Curve.
22. Select "use external" from the drop-down menu.
23. Select the most current and then click OK.
24. Look at each curve under the Absolute Quantification menu to ensure that curves are present and not flat line if a concentration is assigned (Fig. 1, see Note 13).
25. Print a copy of the graph.
26. The Absolute Quantification for the 705/Back 530 is automatically analyzed.
27. Generate a report and print.

3.7 Interpretation of the Results

The interpretation of the results is always done in conjunction with results from internal control (see Note 14). If no signal is detected in either channel 530 or in channel 705/Back 530, the test is invalid due to nonworking internal positive control.

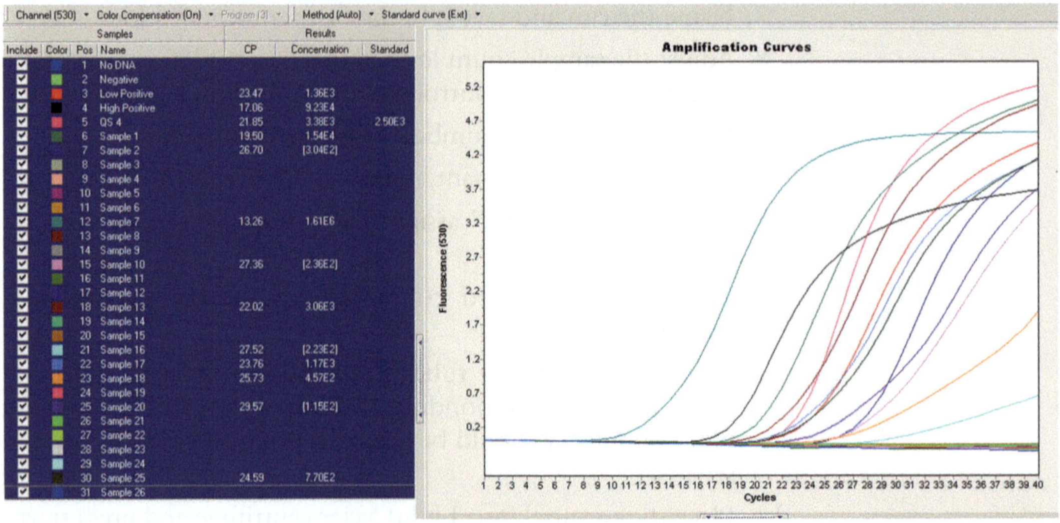

Fig. 1 Amplification curves generated by the LightCycler 2.0

If internal control is acceptable, the following conclusive reports can be issued:

1. Interpretation: The sample contains CMV DNA, if a signal is detected in fluorimeter channel 530 with a crossing point before the 26th cycle of amplification. In this case, the detection of a signal in 705/Back 530 is dispensable because high CMV viral load can out-compete the internal control and result in a reduced or absent Internal Control reading (see Note 15).
2. Interpretation: No CMV DNA is detected. The sample can be considered negative. No signal is detected in fluorimeter channel 530 or a signal is detected in cycle 26 or greater. A signal from the Internal Control is detected in 705/Back 530 channel at the 14th ± 3 cycles of amplification. The presence of Internal Control rules out the possibility of PCR inhibition.

4 Notes

1. The following performance characteristics were determined by the IU Health Molecular Pathology Laboratory during the validation of this procedure.

   Dynamic range of the assay: 250–500,000 copies/mL

   Limit of Detection: 250 copies/mL

   Linearity over the dynamic range: $R^2 = 0.9969$

   Analytical sensitivity: 94.1%

   Analytical specificity: 97.7%

   Predictive value of a positive test: 97%

Predictive value of a negative test: 95.5%

Accuracy of the test: 96.1%

2. Heparin inhibits the polymerase chain reaction, thus heparin tubes are not recommended. Elevated levels of bilirubin (≤4.5 mg/dL), elevated lipids (≤1,100 mg/dL) and hemolytic samples *do not* influence the CMV results.
3. Repeated thawing and freezing of reagents should be avoided. If reagents are used intermittently, they should be frozen in aliquots. Storage at +4 °C should not exceed a period of 5 h.
4. A new standard curve must be generated whenever a new lot number of reagents is received or every six months. The standards included with the kit should be considered as previously extracted DNA. Ten μL of each standard is added to the master mix. Three replicates of Quantitation Standards QS 4,3,2,1, and a 1:10 dilution of QS4 are included in the run to generate the standard curve. The results of this run must be graphed. The resulting linearity coefficient must be ≥0.81. In order to assure accurate Quantitation, add 1 μL of IC for each standard to the master mix used in generating the standard curve. The current external standard curve may be imported into the run during the analysis phase.
5. If multiple instruments are used to run the CMV quantitative assay a comparability study must be conducted at least every six months to evaluate the performance of all instruments. A run of at least six samples should be performed and analyzed on all the instruments and the results must be within 0.5 Log_{10} difference of each other to be considered acceptable. Patient samples, Acrometrix controls or Acrometrix standards are acceptable sample types to be used for the correlation study.
6. We have performed validation for samples within 6 h of procurement. This reflects an internal laboratory policy related to the uniform handling of all samples submitted for viral load studies, some of which are RNA-based. Individual clinical laboratories should validate the specimen requirements independently. As previously published, CMV DNA, when EDTA anticoagulated samples are stored at a temperature of 4 °C, is stable up to 14 days after collection (22).
7. The diagnostic challenge with CMV disease is to distinguish asymptomatic latent or low level persistent infection from clinically significant disease since viral nucleic acid can be detected in patients without clinically significant disease. The use of plasma may provide a better correlation with clinically significant infection than detection of CMV DNA from whole blood or leukocytes because it measures CMV DNA circulating in the blood stream which is a direct result of active viral replication rather than the latent intracellular CMV DNA. Patients with

active CMV disease have consistently higher CMV viral loads than patients with asymptomatic infection (23).

8. Various DNA extraction methods and kits are available. In our laboratory, we routinely use the Maxwell®16 Viral Total Nucleic Acid Purification for automated DNA extraction (Promega, Madison, WI). We have also tested QIAamp DNA Blood Mini Kit as a manual backup DNA extraction method (Qiagen, Valencia, CA). We included the procedures as used in our laboratory for completeness. Alternatively, the detailed descriptions of the methods are provided with the kits (24, 25).
9. Standard precautions are used when working with nucleic acids and PCR methodologies. All DNA extractions are to be performed in the extraction room separated from the post-amplification area. Uncontained amplicons pose the potential for contamination of specimens and false positive results. To prevent this from occurring molecular assays should be performed in designated areas. Separated areas should be dedicated for master mix setup, specimen extractions, and amplification/detection. Each of these areas should have dedicated supplies such as pipettes, tips, racks, coats, etc. and should not be taken into the other areas. If supplies are moved into an area they should be bleached before taking back into original area. Gloves should be changed at any sign of potential contamination to prevent carryover during extraction and PCR setup and when moving from one area of the lab to another unless moving in a unidirectional workflow starting in the cleanest area.
10. After extraction the DNA quality does not need to be assessed or spectrophotometric determination of DNA concentration is not routinely performed following DNA isolation. The internal control added prior to DNA extraction acts as a control for the extraction process. Alternatively, 1 μL of Internal Control may be added to each Master vial. If added to the master mix, the Internal Control acts only as an amplification control.
11. We prepare a CMV Excel worksheet listing all patient samples and controls and including the date of the run, reagent kit lot numbers, verification of growth curves, and working control limits. This Excel worksheet calculates the total amount of each reagent needed to make up the master mix. The worksheet should multiply the amount of each reagent needed per sample times the number of samples and controls plus one (to compensate for loss due to pipetting). A copy of the LightCycler run report is included with the run.
12. Every assay run must include a no DNA control, negative control, a low positive control, a high positive control, either QS3 or QS4 and all patient samples. The capillaries must be set up in the following order:

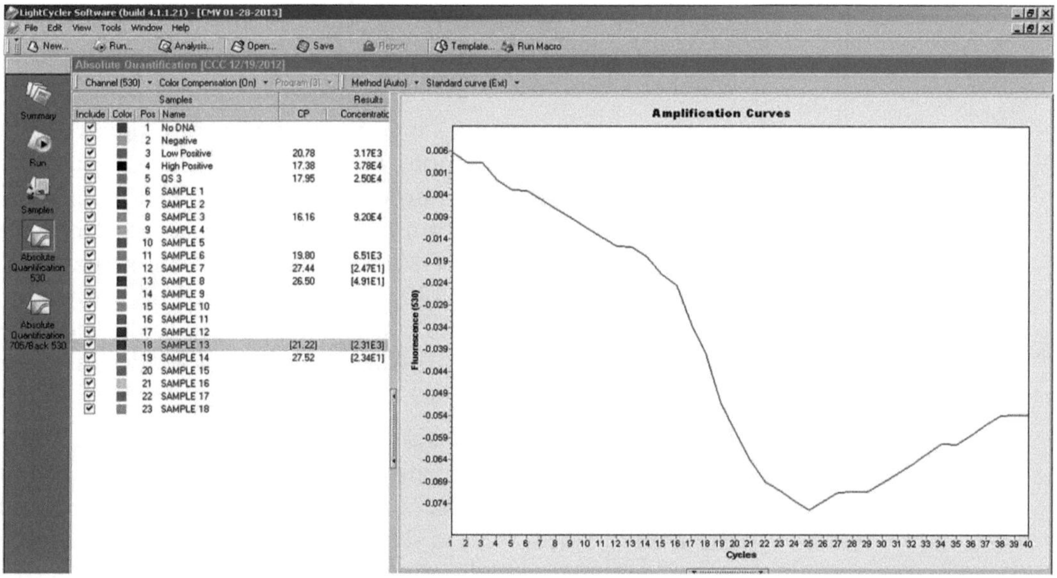

Fig. 2 LightCycler 2.0 generates a viral load for a sample even though the amplification curve of the sample is a flat line indicating that no amplification actually occurred and the sample has no CMV viral load

(a) No DNA control—contamination control: All reagents are included except the DNA template.

(b) Negative control, Acrometrix Optiqual CMV negative control.

(c) Low positive control, Acrometrix CMV Low Positive Control. Expected viral load is determined and adjusted for each lot number.

(d) High positive control, Acrometrix CMV High Positive Control. Expected viral load is determined and adjusted for each lot number.

(e) Standard Control.

If any of the controls fall out of range, the unacceptable results are recorded and attached to the assay results. A control flow chart can be developed to help determine the parts of the assay that need to be repeated.

13. In some instances the LightCycler 2.0 generates a viral load for a sample even though the amplification curve of the sample is a flat line indicating that no amplification actually occurred and the sample has no CMV viral load(Fig. 2). Therefore, one should always look at the amplification curves of all viral load samples to verify that amplification did in fact occur. In a clinical laboratory, the second technologist should also verify all amplification curves before results are verified. In our laboratory, for any given sample, if the Crossing Point (CP) occurs at 26 cycles or above, the signal is considered due to nonspecific

amplification as determined during the test validation. Therefore, the result is considered "not detected" regardless of whether a viral load is generated or not.

14. An Internal Control (IC) is added to each sample and control during the DNA extraction. Therefore, it acts as a control for both the extraction process and amplification. The amplification and detection of the IC does not interfere with the amplification of the CMV because detection of the CMV virus occurs in channel 530, whereas the detection of the IC occurs in channel 705. For any given sample or control, the IC signal must have a crossing point of 14 ± 3 cycles to be considered valid.
15. In the past there was a lack of standardization among CMV PCR assays; however, recently the World Health Organization has released for purchase a CMV standard. Laboratories in the United States start to switch to reporting in international units per mL which allows for the comparison across methods.

References

1. Sinzger C, Digel M, Jahn G (2008) Cytomegalovirus cell tropism. Curr Top Microbiol Immunol 325:63–83
2. Bolovan-Fritts CA, Mocarski ES, Wiedeman JA (1999) Peripheral blood CD14(+) cells from healthy subjects carry a circular conformation of latent cytomegalovirus genome. Blood 93:394–398
3. Kondo K, Kaneshima H, Mocarski ES (1994) Human cytomegalovirus latent infection of granulocyte-macrophage progenitors. Proc Natl Acad Sci USA 91:11879–11883
4. Taylor-Wiedeman J, Sissons JG, Borysiewicz LK, Sinclair JH (1991) Monocytes are a major site of persistence of human cytomegalovirus in peripheral blood mononuclear cells. J Gen Virol 72:2059–2064
5. Ljungman P, Hakki M, Boeckh M (2011) Cytomegalovirus in hematopoietic stem cell transplant recipients. Hematol Oncol Clin North Am 25:151–169
6. Lautenschlager I (2009) CMV infection, diagnosis and antiviral strategies after liver transplantation. Transpl Int 22:1031–1040
7. Husain S, Pietrangeli CE, Zeevi A (2009) Delayed onset CMV disease in solid organ transplant recipients. Transpl Immunol 21:1–9
8. Emery VC, Sabin CA, Cope AV, Gor D, Hassan-Walker AF, Griffiths PD (2000) Application of viral-load kinetics to identify patients who develop cytomegalovirus disease after transplantation. Lancet 10:2032–2036
9. Piiparinen H, Höckerstedt K, Grönhagen-Riska C, Lautenschlager I (2004) Comparison of two quantitative CMV PCR tests, Cobas Amplicor CMV Monitor and TaqMan assay, and pp 65-antigenemia assay in the determination of viral loads from peripheral blood of organ transplant patients. J Clin Virol 30: 258–266
10. Cortez KJ, Fisher SH, Fahle GA, Calhoun LB, Childs RW, Barrett AJ et al (2003) Clinical trial of quantitative real-time polymerase chain reaction for detection of cytomegalovirus in peripheral blood of allogeneic hematopoietic stem cell transplant patients. J Infect Dis 188:967–972
11. Gault E, Michel Y, Dehée A, Belabani C, Nicolas JC, Garbarg-Chenon A (2001) Quantification of human cytomegalovirus DNA by real-time PCR. J Clin Microbiol 39:772–775
12. Gourlain K, Salmon D, Gault E, Leport C, Katlama C, Matheron S et al (2003) Quantitation of cytomegalovirus (CMV) DNA by real-time PCR for occurrence of CMV disease in HIV-infected patients receiving highly active antiretroviral therapy. J Med Virol 69:401–407
13. Griscelli F, Barrois M, Chauvin S, Lastere S, Bellet D, Bourhis JH (2001) Quantification of human cytomegalovirus DNA in bone marrow transplant recipients by real-time PCR. J Clin Microbiol 39:4362–4369
14. Schaade L, Kockelkorn P, Ritter K, Kleines M (2000) Detection of cytomegalovirus DNA in human specimens by LightCycler PCR. J Clin Microbiol 38:4006–4009
15. Andrews PA, Emery VC, Newstead C (2011) Summary of the British transplantation society guidelines for the prevention and management of CMV disease after solid organ transplantation. Transplantation 15:1181–1187

16. Pang XL, Fox JD, Fenton JM, Miller GG, Caliendo AM, Preiksaitis JK (2009) Interlaboratory comparison of cytomegalovirus viral load assays. American Society of Transplantation Infectious Diseases Community of Practice; Canadian Society of Transplantation. Am J Transplant 9:258–68
17. Hayden RT, Yan X, Wick MT, Rodriguez AB, Xiong X, Ginocchio CC et al (2012) Factors contributing to variability of quantitative viral PCR results in proficiency testing samples: a multivariate analysis. for the College of American Pathologists Microbiology Resource Committee. J Clin Microbiol 50(2):337–345
18. Fryer JF, Baylis SA, Gottlieb AL, Ferguson M, Vincini GA, Bevan VM et al (2008) Development of working reference materials for clinical virology. J Clin Virol 43:367–371
19. Fryer JF, Minor PD (2009) Standardisation of nucleic acid amplification assays used in clinical diagnostics: a report of the first meeting of the SoGAT Clinical Diagnostics Working Group. J Clin Virol 44:103–105
20. Artus CMV LC PCR Kit Handbook. Qiagen Sample and Assay Technologies. April 2007.
21. Caliendo AM, Ingersoll J, Fox-Canale AM, Pargman S, Bythwood T, Hayden MK et al (2007) Evaluation of real-time PCR laboratory-developed tests using analyte-specific reagents for cytomegalovirus quantification. J Clin Microbiol 45:1723–1727
22. Abdul-Ali D, Kraft CS, Ingersoll J, Frempong M, Caliendo AM (2011) Cytomegalovirus DNA stability in EDTA anti-coagulated whole blood and plasma samples. J Clin Virol 52:222–224
23. Wolf DG, Spector SA (1993) Early diagnosis of human cytomegalovirus disease in transplant recipients by DNA amplification in plasma. Transplantation 56:330–334
24. Technical Bulletin. (2010) Maxwell® 16 Viral Total Nucleic Acid Purification Kit. Instruction for use of product AS1150. Promega January 2010
25. QIAamp® DNA Mini and Blood Mini Handbook Qiagen, 3rd Edition, April 2010

Chapter 20

Thiopurine S-Methyltransferase Pharmacogenetics in Childhood Acute Lymphoblastic Leukemia

Jun J. Yang and Deepa Bhojwani

Abstract

Pharmacogenetics is the growing field of study of genetic variations underlying interindividual differences in drug response. Inherited polymorphisms in genes coding for drug-metabolizing enzymes, transporters, and targets influence toxicity as well as efficacy associated with the medication. Thiopurines are agents widely used in hematologic malignancies, transplantation, and chronic inflammatory conditions. Myelosuppression is the commonly encountered dose-limiting toxicity. Polymorphisms in the thiopurine S-methyltransferase gene (*TPMT*), the predominant inactivating enzyme for thiopurines in hematopoietic tissue, are correlated with enzymatic activity of TPMT, thiopurine metabolism, and risk of clinical toxicity. In this chapter, we present *TPMT* genotype assessment that allows for prescribing pharmacogenetically guided doses to enhance patient safety and drug efficacy.

Key words Acute lymphoblastic leukemia, Thiopurine, TPMT, Pharmacogenetics, Genotyping

1 Introduction

Childhood acute lymphoblastic leukemia (ALL), the most common childhood cancer, is a prototype for a malignancy that is highly curable with multi-agent chemotherapy (1). Genetic variations in drug-metabolizing enzymes, drug transporters, and drug targets can significantly modify disposition and therapeutic effects of anti-leukemic medications (2, 3). In particular, germline polymorphisms in genes involved in metabolism of thiopurines have been well characterized (4) and the clinical application of thiopurine pharmacogenetics is among the few examples of genetics-guided treatment individualization (5, 6).

The thiopurines, namely, 6-thioguanine (6-TG) and 6-mercaptopurine (6-MP), are integral components of multi-agent chemotherapeutic regimens for childhood ALL. Higher dose intensity of 6-MP is associated with improved outcome (7). Anticancer activity of thiopurines depends in part upon the

Magdalena Czader (ed.), *Hematological Malignancies*, Methods in Molecular Biology, vol. 999,
DOI 10.1007/978-1-62703-357-2_20, © Springer Science+Business Media New York 2013

metabolism of 6-TG and 6-MP and conversion to thioguanine nucleotides (e.g., 6-thio-dGTP) (Fig. 1) (8). Incorporation of such nucleotide analogues during DNA replication introduces anomalous DNA structure, triggering futile mismatch repair, and eventually apoptosis (9, 10). Evidence also exists that disruption of de novo purine synthesis is a possible mechanism of action for thiopurines (11). Inactivation of both 6-MP and 6-TG is mediated by thiopurine S-methyltransferase (TPMT) that transfers the methyl group from S-adenosyl methionine to the sulfur atom of thiopurines (4). TPMT also catalyzes methylation of thioguanine nucleotides (12).

The thiopurines have a relatively narrow therapeutic index and the major dose-limiting toxicity is bone marrow suppression. Hematopoietic toxicity necessitates reduction in dose or temporary suspension of administration of thiopurines as well as other essential drugs, obligates platelet and red blood cell transfusions, and increases infections risk associated with neutropenia. Hematopoietic toxicity consequent to thiopurines is inversely correlated with TPMT activity as S-methylation is the primary inactivation pathway for thiopurines in this tissue (13). While the majority of patients exhibit normal to high TPMT activity, TPMT deficiency is noted in about 5–10% of individuals (14, 15) leading to excessive cellular accumulation of active thioguanine nucleotides (e.g., up to tenfold higher concentrations of erythrocyte thioguanine nucleotides (12)). The large interindividual differences of TPMT activity are inherited and attributable to a small number of germline polymorphisms of this gene. Thus, the three most frequent inactivating variant alleles (*TPMT*2*: G238C; *TPMT*3A*: G460A and A719G; and *TPMT*3C*: A719G) account for more than 95% of the variability in enzyme activity (16). Significant ethnic differences in the frequency of *TPMT* variant alleles are noted (17, 18). In a comprehensive analysis of *TPMT* status in 180 children with ALL receiving conventional doses of 6-MP, it was noted that the cumulative incidence of 6-MP-related toxicity was 100%, 35%, and 7% for patients with homozygous deficiency, heterozygous deficiency, and wild type, respectively (19). In fact, these patients homozygous for the *TPMT* mutant allele required a reduction of more than 90% of the conventional dose (75 $mg/m^2/day$). When 6-MP dosing is individualized based on *TPMT* genotype, equivalent systemic exposure and tolerance can be achieved in patients with different TPMT activity levels (20). Therefore, *TPMT* genotype assessment allows for prescribing pharmacogenetically guided doses to enhance safety and efficacy (Fig. 2). In this chapter, we have detailed *TPMT* genotyping for common variant alleles (*TPMT*2* and *TPMT*3*). *TPMT* genotyping is based on PCR amplification that is specific to genetic variants of interest and restriction fragment length polymorphism (RFLP) methods (16, 18, 21). Evaluation of toxicity and dose adjustments are clinically determined in conjunction with measurements of TPMT activity and levels of thioguanine nucleotides.

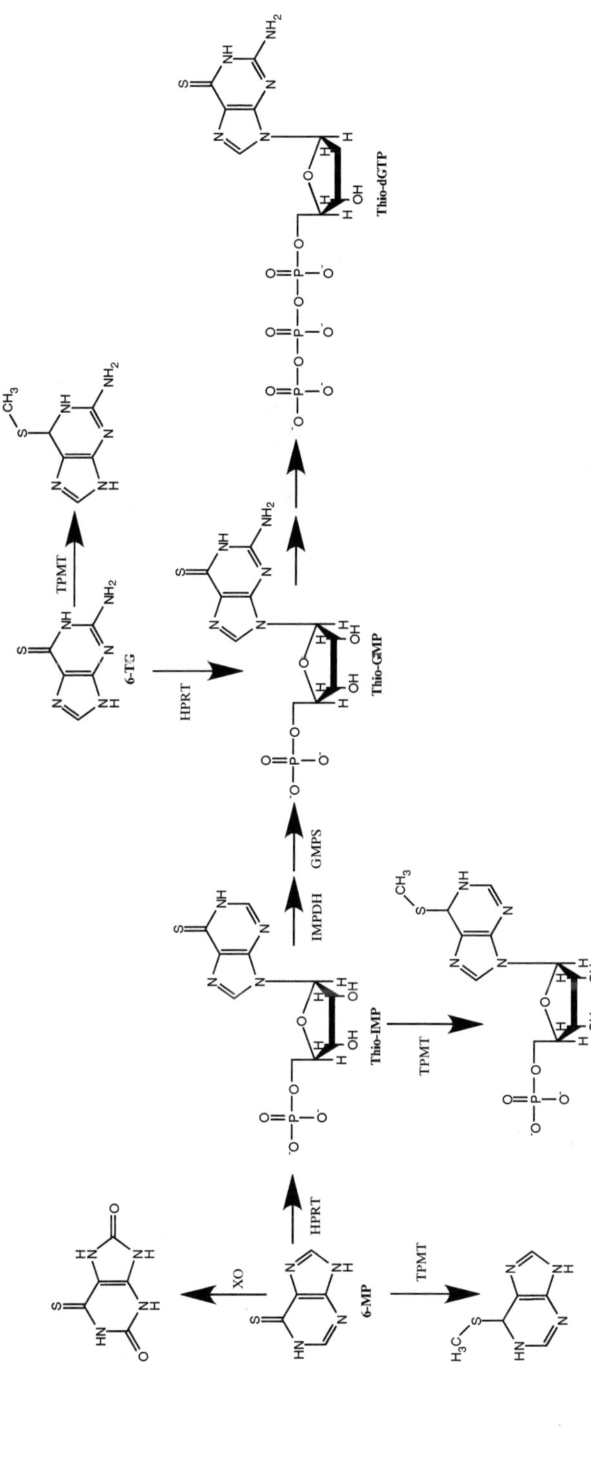

Fig. 1 Metabolism of thiopurines. 6-MP and 6-TG are prodrugs that require conversion to active metabolites through multiple enzyme-mediated reactions. TPMT inactivates both thiopurines and their metabolites via S-methylation. *6*-MP, 6-mercaptopurine; *6*-TG, 6-thioguanine; IMP, inosine monophosphate; *GMP*, guanosine monophosphate; GTP, guanosine triphosphate, *TPMT*, thiopurine S-methyltransferase, *HPRT*, hypoxanthine-guanine phosphoribosyltranferase, *XO*, xanthine oxidase; *IMPDH*, inosine monophosphate dehydrogenase; *GMPS*, guanine monophosphate synthetase

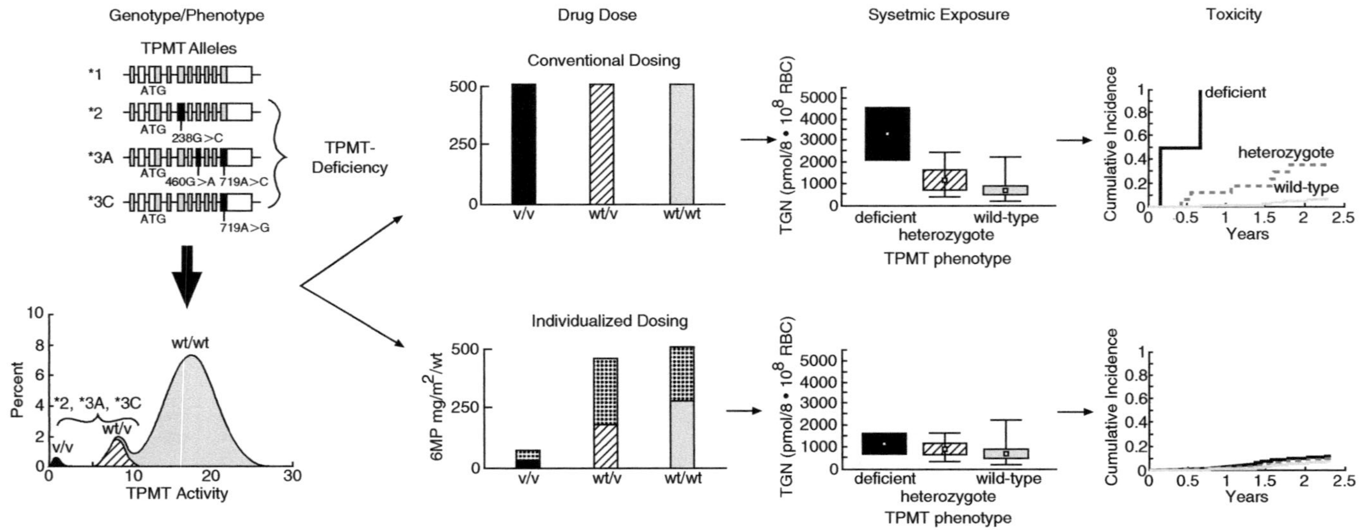

Fig. 2 *TPMT* pharmacogenetics-guided thiopurine dosing genotypes at polymorphisms within the *TPMT* gene (*top left panel*) are correlated with TPMT enzyme activity (*bottom left panel*). With conventional dosages of thiopurines, patients carrying *TPMT* mutant allele accumulate excessive levels of active metabolites (*top middle*) and are associated with excessive toxicity (*top right*). *TPMT* genotype-based dosing normalizes exposure of thiopurine metabolites (*bottom middle*) and effectively eliminates the excessive drug-related toxicity in patients with mutant *TPMT* (*bottom right*) (Reproduced with permission from Evans et al. Pharmacogenetics 2002)

2 Materials

2.1 Primers

1. *TPMT**2 (G238C):

Forward primer (wildtype)	5′-GTATGATTTTATGCAGGTTTG-3′
Forward primer (mutant)	5′-GTATGATTTTATGCAGGTTTC-3′
Reverse primer	5′-TAAATAGGAACCATCGGACAC-3′

2. *TPMT**3 (A719G and G460A):

A719G	
Forward primer	5′-GAG ACA GAG TTT CAC CAT CTT GG-3′
Reverse primer	5′-CAG GCT TTAGCA TAA TTT TCA ATT CCT C-3′

G460A	
Forward primer	5′-AGG CAG CTA GGG AAA AAG AAA GGT G-3′
Reverse primer	5′-CAA GCC TTA TAG CCT TAC ACC CAG G-3′

2.2 PCR

1. Expand High Fidelity PCR system (Roche, Basel, Switzerland): Expand HF buffer 10× (1.5 mM $MgCl_2$) and Taq polymerase (3.5 U/μl).
2. PCR Nucleotide Mix (Roche, Basel, Switzerland): premixed dNTP (10 mM each).
3. Nuclease-free water (Promega, WI, USA).
4. PCR tubes (0.2 ml).
5. Eppendorf Mastercycler thermocycler (Eppendorf, Hamburg, Germany).
6. True Allele PCR Premix (Applied Biosystem, Foster city, CA, USA).

2.3 Electrophoresis and RFLP

1. Restriction enzymes: *Acc*I and *MWO*I (New England Biolabs, MA, USA).
2. Agarose (Sigma, MO, USA).
3. Electrophoresis chamber (Biorad, CA, USA).
4. Loading buffer (New England Biolabs, MA, USA).
5. 100 bp DNA ladder (New England Biolabs, MA, USA).
6. Ethidium bromide (Sigma, MO, USA).
7. TBE buffer (Fisher Scientific, MA, USA).

2.4 Genomic DNA Preparation

1. FlexiGene DNA Kit (Qiagen, Venlo, Netherlands).

3 Methods

3.1 PCR Experiments (see Note 1)

1. Decontaminate all the tubes, pipettes, and tips to be used for PCR under the UV within 15–20 min prior to the experiment.
2. Resuspend the primers with nuclease-free water to obtain a final concentration of 300 pmol/μl, and confirm the concentration of the solution by UV at 260 nm.
3. Prepare PCR master mix as presented in Table 1.
4. Prepare genomic DNA by placing 5 ng of genomic DNA (prepared following manufacture's instruction) and 2 μl nuclease-free water in a 0.2 ml PCR tube.
5. Add 48 μl PCR master mix and spin briefly.
6. Place tubes into the thermocycler and run the PCR programs using parameters listed in Table 2.

Table 1
PCR master mix preparation

***TPMT*2 (G238C)**	
Forward primer (300 pmol/μl)	0.43 μl
Reverse primer (300 pmol/μl)	0.43 μl
True allele PCR premix	22.14 μl

***TPMP*3* (A719G)**	
Forward primer (300 pmol/1 μl)	0.4 μl
Reverse primer (300 pmol/1 μl)	0.4 μl
Buffer 10×	5 μl
dNTPs (10 mM)	1 μl
PCR water	40.8 μl
Taq polymerase	0.4 μl

***TPMT*3* (G460A)**	
Forward primer (300 pmol/μl)	0.4 μl
Reverse primer (300 pmol/μl)	0.4 μl
Buffer 10×	5 μl
dNTPs (10 mM)	1 μl
PCR water	40.8 μl
Taq polymerase	0.4 μl

Table 2
PCR amplification steps for *TPMT*2* (G238C), *TPMP*3* (A719G), and *TPMT*3* (G460A)

***TPMT*2* (G238C)**			
1	Initial denaturation	94 °C	04:00 min
2	Denaturation step	94 °C	00:30 min
3	Annealing	56 °C	01:00 min
4	Extension	72 °C	01:00 min
5	Go to step 2, $n=34$		
6	Final extension	72 °C	10:00 min

Note: The run time is 2 h 15 min

***TPMP*3* (A719G)**			
1	Initial denaturation	94 °C	04:00 min
2	Denaturation step	94 °C	00:30 min
3	Annealing	60 °C	01:00 min
4	Extension	72 °C	01:00 min
5	Go to step 2, $n=34$		
6	Final extension	72 °C	10:00 min

Note: The run time is 2 h 10 min

***TPMT*3* (G460A)**			
1	Initial denaturation	94 °C	04:00 min
2	Denaturation step	94 °C	00:30 min
3	Annealing	63 °C	01:00 min
4	Extension	72 °C	01:00 min
5	Go to step 2 $n=34$		
6	Final extension	72 °C	10:00 min

Note: The run time is 2 h 10 min

*3.2 TPMT*2 (G238C) Genotype Detection (See Notes 2 and 3)*

The detection of the G238C genotype is based on selective amplification of the DNA by two different forward primers having either a guanosine (238G; wild type) or a cytosine (238C; mutant) at the 3′ end of the primer. The absence or presence of the amplification product is determined by electrophoresis (steps 1–7 below). Example of the results is presented in Fig. 3.

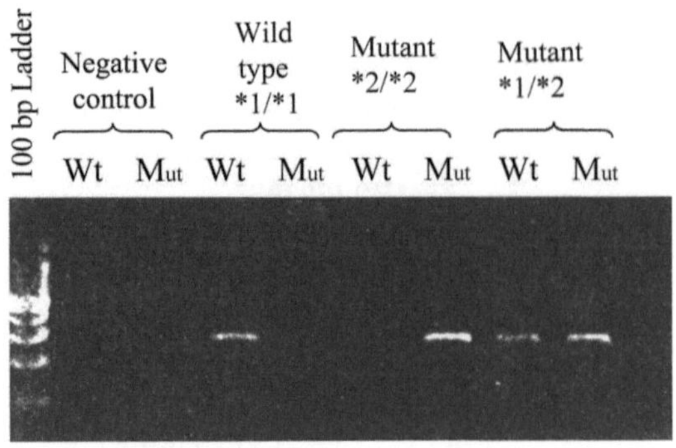

Fig. 3 *TPMT**2 (G238C) genotype detection. (1) Wildtype: only one visible band for the forward primer wild type (Wt). (2) Homozygous mutant: only one visible band for the forward primer mutant (Mut). (3) Heterozygous mutant: Two bands are visible (one amplification for each allele)

1. Weigh 2.0 g agarose and dissolve in 100 ml 1× TBE buffer.
2. Add 5 μl ethidium bromide.
3. Heat the solution for 5 min in the microwave oven until completely dissolved.
4. Pour the gel on a rack.
5. Load 3 μl of 6× loading buffer into PCR reaction.
6. Load negative control (water in place of genomic DNA), 100 bp DNA ladder, and PCR reactions into wells of the gel.
7. Run at 100 V for 60–90 min.
8. Results are interpreted as following (Fig. 3, see Note 4):
   (a) The wild-type genotype is found when only one band is visible for the forward primer wildtype (Wt).
   (b) Homozygous mutant: Only one visible band for the forward primer mutant (Mut).
   (c) Heterozygous mutant: Two bands are visible (one amplification for each allele).

3.3 TPMT*3 (A719G) Genotype Detection

The detection of the A719G genotype is based on selective amplification of the DNA by the forward primer specific to nucleotides 401–423 of intron 9 and the reverse primer specific to nucleotides 746–773 of exon 10 of the *TPMT* gene. Genotypes are then determined by the RFLP method. Thus, the amplified products (expected size 373 bp) are subjected to *Acc*I enzyme digestion. Amplicons with the mutant genotype (G) are digested after *Acc*I treatment while the wild-type samples remain intact, which is distinguished by electrophoresis.

1. Prepare the following mixture for *Acc*I digestion: 10 μl of PCR amplification product, 1.2 μl digestion buffer 10×, and 1 μl *Acc*I.

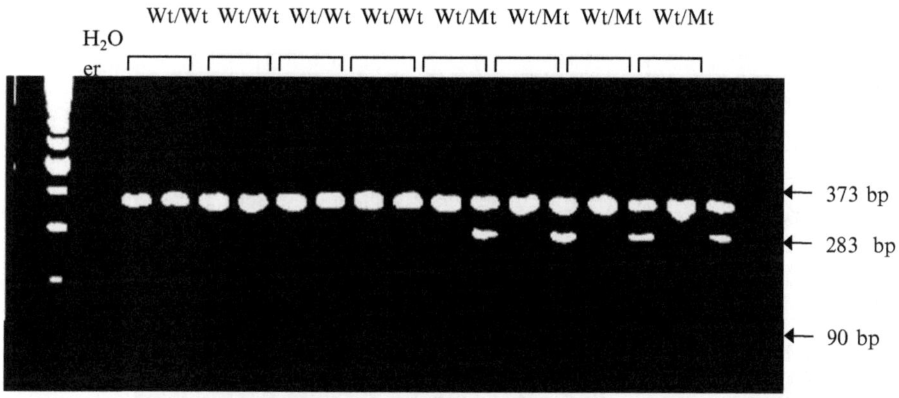

Fig. 4 *TPMT**3 (A719G) genotype detection. Wildtype: no cut, a single band of 373 bp; heterozygous mutant: 373 + 283 + 90 bp, three bands. Note that the 90 bp band for Wt/*3A patient is not visible because of low resolution of the scanner

2. Incubate at 37° for 2 h.
3. Run electrophoresis as in Subheading 3.2, steps 1–7.
4. The results are interpreted as follows (Fig. 4):
   (a) Wild type: A single band of 373 bp.
   (b) Homozygous mutant: Two bands of 283 and 90 bp.
   (c) Heterozygous mutant: Three bands of 373, 283, and 90 bp.

3.4 TPMT*3 (G460A) Genotype Detection

The detection of the G460A genotype is based on selective amplification of the DNA by the forward primer specific to nucleotides 756–780 of intron 6 and the reverse primer specific to nucleotides 1425–1449 of exon 7 of the *TPMT* gene. Genotypes are then determined by the RFLP method. Thus, the amplified products (expected size 694 bp) are subjected to *MWO*I enzyme digestion. Amplicons with the wild-type genotype (A) are digested after *MWO*I treatment while samples with the mutant genotype remain intact, which is resolved by electrophoresis.

1. Prepare the following mixture for *MWO*I digestion: 10 μl PCR amplification product, 1.2 μl digestion buffer 10×, and 1 μl *MWO*I.
2. Incubate at 37° for 2 h.
3. Run electrophoresis as in Subheading 3.2, steps 1–7.
4. The results are interpreted as follows (Fig. 5):
   (a) Wild type: Two bands of 251 and 453 bp.
   (b) Homozygous mutant: A single band of 694 bp.
   (c) Heterozygous mutant: Three bands of 251, 453, and 694 bp.

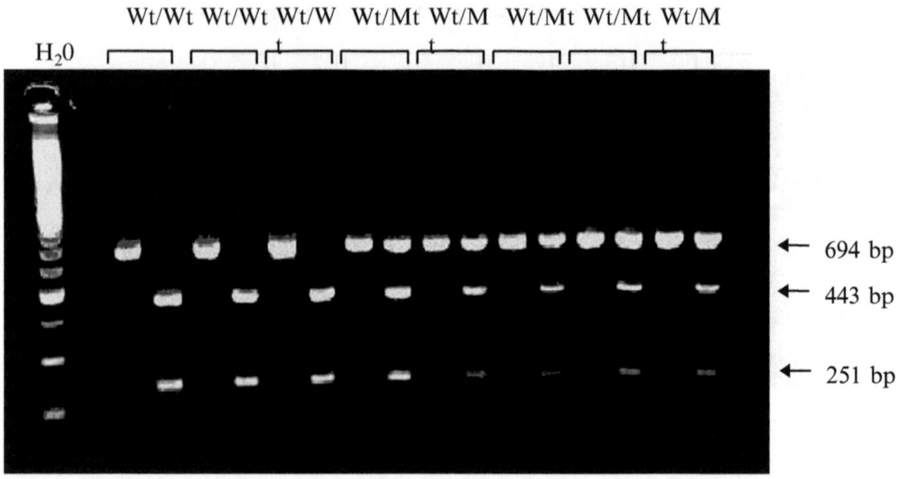

Fig. 5 Detection of *TPMT**3 (G460A) genotype. Wildtype: 251 + 453 bp, two bands; homozygous mutant: a single band of 694 bp; heterozygous mutant: 251 + 453 + 694 bp, three bands

4 Notes

1. Always wear gloves, and change them frequently to avoid contamination. All experiments should be conducted wearing gloves. All genotyping PCRs include negative controls (water in place of genomic DNA templates).
2. *2 and *3 are the most common variants observed in the human *TPMT* gene. However, many other sequence variations have been reported and linked to reduced TPMT function. A complete listing of *TPMT* variants can be found at www.pharmgkb.org and is updated on a regular basis. Also, TPMT genotyping as described herein cannot detect previously unknown variants which can be identified only through resequencing.
3. Other genes, such as *ITPA* (22) and *ABCC4* (23), have also been associated with variability in thiopurine metabolism and disposition, and can affect thiopurine response independent of *TPMT*.
4. Thiopurine dose recommendations based on preemptive TPMT genotyping are as follows:
   (a) Homozygous wild type: Normal starting dose.
   (b) Heterozygous: 30–70% of normal starting dose.
   (c) Homozygous variant: 10% of normal starting dose and monitor toxicity (myelosuppression) carefully for further adjustment.

Acknowledgments

We would like to acknowledge Drs. William Evans, Mary Relling, and Kristine Crews for establishing clinical procedures for *TPMT* genotyping. We also thank Dr. Gabriele Stocco for reading the manuscript and insightful discussions, and Pam McGill for her technical assistance.

References

1. Pui CH, Evans WE (2006) Treatment of acute lymphoblastic leukemia. N Engl J Med 354: 166–178
2. Relling MV, Dervieux T (2001) Pharmacogenetics and cancer therapy. Nat Rev Cancer 1:99–108
3. Meeker ND, Yang JJ, Schiffman JD (2010) Pharmacogenomics of pediatric acute lymphoblastic leukemia. Expert Opin Pharmacother 11:1621–1632
4. Krynetski E, Evans WE (2003) Drug methylation in cancer therapy: lessons from the TPMT polymorphism. Oncogene 22:7403–7413
5. Weiss ST, McLeod HL, Flockhart DA et al (2008) Creating and evaluating genetic tests predictive of drug response. Nat Rev Drug Discov 7:568–574
6. Relling MV, Gardner EE, Sandborn WJ et al (2011) Clinical Pharmacogenetics Imple mentation Consortium guidelines for thiopurine methyltransferase genotype and thiopurine dosing. Clin Pharmacol Ther 89:387–391
7. Relling MV, Hancock ML, Boyett JM et al (1999) Prognostic importance of 6-mercaptopurine dose intensity in acute lymphoblastic leukemia. Blood 93:2817–2823
8. Aarbakke J, Janka-Schaub G, Elion GB (1997) Thiopurine biology and pharmacology. Trends Pharmacol Sci 18:3–7
9. Tidd DM, Paterson AR (1974) Distinction between inhibition of purine nucleotide synthesis and the delayed cytotoxic reaction of 6-mercaptopurine. Cancer Res 34:733–737
10. Yan T, Berry SE, Desai AB et al (2003) DNA mismatch repair (MMR) mediates 6-thioguanine genotoxicity by introducing single-strand breaks to signal a G2-M arrest in MMR-proficient RKO cells. Clin Cancer Res 9:2327–2334
11. Tay BS, Lilley RM, Murray AW et al (1969) Inhibition of phosphoribosyl pyrophosphate amidotransferase from Ehrlich ascites-tumour cells by thiopurine nucleotides. Biochem Pharmacol 18:936–938
12. Krynetski EY, Krynetskaia NF, Yanishevski Y et al (1995) Methylation of mercaptopurine, thioguanine, and their nucleotide metabolites by heterologously expressed human thiopurine S-methyltransferase. Mol Pharmacol 47: 1141–1147
13. Evans WE, Hon YY, Bomgaars L et al (2001) Preponderance of thiopurine S-methy ltransferase deficiency and heterozygosity among patients intolerant to mercaptopurine or azathioprine. J Clin Oncol 19:2293–2301
14. Weinshilboum RM, Sladek SL (1980) Mercaptopurine pharmacogenetics: monogenic inheritance of erythrocyte thiopurine methyltransferase activity. Am J Hum Genet 32:651–662
15. McLeod HL, Lin JS, Scott EP et al (1994) Thiopurine methyltransferase activity in American white subjects and black subjects. Clin Pharmacol Ther 55:15–20
16. Yates CR, Krynetski EY, Loennechen T et al (1997) Molecular diagnosis of thiopurine S-methyltransferase deficiency: genetic basis for azathioprine and mercaptopurine intolerance. Ann Intern Med 126:608–614
17. McLeod HL, Pritchard SC, Githang'a J et al (1999) Ethnic differences in thiopurine methyltransferase pharmacogenetics: evidence for allele specificity in Caucasian and Kenyan individuals. Pharmacogenetics 9: 773–776
18. Collie-Duguid ES, Pritchard SC, Powrie RH et al (1999) The frequency and distribution of thiopurine methyltransferase alleles in Caucasian and Asian populations. Pharmacogenetics 9:37–42
19. Relling MV, Hancock ML, Rivera GK et al (1999) Mercaptopurine therapy intolerance and heterozygosity at the thiopurine S-methyltransferase gene locus. J Natl Cancer Inst 91:2001–2008
20. Evans WE (2002) Thiopurine S-methyltransferase: a genetic polymorphism that affects a small number of drugs in a big way. Pharmacogenetics 12:421–423
21. Ameyaw MM, Collie-Duguid ES, Powrie RH et al (1999) Thiopurine methyltransferase

alleles in British and Ghanaian populations. Hum Mol Genet 8:367–370

22. Stocco G, Cheok MH, Crews KR et al (2009) Genetic polymorphism of inosine triphosphate pyrophosphatase is a determinant of mercaptopurine metabolism and toxicity during treatment for acute lymphoblastic leukemia. Clin Pharmacol Ther 85:164–172
23. Krishnamurthy P, Schwab M, Takenaka K et al (2008) Transporter-mediated protection against thiopurine-induced hematopoietic toxicity. Cancer Res 68:4983–4989

Chapter 21

MicroRNA Expression Profiling Using Microarrays

Cassandra Love and Sandeep Dave

Abstract

MicroRNAs are small noncoding RNAs which are able to regulate gene expression at both the transcriptional and translational levels. There is a growing recognition of the role of microRNAs in nearly every tissue type and cellular process. Thus there is an increasing need for accurate quantitation of microRNA expression in a variety of tissues. Microarrays provide a robust method for the examination of microRNA expression. In this chapter, we describe detailed methods for the use of microarrays to measure microRNA expression and discuss methods for the analysis of microRNA expression data.

Key words MicroRNA, miRNA, Microarray, Expression profiling, Gene regulation

1 Introduction

MicroRNAs are small 18–22-mer noncoding RNAs which regulate gene expression at either the transcriptional or translational level. Since their discovery, hundreds of microRNAs have been found in a number of plant and animal species suggesting conserved function in gene regulation spanning millions of years in evolution. MicroRNAs have been found to play important roles in many cellular processes including development, differentiation and oncogenesis (1–3). Their differential expression has been associated with prognosis and survival of important malignancies including chronic lymphocytic leukemia, colorectal carcinoma, and lung cancer (4–8).

The ability to measure microRNA expression in different cell types is essential for understanding their biological roles. This chapter provides detailed procedures for the measurement of microRNA expression using microarrays. Although the methods we describe use materials and modified protocols from Ambion and Exiqon, the general methods are adaptable to those from most suppliers. This procedure delivers robust expression data, which can be further analyzed using standard statistical approaches.

Magdalena Czader (ed.), *Hematological Malignancies*, Methods in Molecular Biology, vol. 999,
DOI 10.1007/978-1-62703-357-2_21,

We describe a step-by-step approach to RNA isolation, microarray labeling, microarray hybridization and scanning, and normalization of data.

2 Materials

2.1 Isolation of RNA Using Ambion Method (see note 1)

1. 2× denaturing solution stored at 4°C (Ambion, Austin, TX).
2. Tissue homogenizer (see Note 2).
3. ASC grade 100% ethanol.
4. Acid-phenol–chloroform: 30-40% phenol, 10–20% chloroform, 45–55% citric acid buffer. Store at 4°C (Ambion, Austin, TX).
5. Wash solutions 1 and 2/3 (Ambion, Austin, TX).
6. RNase-free water.
7. Cell disruption buffer (Ambion Austin, TX).
8. RNA cleanup filter cartridge (Ambion Austin, TX).

2.2 Isolation of RNA Using Trizol Method

1. Trizol.
2. Tissue homogenizer (see Note 2).
3. Chloroform.
4. Isopropanol.
5. 75% ASC grade ethanol in RNase-free water.
6. RNase-free water.

2.3 Microarray Labeling Total RNA with Cy5 and Cy3

1. MirCURY LNA microRNA labeling kit (Exiqon, Woburn, MA).
2. 2× Hybridization buffer (Exiqon, Woburn, MA).

2.4 Microarray Slide Preparation and Hybridization of Labeled microRNA to Microarray Slides

1. Pre-hybridization buffer: 5× SSC, 0.1% SDS, and 0.5% Bovine Serum Albumin in RNase-free water. Store at 4°C (see Note 3).
2. 0.22 μm bottle top filter.
3. Lifter slips that fit the dimensions of the array being used.
4. Wash buffer 1: 1× SSC and 0.2% SDS in RNase-free water. Filter through the 0.22 μm bottle top filter preheated to 45°C.
5. Wash buffer 2: 0.2× SSC and 0.1% SDS in RNase-free water. Filter through the 0.22 μm bottle top filter.
6. Wash buffer 3: 0.2× SSC in RNase-free water. Filter through the 0.22 μm bottle top filter.
7. Wash buffer 4: 0.05× SSC in RNase-free water. Filter through the 0.22 μm bottle top filter.
8. Water bath set at 42°C.

2.5 Scanning Microarray Slides and Normalization of Raw Expression Values

1. Genepix scanner (Molecular Devices, Sunnyvale, CA).
2. Genespring (Agilent, Santa Clara CA) expression analysis software (or similar).

3 Methods

3.1 Isolation of RNA Using Ambion Method

1. Use a scalpel to carefully cut a frozen specimen on dry ice, ensuring that the sample remains frozen. The freshly cut sample is placed into a 1.5 ml tube and kept on dry ice until the next step. If the sample is embedded in OCT, then the OCT should be removed as much as possible.
2. Lyze the samples by adding 100–600 μl of ice-cold cell disruption buffer. About 300 μl of cell disruption buffer should be added for every 1,000,000 cells.
3. Homogenize the sample thoroughly (10–30 s). There should be no solid tissue left in the lysate and the solution should be homogenous. (see Notes 4 and 5).
4. Mix the lysate in an equal volume of 2× denaturing solution and pipette up and down thoroughly.
5. Incubate sample on ice for 5 min.
6. Double the existing volume with Acid-phenol–chloroform. Vortex the sample for 30–60 s and centrifuge for 5 min at maximum speed (at least 10,000 ×*g*).
7. Pipette the aqueous (upper) phase into a new 1.5 ml centrifuge tube, noting the volume of the sample.
8. Precipitate the RNA by adding 1.25 times the volume of the sample of 100% ethanol and mix thoroughly by pipetting up and down several times. The solution should be completely homogenous.
9. Pass the sample through a filter cartridge placed in a collection tube by adding up to 700 μl of the sample and spinning at 10,000 ×*g* for about 30 s.
10. Discard the flow through and repeat until the entire sample has been passed through the filter.
11. Wash the RNA bound to the filter with 700 μl of wash buffer 1 and centrifuge at 10,000 ×*g* for 30 s.
12. Discard the flow through after the wash.
13. Wash the sample twice with 500 μl of wash buffer 2/3 and centrifuge at 10,000 ×*g*, discarding the flow through after each wash.
14. Remove any residual buffer by centrifuging the column in an empty collection tube at 10,000 ×*g* for 1 min.

15. Transfer the column to a new 1.5 ml RNase-free tube and add 50–100 μl of the RNase-free water, preheated to 95°C.
16. Let the sample stand for 30 s and then centrifuge for 30 s at full speed.
17. Measure the concentration of the sample by NanoDrop. The sample can be concentrated to a desired concentration by speed vacuum. Store the sample at −80°C.

3.2 Isolation of RNA Using Trizol Method

1. Obtain a frozen specimen following the same directions as described in step 1 of Subheading 3.1.
2. Lyse the tissue by adding 1 ml of Trizol.
3. Homogenize the sample following the same directions as described in step 3 of Subheading 3.1.
4. Add 200 μl of chloroform to the sample and shake tubes vigorously for 15 s.
5. Centrifuge the sample at 13,000 × *g* for 15 min at 4°C.
6. Pipette the aqueous (upper) phase into a new 1.5 ml centrifuge tube, taking care to avoid the interphase.
7. Precipitate the RNA by adding 500 μl of isopropanol and vortex the sample until the solution is homogenous.
8. Incubate the mixture at room temperature for 5 min.
9. Centrifuge the sample at 13,000 × *g* for 10 min at 4°C.
10. Pipette the supernatant from the sample and discard. Gently invert the open mouth of the tube on a paper towel to remove any residual liquid from the sample.
11. Wash the pellet with 1,000 μl of 75% ethanol. Centrifuge at 6,500 × *g* for 5 min at 4°C.
12. Pipette the ethanol and gently invert the tube on a paper towel to remove any residual ethanol from the sample.
13. Dry the rim of the tube with a sterile cotton swab, taking care to avoid the RNA pellet.
14. Dissolve the RNA in 25–45 μl of RNase-free water and incubate at 42°C for 5 min. Immediately place the RNA on ice following incubation.
15. Directions for measuring, concentration and storage of sample are described in step 17 of Subheading 3.1.

3.3 Labeling of Total RNA with Cy5 and Cy3 Using miRCURY LNA Labeling Kit

1. Dilute 250–1,000 μg of the total RNA sample to a total volume of 2 μl in RNase-free water. The same amount of total RNA should be used for both the test sample and control reference sample (RNA from benign lymph node).

Table 1
Guidelines to preparing the CIP mixture for RNA during the miRNA labeling procedure

Reagent	1× Reaction (μl)
Spike-in controls	1.0
CIP buffer	0.5
CIP enzyme	0.5
Total	2.0

2. Prepare a master mix for the CIP reaction as follows (Table 1): Spike in controls (1.0 μl), CIP buffer (0.5 μl) and CIP enzyme (0.5 μl).
3. Add 2 μl of the master CIP mix into each RNA sample (test and control separately) for a total reaction volume of 4 μl.
4. Incubate the reaction in a thermal cycler with a heated lid using the following program:
   (a) 1 cycle at 37°C for 30 min.
   (b) 1 cycle at 95°C for 5 min.
   (c) Hold at 4°C.
5. Place the sample on ice for 2–15 min.
6. For the remainder of the experiment, the overhead lights should remain off in order to prevent bleaching of the dyes. Prepare a labeling master mix for each Cy3 or Cy5 dye as follows (Table 2): Labeling buffer (3 μl), Cy3 fluorescent label or Cy5 fluorescent label (1.5 μl), DMSO (2 μl), and labeling enzyme (2 μl).
7. Add 8.5 μl of the Cy5 master labeling reaction to the test sample and Cy3 master labeling reaction to the reference sample for a total volume of 12.5 μl.
8. Incubate the reaction in a thermal cycler with a heated lid using the following program:
   (a) 1 cycle at 16°C for 1 h.
   (b) 1 cycle at 65°C for 15 min.
   (c) Hold at 4°C.
9. Briefly spin the reaction and store the samples at 4°C until ready for the hybridization step. The samples should be hybridized within 1–2 h from labeling.

Table 2
Guidelines to preparing the labeling mixture for RNA during the miRNA labeling procedure

Reagent	1× Reaction (μl)
Labeling buffer	3.0
Cy3 Fluorescent label	1.5
Cy5 Fluorescent label	1.5
DMSO	2.0
Labeling enzyme	2.0
Total	8.5

3.4 Microarray Slide Preparation

1. Pre-warm the pre-hybridization buffer to 42°C.
2. Bake the slides in an oven at 80°C for 80 min.
3. Place the slides in a UV link set for 2000× 100 μJ.
4. Draw a line outlining where the printed spots are using a diamond tip pencil. This will be useful to guiding where the lifter slip is placed on the slide.
5. Place the slides in a glass chamber containing pre-hybridization buffer and incubate at 42°C for 60 min.
6. Wash the slides two times for 1 min each time in RNase-free water.
7. Spin the slides to dry at 1,500 ×*g* for 3 min.
8. Store the slides in a desiccator until they are ready to be used.

3.5 Hybridization of Labeled MicroRNA to Microarrays

1. Heat the 2× hybridization buffer to 55°C. Vortex the sample and ensure that there is no precipitate in the solution. If there is precipitation, heat the buffer for a longer period time.
2. Mix the Cy3 sample and the Cy5 reference sample together in a 1.5 ml tube.
3. Add 25 μl of the 2× hybridization buffer to each sample and mix by vortexing followed by a 10 s centrifugation.
4. Denature the sample by incubating at 95°C for 3 min.
5. Spin the sample briefly and place on ice for 2–15 min.
6. Obtain a freshly prepared slide and place it into a slide chamber. Carefully place a lifter slip over the spotted portion of the slide.
7. Slowly pipette the entire sample to the bottom edge of the lifter slip and allow the sample to move under the slip by capillary action.

8. Add about 500 μl of 1X salt solution to each end of the slide chamber to prevent the sample from drying up during hybridization.
9. Carefully assemble the slide chamber so that it is air tight. Reinforce the screws using a wrench to ensure that no water can leak through during hybridization.
10. Carefully submerge the slide chamber in a water bath heated to 56°C. Allow the sample to hybridize for 16 h.
11. Preheat wash buffer 1–56°C. Take the slides out of the chamber and remove the lifter slips by dipping the slide in wash buffer 1.
12. Wash the slides in wash buffer 1 at 56°C for 2 min, agitating the buffer by shaking.
13. Wash the slides in wash buffer 1 at room temperature for 1 min, wash buffer 2 for 1 min, wash buffer 3 for 2 min, and wash buffer 4 for 2 min.
14. Dry the slides by centrifuging for 5 min at 1,500 × *g*. Place the slides in a light protective slide holder and scan within 1–2 h.

3.6 Scanning MicroRNA Microarray Slides Using Genepix Pro

These directions assume the use of Genepix pro for scanning the two color arrays.

1. Place the slides in the Genepix scanner and perform a quick-scan. Adjust the red (610 nm) and green (520 nm) PMT gain accordingly, thus that the spike-in controls have equal red and green emission wavelengths.
2. Upload the appropriate GAL file containing the information which correlates the spots on the grid to the correct probes for each spot (see Note 6).
3. Inspect the entire scan under magnification to see if the microarray is of good quality. A good quality scan will have a good representation of red, green and yellow spots. A poor quality microarray may have many splotches and smudges which may indicate that the array may need to be discarded (Fig. 1).
4. Align each block onto the appropriate array such that the four corners of the array line up. Most arrays have control probes which always fluoresce in the corners of the array to make it easier for one to align each block correctly (Fig. 2).
5. Using the cursor, highlight every block on the slide and press F5 in order to update flags between each scan. Under high magnification, go through each block and flag spots which appear to have poor quality as "bad."
6. Save scanned image as a TIFF file and the raw expression data as a GPR file. The image files can be used as a reference of the quality of the microarray. The GPR files can be opened in Excel as well as directly uploaded into expression analysis programs.

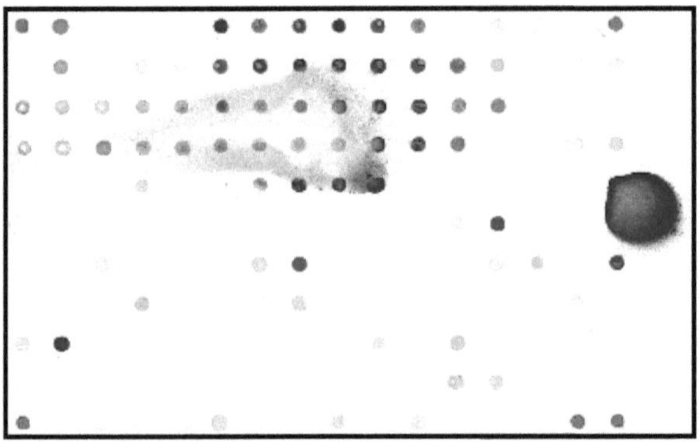

Fig. 1 Shown is an example of an array displaying poor quality. There is an area where the array seems splotchy and the spots are not defined well. There is also a large bright spot which is clearly not a probe

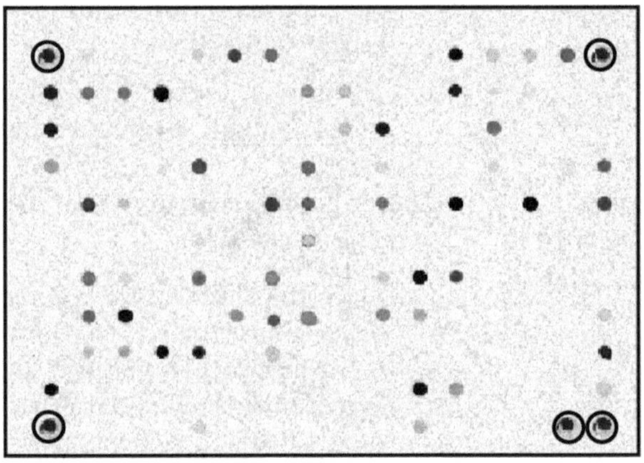

Fig. 2 Shown is an example of one block of an array. Outlined in bold are the control corner spots which are used to guide the user to correctly place the blocks

3.7 Normalization of Raw Expression Data

1. Upload the GPR files containing the raw expression data for each sample into an expression analysis software program. The appropriate GAL file containing the probe name and ID should also be uploaded and saved as a genelist (see Note 7). Choose the appropriate genelist for your arrays and import the raw data.
2. Before analysis, the data must always be normalized. The raw data tends to have many sources of variables and the goal of normalization is to reduce that variability. The data should be subject to per spot and per chip intensity dependent locally weighted scatterplot smoothening (LOWESS) normalization. LOWESS normalization will reduce the variability observed between the dyes and calculates the locally weighted regression as a function of the log2(ratio) of the intensity values (9). Figure 3 shows Cy5 and Cy3 data plotted before and after normalization.

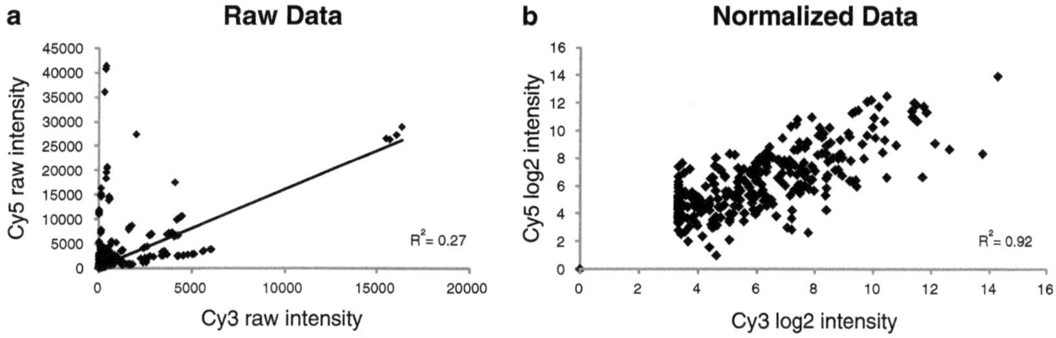

Fig. 3 Shown are examples of plotted intensities of Cy5 and Cy3. (**a**) The raw intensity values for Cy5 and Cy3. This data was directly taken from the GPR file obtained after scanning the image and flagging probes. There is little correlation observed ($R^2 = 0.21$) and it is clear that there is a lot of variance. (**b**) The Lowess normalized intensity values for Cy5 and Cy3 were plotted and are shown to have very high correlation ($R^2 = 0.92$) and little variance. The variance that is observed is due to miRNAs which are differentially expressed and therefore are seen as outliers on the scatterplot

3. The normalized expression values should be exported to Excel where they are subject to log2 transformation.
4. As a quality control method, the test sample (Cy3) and control sample (Cy5) intensity values should be plotted against each other. A high degree of correlation should be observed as compared to the raw intensity values plotted before normalization.

3.8 Unsupervised Statistical Analysis of Expression Data

1. The expression data can be reformatted as a tab delimited (txt) file and directly uploaded into a clustering program were probe expression values are median centered.
2. The arrays may then be clustered to the correlation of gene expression, sample type, or both. You would expect that similar samples will cluster together and that genes will cluster together if they have a high degree of correlation. Seen in Fig. 4 is an example of hierarchical clustering of two different lymphoma types using a freely available program published previously (10).

3.9 Supervised Statistical Analysis of Expression Data

1. A complete description of supervised analysis is beyond the scope of this chapter. Key issues related to microarray analysis include a correction for false discovery, and the need for cross-validation.
2. A significant source of bias in microarray experiments is the sheer number of simultaneous measurements generated. Thus, the number of measured variables (e.g., all the microRNAs present in a tissue) typically far exceed the outcome variables examined (e.g., microRNAs associated with progression of cancer), leading to a high likelihood that some measured variables may be highly associated with the outcome variable by

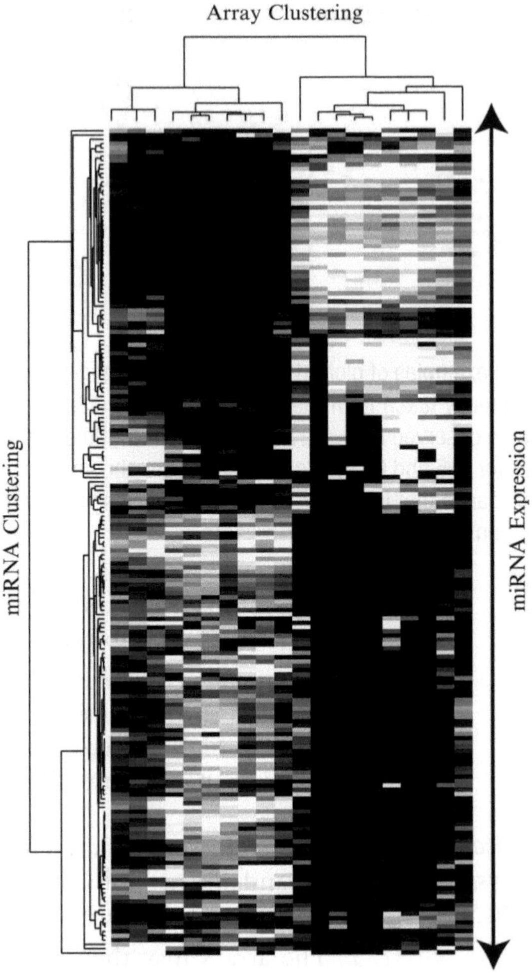

Fig. 4 An example of hierarchical clustering of miRNA expression between two lymphoma types: chronic lymphocytic leukemia and Burkitt lymphoma. The array cluster clearly shows that there the two lymphoma types are clearly distinguished from each other in that there is only one node separating the two classes. The miRNA expression cluster is able to group the miRNAs based on their expected correlation of expression. Those miRNAs which appear in tight nodes are highly correlated to each other

chance alone. In order to mitigate these risks, results obtained by microarray analysis are typically corrected for false discovery rates using methods such as significance analysis of microarrays (SAM) (11) or Bonferroni correction for multiple hypothesis testing (12). Additionally, cross-validation of results using leave out one cross-validation or testing the conclusions in an independent validation set of cases provides further confirmation of whether the findings are likely to be robust (12).

4 Notes

1. Not all standard RNA extraction methods will preserve microRNA, refer to the informational sheet or contact the manufacturer for the specific reagents being used. Filter-based methods may also present problems by either not retaining small RNAs, or when using frozen specimens embedded in OCT. Review the manufacturer specifications carefully for the size of RNAs retained by the filter. If using a filter-based method on OCT, be sure to remove as much of the OCT from the sample as possible to avoid clogging the filter.
2. There are several ways to homogenize tissue for RNA extraction. The simplest way in this protocol is to use a hand held tissue shredder so that the tissue can be shredded while in the lysis buffer solution. If this instrument is not available it is also possible to grind the tissue using a mortar and pestle while keeping the tissue cold on dry ice and grinding it into a powder.
3. Pre-hybridization buffer is stored at 4°C which can cause precipitation. It is important to preheat the solution well before the start of the experiment so that the precipitate will dissolve in time for pre-hybridization of the microarray slides. In some instances the solution may have to be stirred on a heated plate at 50°C.
4. Both the Ambion and Trizol RNA extraction protocols can be used on suspension cells as well. When preparing suspension cells, they should be pelleted followed by aspiration of the medium. After adding the lysis buffer, no homogenization is needed. To lyse the cells, simply pipette up and down until the solution is homogenous.
5. If multiple samples are being processed, then the homogenizer should be cleaned and sterilized by mixing in the following solutions for 30 s each in the order described: 100% ethanol, RNase-free water, 10% bleach, RNase-free water, and 100% ethanol.
6. The GAL files are usually provided on a CD or a download by the microarray manufacturer.
7. Students *T*-test is a good application to obtain an initial idea of how your expression data looks. It can be used as a filter for later applications such as SAM and binary regression analysis as well as hierarchical clustering. It should not however be used as the only statistical application for expression profiling.

References

1. Nana-Sinkam SP, Croce CM (2010) MicroRNA in chronic lymphocytic leukemia: transitioning from laboratory-based investigation to clinical application. Cancer Genet Cytogenet 203:127–133
2. Zhang J, Jima DD, Jacobs C, Fischer R, Gottwein E, Huang G et al (2009) Patterns of microRNA expression characterize stages of human B cell differentiation. Blood 113:4586–4594
3. Jima DD, Zhang J, Jacobs C, Richards KL, Dunphy CH, Choi WW et al (2010) Deep sequencing of the small RNA transcriptome of normal and malignant human B cells identifies hundreds of novel microRNAs. Blood 116:118–127
4. Marcucci G, Haferlach T, Döhner H (2011) The prognostic and functional role of microRNAs in acute myeloid leukemia. Blood 117:1121–1129
5. Zhai H, Ju J (2011) Implications of microRNAs in colorectal cancer development, diagnosis, prognosis, and therapeutics. Front Genet 2:pii:00078
6. De Preter K, Mestdagh P, Vermeulen J, Zeka F, Naranjo A, Bray I et al (2011) miRNA expression profiling enables risk stratification in archived and fresh neuroblastoma tumor samples. Clin Cancer Res 17:7684–7692
7. Calin GA, Ferracin M, Cimmino A, Di Leva G, Shimizu M, Wojcik SE et al (2005) A MicroRNA signature associated with prognosis and progression in chronic lymphocytic leukemia. N Engl J Med 353:1793–1801
8. Yu SL, Chen HY, Chang GC, Chen CY, Chen HW, Singh S et al (2008) MicroRNA signature predicts survival and relapse in lung cancer. Cancer Cell 13:48–57
9. Yang YH, Dudoit S, Luu P, Lin DM, Peng V, Ngai J et al (2002) Normalization for cDNA microarray data: a robust composite method addressing single and multiple slide systematic variation. Nucleic Acids Res 30:e15
10. Eisen MB, Spellman PT, Brown PO, Botstein D (1998) Cluster analysis and display of genome-wide expression patterns. Proc Natl Acad Sci USA 95:14863–14868
11. Tusher VG, Tibshirani R, Chu G (2001) Significance analysis of microarrays applied to the ionizing radiation response. Proc Natl Acad Sci USA 98:5116–5121
12. Radmacher MD, McShane LM, Simon R (2002) A paradigm for class prediction using gene expression profiles. J Comput Biol 9:505–511

INDEX

Magdalena Czader (ed.), *Hematological Malignancies*, Methods in Molecular Biology, vol. 999,
DOI 10.1007/978-1-62703-357-2, © Springer Science+Business Media New York 2013

D

E

F

G

H

L

M

N

P

MIX
Papier aus verantwortungsvollen Quellen
Paper from responsible sources
FSC® C105338

If you have any concerns about our products,
you can contact us on
ProductSafety@springernature.com

In case Publisher is established outside the EU,
the EU authorized representative is:
Springer Nature Customer Service Center GmbH
Europaplatz 3, 69115 Heidelberg, Germany

Printed by Libri Plureos GmbH
in Hamburg, Germany